Butterworths International Medical Reviews

Surgery 2

Endocrine Surgery

Butterworths International Medical Reviews

Surgery 2

Editorial Board
R. W. Beart
P. F. Bell
D. C. Carter
A. Cuschieri
M. H. Irving
I. D. A. Johnston
H. C. Polk
D. B. Skinner
N. W. Thompson
N. L. Tilney

Published in this Series

Volume 1 Trauma

Edited by David C. Carter and Hiram C. Polk, Jr

Future volumes to include

Gastroenterological Surgery

Butterworths
International
Medical
Reviews

Surgery 2

Endocrine Surgery

Edited by
I. D. A. Johnston, FRCS
Professor of Surgery
University of Newcastle upon Tyne, UK

and

Norman W. Thompson, MD, FACS
Henry King Ransom Professor of Surgery
University of Michigan
Ann Arbor
Michigan, USA

Butterworths
London Boston Durban
Singapore Sydney Toronto Wellington

All rights reserved. No part of this publication may be reproduced
or transmitted in any form or by any means, including
photocopying and recording, without the written permission of
the copyright holder, application for which should be addressed to
the Publishers. Such written permission must also be obtained
before any part of this publication is stored in a retrieval system of
any nature.

This book is sold subject to the Standard Conditions of Sale of
Net Books and may not be re-sold in the UK below the net price
given by the Publishers in their current price list.

First published 1983

© Butterworth & Co (Publishers) Ltd. 1983

British Library Cataloguing in Publication Data

Endocrine surgery. – (Butterworths international
  medical reviews. Surgery ISSN 0260-0188; 2)
  1. Glands, Ductless – Surgery
  I. Johnston, I.D.A.   II. Thompson, Norman W.
  617'.44   RD599

ISBN 0-407-02317-8

Photoset by Butterworths Litho Preparation Department
Printed and bound in England by Robert Hartnoll Ltd., Bodmin,
Cornwall

Foreword

Endocrine Surgery is a new, rapidly growing discipline. Until recently, individual surgeons concentrated on particular glands, such as the thyroid, pituitary, adrenals or parathyroids, and some have written monographs about them. An increasing number of surgeons, however, now see the endocrine system as a whole. Very few devote themselves entirely to endocrine surgery but many are interested in the endocrinology, pathology, radiology and surgery of all the glands, in their inter-relationships, and in the endocrine aspects of such phenomena as the response of the body to injury and the growth and control of cancer. They are establishing themselves as *endocrine surgeons* to improve their understanding, techniques and standards of care, to teach and to undertake research. National and international associations have been formed, postgraduate courses are popular and several books on endocrine surgery as a whole have been written. At the same time these surgeons co-operate closely with colleagues in other relevant medical and surgical fields for the benefit of all. Advances are often rapid and growing points – involving several disciplines – change every few years, the stimuli coming from different sources.

It is entirely appropriate that *Endocrine Surgery* should be the topic of this second volume in Butterworths International Medical Reviews and the publishers could not have chosen two better editors than my good friends Professors Ivan Johnston and Norman Thompson, one from each side of the Atlantic. I welcome the book and am honoured to have been invited to contribute a chapter and to write this foreword. Twelve topics of current interest have been chosen and an international team of active workers representing surgery, internal medicine, radiology and anatomy has been assembled, each member writing on his own particular field. The editors have written some of the chapters themselves and have provided commentaries on several others, adding greatly to the value of the book.

The result makes fascinating reading and provides a happy blend of laboratory work, clinical research and practical surgery. It is a major contribution to current practice in endocrine surgery, illustrating well how fast the subject is advancing.

I commend this book warmly to all endocrine surgeons, established or in training, to endocrinologists and those in other disciplines, including radiology and pathology, whose work is related to endocrine surgery.

Richard Welbourn

List of Contributors

Helene P. Ayres, BA
Columbus, Ohio, USA

Murray F. Brennan, MD
Professor of Surgery, Cornell University Medical School; Chief of the Gastric and Mixed Tumor Service, Memorial Sloan-Kettering Cancer Center, New York, USA

Kyung J. Cho, MD
Associate Professor, Department of Radiology, The University of Michigan, Ann Arbor, Michigan, USA

P. R. Daggett, MRCP
Physician, Mid-Staffordshire Health District, UK

Stefan S. Fajans, MD
Professor, Internal Medicine and Head, Division of Endocrinology and Metabolism; Director, Michigan Diabetes Research and Training Center, The University of Michigan, Ann Arbor, Michigan, USA

John R. Farndon, MD, FRCS
Senior Lecturer in Surgery, University of Newcastle upon Tyne; Newcastle Area Health Authority (Teaching), Central Sector, The Royal Victoria Infirmary, Newcastle upon Tyne, UK

Lennart Fagraeus, MD, PhD
Associate Professor of Anesthesiology, Duke University Medical Center, Durham, North Carolina, USA

List of contributors

Akihiro Funakoshi, MD
Research Fellow, Internal Medicine, Division of Endocrinology and Metabolism, The University of Michigan, Ann Arbor, Michigan, USA

Ben Glaser, MD
Research Fellow in Internal Medicine, The University of Michigan, Ann Arbor, Michigan, USA

Jerry Glowniak, MD
Research Fellow in Internal Medicine, The University of Michigan, Ann Arbor, Michigan, USA

I. D. A. Johnston, FRCS
Professor of Surgery, Royal Victoria Infirmary, Newcastle upon Tyne, UK

J. H. Lazarus, MA, MD, FRCP
Senior Lecturer in Medicine and Honorary Consultant Physician, Department of Medicine, Welsh National School of Medicine, Cardiff, UK

L. P. Le Quesne, DM, MCh, FRCS
Professor of Surgery, The Middlesex Hospital Medical School, London, UK

Paul McMaster, MA, ChM, FRCS
Consultant Surgeon, Queen Elizabeth Hospital, Birmingham, UK

K. J. Manolas, MD(Athens)
Research Fellow, Royal Postgraduate Medical School and Honorary Senior Registrar, Hammersmith Hospital, London, UK

Mikael E. Romanus, MD, PhD
Assistant Professor in Anatomy and Resident, Department of Surgery I, University of Gothenburg, Sweden

Brahm Shapiro, MB, BCh, PhD
Assistant Professor, Department of Internal Medicine, The University of Michigan, Ann Arbor, Michigan, USA

Norman W. Thompson, MD, FACS
Henry King Ransom Professor of Surgery, The University of Michigan, Ann Arbor, Michigan, USA

Aaron I. Vinik, MB, BCh, FCP, MDFACP
Professor, Internal Medicine and Surgery, The University of Michigan, Ann Arbor, Michigan, USA

List of contributors

J. S. H. Wade, MC, TD, FRCS
Consultant Surgeon, Department of Surgery, Welsh National School of Medicine, Cardiff, UK

R. B. Welbourn, MA, MD(Cantab), Hon MD(Karolinska), FRCS(Eng), FCS(W Africa), Hon MRCS(Denmark)
Professor of Surgical Endocrinology, Department of Surgery, Royal Postgraduate Medical School and Hammersmith Hospital, London, UK

Samuel A. Wells, Jr, MD
Bixby Professor of Surgery and Chairman, Department of Surgery, Washington University School of Medicine at Barnes Hospital, St Louis, Missouri, USA

Robert M. Zollinger, MD, DSc(Hon), FACS(Hon)
Emeritus Regents Professor and Chairman of the Department of Surgery, The Ohio State University College of Medicine; Chief of Surgical Service, University Hospitals, University Hospital, Columbus, Ohio, USA

Contents

1 The role of surgery in the management of thyrotoxicosis   1
  J. H. Lazarus and J. S. H. Wade

2 The thyroid nodule – surgical management   14
  Norman W. Thompson

3 Transplantation of the parathyroid glands   25
  Mikael E. Romanus, J. R. Farndon and Samuel A. Wells

4 Reoperation for suspected hyperparathyroidism   41
  Murray F. Brennan and Samuel A. Wells

5 The role of adrenalectomy in the management of Cushing's syndrome   53
  R. B. Welbourn and K. J. Manolas

6 Localization of gastroentero-pancreatic (GEP) tumors   76
  A. I. Vinik, J. Glowniak, B. Glaser, B. Shapiro, A. Funakoshi, K. J. Cho, N. W. Thompson and S. S. Fajans

7 Insulin tumors of the pancreas   104
  L. P. Le Quesne and P. R. Daggett

8 Pancreatic transplantation   125
  Paul McMaster

9 Surgical considerations in the MEA I syndrome   144
  Norman W. Thompson

10 Current views on the surgery of gastrinoma in the post-cimetidine era   164
   Robert M. Zollinger and Helene P. Ayres

Contents

11 Surgery of primary aldosteronism   182
   I. D. A. Johnston

12 Recent developments in the management of phaeochromocytoma   189
   John R. Farndon, Lennart Fagraeus and Samuel A. Wells

   Index   203

1
The role of surgery in the management of thyrotoxicosis

J. H. Lazarus and J. S. H. Wade

The syndromes of thyrotoxicosis for which surgery is often the treatment of choice are:

(1) hyperthyroidism due to thyroid stimulating antibodies (TsAb)
    (a) diffuse toxic goitre (Graves' disease)
    (b) toxic multinodular goitre with internodular hyperplasia (or nodular overactivity)
(2) hyperthyroidism due to autonomous overactive thyroid tissue
    (a) toxic adenoma (Plummer's disease)
    (b) toxic multinodular goitre with nodular overactivity

Other, rarer causes of thyrotoxicosis suitable for surgery are struma ovarii with hyperthyroidism, hyperthyroidism associated with a pituitary tumour and elevated thyroid stimulating hormone (TSH) levels, and hyperthyroidism due to metastatic thyroid carcinoma. These are very rare conditions and will not be discussed further. Surgery is contraindicated in the hyperthyroidism associated with the early stages of viral subacute thyroiditis (de Quervain's disease) and when autoimmune thyroiditis presents with hyperthyroidism.

Once the diagnosis of thyrotoxicosis has been made, it is important to establish which syndrome is present, because this will influence the choice of treatment and give an indication of the likelihood of long-term follow up problems.

The identification of the syndrome is made on clinical examination and on laboratory tests. Clinical examination will determine the type of goitre (diffuse, multinodular or uninodular) and also reveal the presence of other manifestations of Graves' disease not due to the hyperthyroidism. Scanning with radio-iodine or technetium is of some value in demonstrating a diffuse toxic goitre; it is essential in the diagnosis of a toxic adenoma and helpful in determining the site of overactivity in a toxic multinodular goitre.

Antibody titres of thyroid microsomes and thyroglobulin should be estimated, as they may give some indication of the long-term result of surgery.

TREATMENT

Thyrotoxicosis may be treated by surgery, by the long-term use of antithyroid drugs, or by one or more therapeutic doses of radio-iodine. There is no place for the routine use of any one of these means of treatment; each patient must be considered individually.

Let us consider the four different syndromes and, in particular, the place of surgery in treatment.

Diffuse toxic goitre (Graves' disease)

Treatment with antithyroid drugs is indicated when the goitre is small and the patient is young. Recent studies have shown that when used in Graves' disease, antithyroid drugs may have a marked immunosuppressive effect on thyroid stimulating antibody production[9]. Attempts have been made to predict which patients might relapse after a 6-month course of antithyroid drugs on the basis of HLA status and the presence of TsAb[14].

Surgery is indicated in young persons when the goitre is large and when there is a recurrence of hyperthyroidism after one or more full doses of treatment with antithyroid drugs.

Although some clinicians are prepared to treat patients over the age of 25 with radio-iodine, in the United Kingdom this treatment is generally reserved for those over the age of 45. Radio-iodine is particularly useful in patients over the age of 60[11].

Toxic adenoma (Plummer's disease)

As the overactive thyroid tissue is autonomous, a permanent cure with antithyroid drugs is impossible: relapse is inevitable when the drugs are withdrawn.

Radio-iodine is excellent treatment for those over the age of 45 because there is no risk of delayed thyroid insufficiency. The normal thyroid tissue is suppressed and takes up none of the isotopes.

Surgery is indicated for those under the age of 45; the adenoma is removed and TSH control of the previously suppressed thyroid tissue is rapidly restored. Recurrence of hyperthyroidism or the development of postoperative thyroid insufficiency is rare following treatment by either radio-iodine or surgery.

Toxic multinodular goitre

In both syndromes of toxic multinodular goitre (internodular hyperplasia or nodular overactivity) the presence of a large goitre which may be responsible for obstructive symptoms influences treatment. Surgery is therefore the treatment of choice unless there are very definite contraindications.

Antithyroid drugs are not useful as a definitive treatment. If autonomous thyroid tissue is present they will fail, and if the overactive thyroid tissue is internodular long-term treatment is likely to increase the size of the goitre.

Treatment with radio-iodine is given if surgery is contraindicated but it has little or no effect on the size of the goitre.

These indications for treatment apply in general. However, every case of thyrotoxicosis must be considered individually, and the wishes and fears of each patient must be taken into account when advising any one of the three forms of treatment. The circumstances of the patient must also be considered: it would, for example, be unwise to start treatment with antithyroid drugs if a patient's job was in an area where adequate supervision was not available. Surgery is also indicated in patients who express a preference for it for social or cosmetic reasons. In the same way, the age of 45 is not a rigid watershed between treatment with radio-iodine and treatment by surgery or antithyroid drugs.

TREATMENT OF SPECIAL CASES

There are certain special cases which will now be considered.

Children

Hyperthyroidism in children is not common and is best managed by antithyroid drugs[1]. Radio-iodine is absolutely contraindicated. If surgery is required because of relapse when antithyroid drugs are withdrawn, the operation should be postponed for as long as possible. It is our impression that the risk of recurrent hyperthyroidism after surgery is higher in children and adolescents than in adults. If surgery has to be undertaken, it must therefore be at least as radical as in the adult, if not more so.

Continuous treatment with antithyroid drugs may therefore be required for many years in some children. A considerable increase in size and vascularity of the goitre may sometimes be prevented during this period by prescribing tri-iodothyronine together with the antithyroid drugs. This will prevent the rise in serum TSH level which is responsible for enlargement of the goitre in some patients on prolonged antithyroid drug treatment.

Pregnancy

Surgery may be performed during the second trimester with no hazard to maternal health[19]. Older series of surgically treated pregnant patients contained an unacceptable rate of foetal loss. This has now been reduced, but is still present, and must be balanced against the modest risks of antithyroid drug therapy in pregnancy. Thyroidectomy during pregnancy may be advised in patients who exhibit poor compliance with antithyroid drugs or develop drug reactions. It is more readily advised when a patient already has a family than when she is expecting her first child, particularly if she is over the age of 30.

Thyrocardiac patients

Many patients with toxic multinodular goitres are elderly and have coexisting heart disease due partly or wholly to the thyrotoxicosis. Surgery is inadvisable unless there are significant obstructive symptoms in the neck. The treatment of choice is a large dose of radio-iodine and antithyroid drugs given either before or after the dose of radio-iodine. Hyperthyroidism in the elderly is as common as in the younger age group, and selection for surgery should be based on medical advice.

Poor compliance and drug reaction

Patients who do not respond to antithyroid drug therapy because of poor compliance or adverse reaction to the drugs should be operated on if under the age of 45.

Recurrent hyperthyroidism after surgery

If an adequate operation has previously been carried out, any further surgery for a recurrence of hyperthyroidism is most inadvisable[15]. Apart from the risk to the recurrent laryngeal nerves and parathyroid glands at a second operation, there can be no guarantee that a further recurrence may not occur unless a total thyroidectomy is carried out.

Exophthalmos

The main objective of treatment is to render the patient euthyroid as quickly as possible. It has been suggested that surgery should be avoided in patients with Graves' disease in whom exophthalmos had recently developed because of the risk of increasing proptosis and causing malignant exophthalmos[4]. It is difficult to be sure whether or not this is a valid argument. There has been little support for the view that total or subtotal thyroidectomy followed by total ablation of thyroid tissue by radio-iodine is of value in the control of severe exophthalmos.

PREOPERATIVE PREPARATION

Antithyroid drugs should be the mainstay of treatment to render the patient euthyroid prior to surgery. The thionamide drugs (carbimazole or methimazole) will lower the serum thyroid hormone levels by 30% in 2 weeks, and nearly all patients should be euthyroid by 6 weeks. Patients should be seen frequently to ensure good drug compliance, and progress should be monitored by estimations of serum triiodothyronine and thyroxine. A dose of carbimazole 30 mg daily is adequate in most patients but, if very toxic, a dose of 60 mg daily may be necessary. If operation has to be delayed once the patient has become euthyroid, a lower maintenance dose may be given.

Patients should be warned that they should stop the drug and report back immediately if a sore throat or any other unusual reaction occurs.

Propranolol, long-acting propranolol or other non-selective β-adrenoreceptor blocking drugs may be used in conjunction with the thionamides. Their beneficial effects in reducing the pulse rate and ameliorating many peripheral manifestations of hyperthyroidism are well known. When given together with carbimazole, propranolol 40 mg three times a day is an adequate dose, but higher doses can be safely given.

β-Blocking drugs given with carbimazole are of great value in the immediate control of patients with severe toxic symptoms, and may be continued throughout the whole preoperative period. In some patients requiring immediate control of symptoms, no previous investigations will have been carried out, and a radio-iodine uptake test or scan is required. β-Blocking drugs do not interfere with iodine uptake by the thyroid gland so that symptoms may be controlled by the drug whilst these investigations are performed. Carbimazole is started once the tests are completed.

Some surgical centres have advocated the sole use of propranolol in preoperative preparation[17]. However, we feel safer if the serum thyroid hormone concentrations are within the normal range at the time of surgery, as they should be in patients pretreated with carbimazole, whereas this is not so in patients treated solely with propranolol.

Some surgeons use iodides together with antithryoid drugs during the two weeks immediately prior to operation on the grounds that the drug reduces the vascularity of the thyroid gland and makes it softer and easier to handle. Iodide sensitivity in the patient is the only contraindication to this practice. However, we do not use iodides preoperatively in this manner because we are not convinced that its administration makes the operation any easier.

The use of iodides alone as a preoperative drug is, in our opinion, unwise. If a patient has hyperthyroidism, then a drug far more effective than iodide should be used to ensure a euthyroid state at the time of operation.

Other investigations

Prior to surgery indirect laryngoscopy should be done, because very occasionally an unsuspected unilateral cord paralysis is present and this is likely to influence the extent of surgery. The serum calcium levels should be estimated because thyroid disease and primary hyperparathyroidism due to either a parathyroid tumour or parathyroid hyperplasia rarely occur together. It is seldom necessary to crossmatch blood for thyroid surgery but the patient certainly should be grouped. Deep venous thrombosis is so rare after thyroidectomy that prophylactic measures are unnecessary.

OPERATION

The aim of surgery when hyperthyroidism is due to a nodule of autonomous overactive thyroid tissue is to resect all the overactive tissue and preserve as much normal thyroid tissue as possible. Unilateral subtotal lobectomy is therefore the operation of choice for a toxic adenoma.

When hyperthyroidism is due to thyroid stimulating antibodies all the functioning thyroid tissue is overactive. The aim now must be to reduce the mass of overactive thyroid tissue to such an extent that a recurrence of hyperthyroidism is improbable yet thyroid insufficiency is unlikely to result. To achieve this the surgeon should aim to preserve between 8 and 10 g of thyroid tissue. Thus, for a diffuse toxic goitre (Graves' disease) a bilateral subtotal lobectomy should be performed, leaving a 4–5 g remnant on each side. For a toxic multinodular goitre a similar bilateral resection is done but care is taken to remove any nodule which has been shown on the scan to be active.

The basic principles of thyroidectomy are those of any other surgical operation, namely good exposure, absolute haemostasis and protection of important structures in the operation field[28]. Good exposure involves mobilization of the sternomastoid muscles, division of the pretracheal muscles, and ligature and division of the superior thyroid vessels in order to free the upper pole of the thyroid lobe. Haemostasis is made more certain by also ligating both inferior thyroid arteries and by suturing the thyroid remnants to the tracheal fascia. The recurrent laryngeal nerves and the parathyroid glands need protection. The nerves should be identified, remembering that the right recurrent nerve is anomalous in 1% of patients and may be mistaken for the right inferior thyroid artery. The parathyroid glands are protected by a knowledge of the common anatomical sites and by careful inspection of the thyroid lobes prior to resection. In this way, the risk of inadvertent removal of a gland or of damage to the vascular pedicle of an identified gland is minimized. A search for unidentified parathyroid glands is inadvisable because it may result in injury to the parathyroid end artery and infarction of the gland.

The surgeon must be flexible not only in the choice of treatment for the individual patient with thyrotoxicosis but, on occasion, also in the scope of his operation. Two examples will be quoted. A young woman of 23 developed Graves' disease. She had been treated for Hodgkins' disease 4 years previously and lymph nodes on the right side of the neck had been irradiated. In view of the risk of a thyroid carcinoma developing as a result of irradiation, a total right lobectomy and near-total left lobectomy was performed.

Another young married woman of 28 presented with Graves' disease. When she was 19 years old a large nodule had been resected from the right lobe of the thyroid. She was anxious to start a family and surgery was advised. In view of the risk of damage to the right recurrent nerve and parathyroid glands, a left lobectomy and limited right subtotal lobectomy was performed.

POSTOPERATIVE CARE AND COMPLICATIONS

The patient should be propped up as soon as possible after the operation to relieve venous congestion. The nursing staff in the recovery room and then in the ward should report immediately any difficulty in breathing, any swelling in the neck, or excessive volume in the drainage bottle. A small collection of blood or serum between the deep fascia and the subcutaneous tissue is not serious, but haemorrhage in the deep cervical space is dangerous: it is likely to produce laryngeal oedema and respiratory obstruction and requires emergency evacuation. Respiratory obstruction, which may also occur in the absence of a haematoma, is usually due to laryngeal oedema in the subglottic area just below the vocal cords. Laryngeal oedema may progress very rapidly and it is wise to intubate a patient who develops any degree of inspiratory stridor.

Nowadays, because of careful preoperative preparation of the thyrotoxic patient, postoperative thyroid crisis is virtually unknown. However, if the patient is prepared for surgery with propranolol, it is important to continue the drug for 5 to 7 days after operation. This is even more essential if propranolol has been the sole antithyroid drug used, because in this event hormone levels in the serum are high at the time of the operation and, although the triiodothyronine level falls rapidly, thyroxine is utilized more slowly and does not reach a normal level for some days after thyroidectomy.

Indirect laryngoscopy may be carried out prior to discharge on the fourth postoperative day. In most cases, if a cord paralysis is present, this is suspected, but occasionally a unilateral paralysis is quite symptomless.

Routine postoperative laryngoscopy shows that transient laryngeal nerve paralysis occurs in 2–4% of nerves at risk. It may be unilateral or bilateral, and recovery occurs within 3 months of operation. If the nerve has been identified, paralysis almost invariably recovers; if it has not been identified, permanent paralysis will occur in one third of nerves injured[27].

A postoperative serum calcium level should also be estimated. Hypocalcaemia almost invariably declares itself with unmistakable symptoms, but very rarely a patient with marked hypocalcaemia is symptom-free.

A postoperative fall in the serum calcium may be transient or permanent and occurs in 3–4% of patients following bilateral subtotal lobectomy for toxic goitre. It has been suggested that the early transient hypocalcaemia is due to damage to the parathyroid glands or their blood supply during operation[5, 20, 29]. However, in some instances there is evidence that an important reason for the fall in the serum calcium is the rapid reversal of an osteodystrophy which may have existed preoperatively in the absence of symptoms[16]. Hyperthyroidism is characterized by an increase in bone turnover, with an increase of bone resorption as well as formation, in addition to a pronounced increase in osteoclastic activity in cortical bones[18]. This metabolic state is consistent with the concept of hungry bones being responsible for the transient hypocalcaemia. The pathogenic role of low vitamin D levels[26], and high[12], normal[3] or low[21] parathyroid hormone levels is not clear.

The symptoms of paraesthesiae and tetany usually appear within 36 hours of operation but are sometimes delayed. If symptoms are severe, treatment with intravenous 10% calcium gluconate is effective. Most cases are transient, but permanent hypocalcaemia follows thyroidectomy for Graves' disease in about 1% of cases. Calcium alone may be given in mild cases, but the majority of patients require additional vitamin D or its active synthetic analogue 1α-hydroxycholecalciferol. Parathyroid autotransplantation has been reported to prevent delayed hypocalcaemia in patients undergoing total thyroidectomy for Graves' disease in one centre[7].

RESULTS OF SURGERY

In experienced hands surgery for thyrotoxicosis carries a negligible mortality and a low morbidity. The negligible mortality entails careful assessment of thyrocardiac cases and conservative treatment rather than surgery for any patient in this group who presents an operative risk.

Surgery for an autonomous toxic adenoma is extremely successful. The operation itself is straightforward, and recurrent hyperthyroidism and postoperative thyroid insufficiency are extremely rare.

An operation on a toxic multinodular goitre is usually no more difficult than on a rather vascular simple multinodular goitre. The result is usually very satisfactory in that the goitre is removed and obstructive symptoms, if present, are relieved. Recurrent hyperthyroidism is rare, but there is a significant incidence of postoperative thyroid insufficiency, although not as high as that which follows operation on the diffuse toxic goitre of Graves' disease.

Surgery for Graves' disease is rarely easy. On occasion the operation is extremely difficult and demanding. A bilateral subtotal lobectomy on a large vascular diffuse goitre, such as may be encountered after prolonged treatment with antithyroid drugs, is not an operation to be undertaken by the occasional thyroid surgeon.

There are a large number of reports on the long-term results of partial thyroidectomy for Graves' disease. Early reports did not have the benefit of accurate measurements of thyroid hormone or TSH levels. A review of a number of these early series, in which 84–1000 patients were observed up to 15 years after thyroid surgery, shows an incidence of 4–43% of thyroid insufficiency and a recurrence rate of hyperthyroidism of 0–28%. More recent studies (*Table 1.1*) suggest a 15–20% incidence of thyroid insufficiency and a 5% incidence of recurrent hyperthyroidism, and these figures are very similar to our own.

Although many factors have been studied in order to try and predict the outcome of surgery for Graves' disease, attention has recently focused on the immunological aspects of this condition. Lundström *et al.*[13] found that the development of hypothyroidism was related to the extent of histological lymphoid infiltration, and to the preoperative titres of antithyroglobulin and antimicrosomal antibodies as well as to the size of the remnant. Van Welsum *et al.*[25] had also noted a higher

Table 1.1 Prevalence of hypothyroidism and recurrent hyperthyroidism after bilateral subtotal lobectomy for Graves' disease

Reference	Number of patients	Follow-up (years)	Hypo-thyroidism %	Hyper-thyroidism %
Evered et al. (1975)[6]	76	1–7	12	4
Heimann and Martinson (1975)[10]	272	1–13	38	2
Lundström et al. (1977)[13]	92	1	15	3
Blichert-Toft et al. (1977)[2]	213	5–15	6	9
Tweedle et al. (1977)[24]	122	>1	15	3
Teng et al. (1980)[22]	30	1	23	10

incidence of autoantibodies against thyroid cytoplasm but found no difference in lymphatic infiltration or in the prevalence of antithyroglobulin antibodies between hypothyroid and euthyroid patients.

As the lymphocytes localized in the thyroid appear to be mainly responsible for the production of thyroid stimulating autoantibodies, their surgical removal eventually allows the titre of thyroid stimulating antibodies to fall, giving a low recurrence rate. Patients may still develop high titres of TsAb after surgery, but will only relapse if their thyroid remnant is large enough to overproduce thyroid hormones under the influence of the stimulating antibodies. The value of measuring TsAb in patients undergoing surgery for Graves' disease has been demonstrated in a prospective study of the changes of these immunoglobulins in 30 patients[22]. Preoperative preparation with antithyroid drugs reduced the positive thyroid stimulating antibody titres in patients who were either persistently positive or became positive after surgery. Hypothyroidism was associated only with negative thyroid stimulating antibody titres.

The remnant size may determine the incidence of hypothyroidism[8], but most observers[24] have not found this to be of prognostic significance.

Why then is surgery as successful as it is, curing hyperthyroidism in 95% of patients operated on for Graves' disease? Certainly removal of a major (but not the only) site of antibody synthesis is important. However, the role of other factors, such as the immunogenetic background of the patient, the iodide status of the patient and the details of thyroid remnant function, remains to be clarified.

FOLLOW-UP

The fact that significant numbers of patients who have been treated for thyrotoxicosis by surgery are at risk of developing postoperative hypothyroidism or recurrence of disease which may not show itself for many years means that all patients should be reviewed regularly and for life. However, attendance at a hospital outpatient clinic is time-consuming and expensive. A variety of semi-automated thyroid follow-up systems have therefore been introduced in the United

Kingdom. The basic principle is that an annual blood sample is obtained from the patient by the family physician. This is sent to a central laboratory for the estimation of serum thyroid hormones. If the result is abnormal the patient is requested to attend the clinic, and appropriate therapy is initiated. Patients should not be entered into this scheme until 18 months to 2 years have elapsed since their operation. This allows recognition of early transient hypothyroidism[23]. There is debate as to the necessity of following up patients with a slightly elevated TSH level, but in our experience it is still cost-effective to do so.

CONCLUSION

Surgery is the treatment of choice in many cases of thyrotoxicosis, notably large diffuse toxic goitres, toxic goitres when previous medical treatment has failed, and most toxic multinodular goitres and toxic adenomas in the younger age group.

In experienced hands, mortality is negligible and morbidity is low. The result of surgery for autonomous toxic adenoma is extremely good and for toxic multinodular goitre is very satisfactory. However, in Graves' disease the incidence of recurrent hyperthyroidism and of postoperative thyroid insufficiency – presenting sometimes many years after operation – is higher than most surgeons were prepared to acknowledge until recent years. A careful follow-up of all patients operated on for thyrotoxicosis is essential. This should be done at least yearly and for an indefinite period.

References

1 BARNES, V. and BLIZZARD, R. M. Antithyroid drug therapy for toxic diffuse goiter (Graves' disease): thirty years experience in children and adolescents. *Paediatric Pharmacology and Therapeutics*, **91**, 313–320 (1977)

2 BLICHERT-TOFT, M., JORGENSEN, S. J., HANSEN, J. B., WATT-BOOLSEN, S., CHRISTIANSEN, C. and IBSEN, J. Long-term observation of thyroid function after surgical treatment of thyrotoxicosis. *Acta Chirurgica Scandinavica*, **143**, 221–227 (1977)

3 BURMAN, K. D., MONCHIK, J. M., EARLL, J. M. and WARTOFSKY, L. Ionized and total serum calcium and parathyroid hormone in hyperthyroidism. *Annals of Internal Medicine*, **84**, 668–671 (1976)

4 CATZ, B., PERZIK, S. L. and LEE, N. *Effect of thyroidectomy for thyrotoxicosis on exophthalmos*. Chicago American Thyroid Association Inc. (1963)

5 DAVIS, R. H., FOURMAN, P. and SMITH, J. W. G. Prevalence of parathyroid insufficiency after thyroidectomy. *Lancet*, **2**, 1432–1435 (1961)

6 EVERED, D., YOUNG, E. T., TUNBRIDGE, W. M. G., ORMSTON, B. J., GREEN, E., PETERSEN, V. B. and DICKINSON, P. H. Thyroid function after subtotal thyroidectomy for hyperthyroidism. *British Medical Journal*, **1**, 25–27 (1975)

7 GANN, D. S. and PAONE, J. F. Delayed hypocalcemia after thyroidectomy for Graves' disease is prevented by parathyroid autotransplantation. *Annals of Surgery*, **190**, 508–513 (1979)

8 GRIFFITHS, N. J., MURLEY, R. S., GULIN, R., SIMPSON, R. D., WOODS, T. F. and BURNETT, D. Thyroid function following partial thyroidectomy. *British Journal of Surgery*, **61**, 626–632 (1974)

9 HALL, R., McGREGOR, A. M., McLACHLAN, S., LAZARUS, J. H. and REES SMITH, B. The treatment of hyperthyroidism. In *Advanced Medicine*, edited by W. M. G. Tunbridge, pp. 32–36. Tunbridge Wells, Pitman (1981)

10 HEIMANN, P. and MARTINSON, J. Surgical treatment of thyrotoxicosis: results of 272 operations with special reference to preoperative treatment with anti-thyroid drugs and L-thyroxine. *British Journal of Surgery*, **62**, 683–688 (1975)

11 LAZARUS, J. H. and HARDEN, R. McG. Thyrotoxicosis in the elderly. *Gerontologia Clinica*, **11**, 371–378 (1969)

12 LERMAN, S., VESELY, D. L., WEINSTEIN, R. S., CANTERBURRY, J. M. and LEVEY, G. S. Elevated serum parathyroid hormone concentrations in hyperthyroidism. (Paper read at the *52nd Meeting of the American Thyroid Association*, Toronto, Canada, September, 1976)

13 LUNDSTRÖM, B., HED, J., JOHANSSON, K.-E. and NORRBY, K. Thyroid function after subtotal thyroidectomy for hyperthyroidism related to some morphological and immunological features. *Acta Chirurgica Scandinavica*, **143**, 215–220 (1977)

14 McGREGOR, A. M., REES SMITH, B., HALL, R., PETERSEN, M. M., MILLER, M. and DEWAR, P. J. Prediction of relapse in hyperthyroid Graves' disease. *Lancet*, **1**, 1101–1103 (1980)

15 McLARTY, D. G., ALEXANDER, W. D., HARDEN, R. Mc.G. and CLARK, D. H. Results of treatment of thyrotoxicosis after postoperative relapse. *British Medical Journal*, **3**, 200–203 (1969)

16 MICHIE, W., STOWERS, J. M., DUNCAN, T., PEGG, C. A. S., HAMER-HODGES, D. W., HEMS, G., BEWSHER, P. D. and HEDLEY, A. J. Mechanism of hypocalcaemia after thyroidectomy for thyrotoxicosis. *Lancet*, **1**, 508–514 (1971)

17 MICHIE, W., HAMER-HODGES, D. W., PEGG, C. A. S., ORR, F. G. G. and BEWSHER, P. D. Beta-blockade and partial thyroidectomy for thyrotoxicosis. *Lancet*, **1**, 1009–1011 (1974)

18 MOSEKILDE, L., MELSEN, F., BAGGER, J. P., MYHRE-JENSEN, O. and SORENSEN, N. S. Bone changes in hyperthyroidism: interrelationships between bone morphometry, thyroid function and calcium–phosphorus metabolism. *Acta Endocrinologica*, **85**, 515–525 (1977)

19 PROUT, T. E. Thyroid disease in pregnancy. *American Journal of Obstetrics and Gynecology*, **122**, 669–676 (1975)

20 RIDDELL, V. Thyrotoxicosis and the surgeon. *British Journal of Surgery*, **49**, 465–496 (1962)

21 RUDE, R. K., OLDHAM, S. B., SINGER, F. R. and NICOLOFF, J. T. Treatment of thyrotoxic hypercalcemia with propranolol. *New England Journal of Medicine*, **294**, 431–433 (1976)

22 TENG, C. S., YEUNG, R. T. T., KHOO, R. K. K. and ALGARATNAM, T. T. A prospective study of the changes in thyrotropin binding inhibitory immunoglobulins in Graves' disease treated by subtotal thyroidectomy or radioactive iodine. *Journal of Clinical Endocrinology and Metabolism*, **50**, 1005–1010 (1980)

23 TOFT, A. D., IRVINE, W. J., McINTOSH, D., SETH, J., CAMERON, E. H. D. and LIDGARD, G. P. Temporary hypothyroidism after surgical treatment of thyrotoxicosis. *Lancet*, **2**, 817–818 (1976)

24 TWEEDLE, D., COLLING, A., SCHARDT, W., GREEN, E. M., EVERED, D. C., DICKINSON, P. H. and JOHNSTON, I. D. A. Hypothyroidism following partial thyroidectomy for thyrotoxicosis and its relationship to thyroid remnant size. *British Journal of Surgery*, **64**, 445–448 (1977)

25 VAN WELSUM, M., FELTKAMP, T. E. W., De VRIES, M. J., DOCTOR, R., HENNEMANN, G. and VAN ZIJL, J. Hypothyroidism after thyroidectomy for Graves' disease: a search for an explanation. *British Medical Journal*, **4**, 755–757 (1974)

26 VELENTZAS, C., OREOPOULOS, D. G., FROM, G., PORRET, B. and RAPOPORT, A. Vitamin-D levels in thyrotoxicosis. *Lancet*, **1**, 370–371 (1977)

27 WADE, J. S. H. Clinical research in thyroid surgery. *Annals of the Royal College of Surgeons*, **50**, 112–117 (1972)

28 WADE, J. S. H. Thyroidectomy. In *Contemporary Operative Surgery*, edited by Adrian Marston, pp. 153–160. Northwood Publications (1979)

29 WADE, J. S. H., GOODALL, P., DEANE, L., DAUNCEY, T. M. and FOURMAN, P. The course of partial parathyroid insufficiency after thyroidectomy. *British Journal of Surgery*, **52**, 497–503 (1965)

Editors' commentary on Chapter 1

The viewpoint of these British authors in managing thyrotoxicosis differs somewhat from that of many clinicians in the United States, particularly as regards the use of radioactive iodine. In some American centers, ^{131}I is given as definitive treatment to children with Graves' disease. In most hospitals ^{131}I is offered to nearly all patients with the disease over the age of 20 years as the preferred treatment, usually after a trial of antithyroid drugs has failed to produce a permanent remission. Women who wish to have children, however, frequently prefer to have a subtotal thyroidectomy when they are fully informed of the alternatives. At the present time it is safe to say that in the United States the majority of the adults with Graves' disease are treated with ^{131}I. For those with thyrotoxicosis due to toxic multinodular goiter, surgery is still considered the treatment of choice unless there are absolute contraindications. This is particularly true of those with any symptoms of compression of either the airway or the esophagus.

The management of the autonomous nodule causing thryotoxicosis continues to be somewhat controversial. The majority of clinicians in the United States would recommend surgical excision rather than treatment with ^{131}I. One of the theoretical reasons for doing so is the fact that the normal thyroid tissue surrounding the hyperfunctioning nodule will be exposed to low dose irradiation. Late sequelae of such treatment as far as the 'normal thyroid' tissue is concerned are a cause for anxiety. The surgical treatment of autonomous nodules is simple excision only. These patients do not require thyroid supplementation postoperatively because their remaining thyroid glands usually respond normally to endogenous TSH.

There are two other debatable areas of management that are worthy of mention. In the United States, although children are usually first treated with antithyroid drugs, long-term remission despite 1 or 2 years of treatment is infrequent. Subtotal thyroidectomy is then considered the definitive treatment of choice. Thyroidectomy in children is more extensive than in adults because regeneration of remnant tissue is more likely to cause recurrence. Consequently, most children are treated with near total thyroidectomy followed by thyroid replacement therapy. The second area of contention concerns the management of patients who are diagnosed as having thyrotoxicosis during pregnancy. If the disease cannot be readily controlled with decreasing doses of antithyroid drugs, thyroidectomy during the second trimester may be performed safely. In order to ensure the best maternal and fetal health, these patients are given thyroid supplement throughout the rest of their pregnancy and then re-evaluated *post partum* for continuing need for replacement therapy. The objective is to avoid antithyroid drugs or maternal hypothyroidism, both harmful to the fetus, during the second half of pregnancy.

2
The thyroid nodule – surgical management

Norman W. Thompson

The thyroid nodule continues to be a major source of concern to physicians and surgeons evaluating patients with thyroid disease. The reasons for this are the relative frequency of benign nodules, the infrequency of malignancy and the difficulty in selecting those needing operations. There has been a lack of consensus as to the use and interpretation of various diagnostic studies. However, sufficient experience has been accumulated to allow some conclusions about the relative value of each diagnostic modality and its use in the study of patients with thyroid nodules. In this chapter, the management of clinically solitary nodules without definite evidence of malignancy, such as lower cervical adenopathy or recurrent laryngeal nerve palsy, will receive major emphasis. The indications for operative intervention will be considered and the intraoperative strategy outlined.

Currently, in most US medical centers, the most common indication for a thyroid operation is the presence of a solitary thyroid nodule and the suspicion that it might be malignant. Although multinodular thyroid glands continue to be referred for surgical consideration, the indications for operation are more often related to symptoms of compression, thyrotoxicosis or cosmesis rather than the possibility of thyroid carcinoma. These indications are usually easily defined and are not controversial. Less clear are the indications for operations in patients with small multinodular thyroid glands but no symptoms or history of head or neck irradiation. This group of patients will also be considered.

INCIDENCE

Because the majority of solitary nodules found on clinical examination and considered for operation are suspected of being malignant neoplasms, the true perspective of the problem can only be appreciated when the incidence of both benign nodules and thyroid carcinoma in the general population is considered. The figures from recent studies in the United States are similar to those from other countries in which there has been no iodine deficiency for at least several generations.

It has been estimated that approximately 4.2% of the United States population between the ages of 30 and 60 years have one or more palpable thyroid nodules. This means that there are about 9 000 000 American adults with thyroid nodules. An additional 250 000 adults develop new nodules each year[21].

The occurrence of thyroid carcinoma, as determined by the American Cancer Society, was 9100 new cases in the United States during 1980. This figure accounted for approximately 1% of all the new cancers diagnosed. There were 1050 deaths due to thyroid cancer during the same year. The thyroid carcinoma occurrence rate was 4.4 per 100 000 per year[18].

It is apparent from these figures that the process of selecting patients for surgery is of great practical importance, particularly when one considers that only 1 of 1000 patients with a nodule is likely to have a malignancy. Obviously many individuals with nodules are never evaluated and many others are not considered surgical candidates. The latter group includes many patients with small multinodular goiters.

The reported incidence of carcinoma in surgically treated solitary nodules has varied considerably[2-7, 13, 19]. Factors such as geographical location, selection of patients, and length of follow-up have influenced the results of such studies. Because the natural history of most differentiated thyroid carcinomas is one of very slow growth, the true incidence of malignancy in patients with known thyroid nodules can only be determined after 10 or more years. A shorter follow-up period will invariably result in an underestimated incidence of malignancy. In our experience, 80% of all thyroid carcinomas seen during the past two decades have been differentiated thyroid cancers (papillary or follicular), which can be almost indolent for long periods of time. Medullary carcinoma of the thyroid, which accounts for approximately 7% of all thyroid cancers, is, although occasionally very aggressive, also frequently slow-growing. Therefore only anaplastic thyroid carcinomas or lymphomas of the thyroid gland, which consistently enlarge rapidly, can be diagnosed with certainty during a relatively short period of observation.

DIAGNOSTIC STUDIES

The history and physical examination are the most important considerations in evaluating thyroid nodules. In many patients an asymptomatic nodule is first discovered during a routine physical examination. Often these patients are completely unaware of any thyroid enlargement or symptoms, even after the nodule has been identified. Nearly half the patients with asymptomatic nodules discover them while looking in the mirror, shaving, or casually palpating their necks[6]. During the past decade, many patients, aware of the relationship between external irradiation exposure during infancy or childhood and the development of thyroid carcinoma, have come to their physician requesting thyroid evaluation. The association of thyroid cancer and previous radiation exposure has been widely publicized in both the lay and medical literature. This question should always be asked when taking the history and, if the answer is not known, investigated further. In our experience, subsequent questioning of parents or personal physicians, or review of old hospital records frequently shows that a patient has had head or neck irradiation during childhood or infancy which has been completely forgotten. Most patients are very happy to cooperate in this investigation and some have done excellent detective work in obtaining the required information. A positive history of low-dose radiation exposure is a factor in favor of a more aggressive approach to the thyroid nodule. Nearly 1 in 5 patients under the age of 30 years found to have thyroid carcinoma have such a history. Another important consideration is the use of thyroid hormones, the duration of their administration, and changes in the nodule during treatment. Thyroid suppression as a diagnostic test will be considered in more detail later. It is emphasized here that growth of a nodule in a patient taking suppressive doses of thyroid hormone is significant and suggests that the nodule is an autonomous neoplasm (malignant).

Results from a careful examination of the neck can often determine the possibility of thyroid carcinoma. Large firm lymph nodes in the lower third of the neck are often present, particularly in children and young adults with papillary carcinoma. Lymphadenopathy with an ipsilateral thyroid nodule should always be considered due to malignancy until proven otherwise. Obvious fixation of a nodule to surrounding structures implies malignancy and merits little further consideration in this discussion. The same cannot be said about the palpable consistency of a solitary nodule, however. Some malignancies are not hard or firm, and an occasional benign nodule may be stony hard with calcification. A firm nodule with an irregular outline or capsule does, however, raise the likelihood of malignancy. Hoarseness, without recurrent laryngeal nerve palsy, may be noted with either benign or malignant nodules. Definite paralysis of the recurrent laryngeal nerve (RLN) on the side on which there is a thyroid nodule indicates a carcinoma in nearly all cases. During the past 10 years we have seen only 3 patients with RLN palsies resulting from benign thyroid nodules. In each case very large nodules (more than 10 cm) had caused the nerves to be stretched over their capsules. It is recognized that an occasional patient will develop spontaneous RLN palsy, unrelated to a benign thyroid nodule. So far we have not encountered this.

An evaluation of the entire thyroid gland is important. A careful search is made for evidence of Hashimoto's disease, diffuse enlargement or other nodules. The presence of other nodules, no adenopathy, normal cord function and no history of irradiation reduces the probability of malignancy. Before recommending observation, thyroid suppression or operation, other diagnostic studies may be needed. Those most commonly used will be considered in more detail.

Isotope scintiscans

Thyroid scintiscans are frequently used to supplement the findings of a physical examination[1, 2, 5, 6, 13, 14, 17, 19]. Palpation, however, is usually more accurate in outlining a thyroid nodule, especially when done by an experienced physician. In most cases the results of scintigraphy should not be considered decisive in determining the treatment of thyroid nodules. A lesion must be at least 1 cm or more in diameter before it can be seen on a thyroid scan[14, 17]. The scintiscan, regardless of the isotope administered, usually fails to delineate a nodule that cannot be palpated on physical examination unless it is substernal. Although many patients are referred for surgical treatment after a thyroid scan has already demonstrated a non-functioning ('cold') nodule, this does not mean that the lesion is malignant[6]. There is considerable evidence, including our own, that the majority of 'cold' thyroid nodules are benign[20]. The presence or absence of function is usually of little value in differentiating benign from malignant nodules. Only when a nodule is hyperfunctioning ('hot'), as determined by a radioactive iodine compound, can it be said with relative certainty that it is benign. Even then an occasional 'hot' nodule may be a well differentiated thyroid carcinoma. Because only 5% of all solitary nodules are 'hot', thyroid scintiscans are of little discriminant value in most cases. Nevertheless, thyroid scintiscans are still commonly obtained in patients referred to surgeons with a thyroid nodule. Therefore, their limitations should be understood by every surgeon treating patients with thyroid nodules.

At present, technetium-99 pertechnetate ($^{99}Tc^m$) is the agent of choice for routine imaging of the thyroid gland[17]. It gives the lowest radiation dose of any of the available radioactive isotopes (absorbed dose to the thyroid 1.02 to 3.4 rad) and permits the use of high-resolution but low-efficiency pinhole imaging techniques with the scintillation camera. The limitations of this agent are related to the fact that the maximum uptake of $^{99}Tc^m$ occurs only 20–30 minutes after the injection and that small 'cold' nodules may therefore be missed because the background level of radiation is still high. The isotope is only trapped by the thyroid gland and is not organified, as is iodine. When a nodule is 'hot' with technetium-99 pertechnetate, the possibility of malignancy, particularly papillary carcinoma, is not excluded. A ^{131}I-labeled compound is necessary to assess functional activity of a nodule.

Until the past decade ^{131}I was the most commonly used agent for thyroid imaging and assessment of the functional activity of thyroid tissue and palpable nodules. Currently ^{123}I is considered the best agent for thyroid scanning for diagnostic purposes, primarily because of its short half-life (only 13 hours), and the fact that it is bound organically within the thyroid, and the absorbed radiation dose of the thyroid is very similar to that of $^{99}Tc^m$ and far lower than that of ^{131}I. Its limitations include its short half-life and the fact that it has to be produced in an accelerator. It is also more expensive and has a shorter shelf-life than the other agents. The major restricting factor when used for evaluating thyroid nodules is the lesser discriminating capacity of the γ-camera compared to the scintillation camera used for technetium scanning. Nodules smaller than 1 cm in diameter will usually be missed.

As emphasized earlier, thyroid scintiscans only supplement the findings of a physical examination, which should be considered as more important for the diagnosis. Thyroid functions studies, however, should be done in all patients, particularly those with large nodules. Most patients will prove to be euthyroid. In some cases a scintiscan may demonstrate a nodule that is hyperfunctioning relative to the rest of the gland. This suggests that it may be autonomous in its function. In our experience fewer than 5% of all solitary nodules are 'hot'. This is the one situation in which a radioactive iodine scan is of value in differentiating benign from malignant nodules, because nearly all 'hot' nodules are benign. Furthermore, when a 'hot' nodule is larger than 3 cm in diameter, it may cause thyrotoxicosis. We have not seen hyperthyroidism in a patient with a solitary nodule smaller than 3.5 cm.

Whether all hyperfunctioning thyroid nodules larger than 2 cm in diameter should be surgically excised is debatable. The indication for surgical removal of a 'hot' nodule differs from that for a 'cold' nodule because of its potential for causing hyperthyroidism if this is not already present. In our experience with solitary nodules, only 1 in 150 has had biochemical evidence of hyperthyroidsm.

Whether the routine use of scintigraphy can be justified by the argument that 'hot' nodules would otherwise remain unrecognized is debatable. If one's philosophy is that these are best treated surgically anyway, there is scant justification for the study.

A scintiscan may be of value when the thyroid gland cannot be completely palpated because of substernal extension. In this circumstance a scan may outline the lower extent of the thyroid gland and also delineate 'cold' or 'hot' nodules that would otherwise escape detection because of the bony thorax.

Ultrasonography (echography)

Sonography of the thyroid gland has been widely used during the past 10 years to supplement the physical examination of the thyroid, scintiscan or both[11,12,13,16]. As instrumentation and skill in interpretation improved it became apparent that sonography was useful in determining the consistency of a nodule. Three basic echo patterns could be delineated: cysts, complex nodules (mixed solid and cystic), and solid nodules could be recognized within the thyroid. In most centers, radiologists reported that ultrasonographic diagnosis was accurate in more than 95% of cases[13,16]. The identification of cystic lesions by ultrasonography, perhaps more than any other factor, encouraged the use of needle aspiration. Cystic lesions comprise about 10–20% of solitary thyroid nodules, and their recognition, confirmation and treatment by needle aspiration eliminated the need for operation in most of these patients. As experience was gained it was found that the incidence of malignancy in thyroid cysts was very low, and treatment by aspiration alone became the definitive treatment in those in whom the cyst could be completely aspirated, leading to its disappearance. The complex lesions, composed of cystic and solid areas, were found to represent degenerative areas or old hemorrhage within a solid nodule. This sonographic pattern could not rule out malignancy.

How useful is sonography in the evaluation of solitary thyroid nodules? In our center it has been virtually abandoned in the evaluation of the palpable thyroid nodule. Since the adoption of fine needle aspiration in virtually all cases, it has been found that there is no need to identify nodules as solid or cystic by ultrasonography. This could easily be accomplished at the time of initial examination with fine needle aspiration. There are still many patients, however, who are referred with sonograms 'in hand'. Because fine needle aspiration is performed regardless, we have found that the information offered by sonography is superfluous. In all cases in which a sonogram demonstrated a cystic lesion, fluid has been readily aspirated from the 'palpable nodule'. Sonography is here discussed because of its historical interest and not because of its current practical use.

Needle biopsy

Needle biopsy techniques, which have been extensively used in Scandinavia for more than 25 years, have recently gained wider acceptance and enthusiastic advocates in the United States[1, 3, 4, 8, 9, 10, 13, 22]. During the past 5 years both fine needle aspiration cytology and large needle biopsy have been used in a number of North American centers. One of the principal reasons for not introducing these techniques earlier was the fear of implanting thyroid carcinoma in the needle tract. The reported world-wide experience has conclusively shown that such fears were for the most part groundless. Crile, an American pioneer in the technique of large needle biopsy with 20 years of experience, reported that in more than 2000 needle biopsies of the thyroid, only one small implant of thyroid carcinoma occurred. He contends that the danger of implantation was greatly exaggerated[3]. This complication has been reported in only a few other instances. In one large series there were no reported implants after the needle aspiration of 900 'cold' nodules, 5% of which were malignant. In over 3000 biopsies, Miller[10] observed no cases of cancer implantation. He used both fine needle aspiration and Tru-Cut needle biopsies. During a 25-year period, in which more than 20 000 fine needle aspiration biopsies of palpable thyroid nodules were carried out at the Karolinska Hospital, implantation of thyroid carcinoma did not occur[9]. Thus, one of the major concerns about this technique has proved to be of no clinical significance. The possibility of implantation of malignant cells is not considered a deterrent today. It has been argued that the most important limitation of needle biopsy is that insufficient tissue is obtained for reliable diagnosis[10–12]. Although there are recognized limitations in the interpretation of thyroid needle aspiration or biopsy, its usefulness and the high degree of accuracy attained by those experienced in its technique are unquestioned today.

The two major techniques of needle biopsy currently in use should not be confused or equated, as they are based on different principles[8]. Large needle biopsy implies that a piece of tissue is cut from a nodule for histological examination, whereas in fine needle aspiration a smear is obtained from the aspirate of a nodule. There are virtually no complications from fine needle aspiration when properly performed[9, 10]. Large needle biopsy, however, can lead to complications such as hemorrhage and recurrent laryngeal nerve palsy. The latter technique is limited to large nodules (2 cm in size or greater), whereas fine needle aspiration can be done on any palpable thyroid nodule. As noted earlier, there have been no reported cases of seeding of cancer cells in thousands of patients undergoing fine needle aspiration. This complication has occurred in only a few cases in which core needle biopsy was done. The technique of aspiration biopsy cytology has been described in detail by Löwhagen et al.[8,9] and Miller[10]. The reported results in large series of patients show that false negative diagnoses were made in less than 10%, and false positive diagnoses in 0–2%[10]. When used by a skilled cytologist, this technique is highly accurate and considered the method of choice in the selection of patients for surgery. Löwhagen et al.[9] claimed that at the Karolinska Hospital nearly 80% of patients with thyroid nodules could be spared surgical exploration as a result of such studies. Because of the risk of false negative diagnoses (10%) even the advocates of this technique emphasize the importance of clinical judgment, in addition to the results of the cytological study, in selecting operative candidates. Löwhagen et al.[9] point out that some patients, particularly those with nodular goiters, may have false negative aspirations if occult papillary carcinomas are included as indicative of failure. They justifiably emphasize that advocating thyroidectomy in every patient with a nodular thyroid lesion, in fear of missing an occult carcinoma, is impractical and absurd. World-wide experience supports the Karolinska's results in that false positive cytological diagnoses of thyroid carcinoma are rare. As a diagnostic method, this technique closely parallels histopathological standards of accuracy. It is concluded that aspiration cytology enables the cytologist to distinguish non-neoplastic from neoplastic nodules. Recognition of the type of tumor is also possible in the majority of cases. Papillary and medullary carcinomas both demonstrate a very typical cytological picture, as does anaplastic thyroid carcinoma. Cytological diagnosis cannot as yet reliably differentiate between a malignant and a benign follicular or Hurthle cell neoplasm[8-10]. A definitive diagnosis in these cases depends on histological examination of the excised tumor.

The disadvantages of fine needle biopsy compared to large needle biopsy have been critically evaluated by Miller[10], who found that the major limitation of fine needle biopsy is that it may not provide a sample of sufficient cellular material for diagnosis. The reasons for this are that the needle may have missed the nodule or too small a needle was used, or that too little suction was applied and suction alone failed to dislodge cellular material. In Miller's experience, when fine needle biopsy did not yield a sufficient aspirate of cellular material this could be successfully obtained by large needle biopsy. This was also used for nodules larger than 3.5 cm and when the cytological diagnosis was questionable. Large needle biopsy was found useful in approximately 15% of patients in whom fine needle biopsy was considered unsatisfactory or in need of further clarification. In Miller's experience with both techniques the chances of a false negative diagnosis were considered to be less than 1% when occult papillary carcinomas were excluded. Miller concluded that needle biopsy of the thyroid is the simplest, most direct and most cost-effective method for determining the diagnosis of a thyroid nodule. The best results were achieved by using a combination of fine and large needle biopsies. Either alone was far superior to any combination of clinical or non-invasive diagnostic approaches.

The introduction of needle biopsies has drastically reduced the number of diagnostic surgical operations for benign lesions in centers where it has been extensively used[3, 9, 10]. In some Scandinavian hospitals, needle aspiration is routinely carried out before operative intervention is considered. At present the major factor limiting the universal use of this technique is a shortage of pathologists or cytologists experienced in the interpretation of thyroid cytology.

Thyroid suppression

It has been claimed that with the administration of exogenous thyroxin and effective suppression of thyroid stimulating hormone (TSH) approximately 50% of benign thyroid nodules will decrease in size or disappear[5, 20]. Thyroid suppression therapy has been advocated for nearly 30 years. Usually thyroid feeding is recommended for a minimal period of 3 to 6 months. Our experience does not support the claims made for thyroid suppression therapy. Some 'nodules' may regress in 6 weeks without any treatment whatsoever. These are invariably hemorrhagic thyroidal cysts, usually appearing acutely, and can be suspected from a careful clinical history. In our opinion the majority of 'nodules' that disappear are lobulations of the thyroid gland, or diffuse enlargement of a thyroid lobe associated with either Hashimoto's disease or colloid goiter. Although an occasional nodule will decrease in size or even disappear, this occurs in fewer than 4% of solitary non-cystic nodules. More frequently, after suppressive therapy, the surrounding parenchyma shrinks and the nodule becomes more discrete to palpation. Suppression of the thyroid gland by thyroxin may help in the selection of patients for operation in a few cases. If TSH suppression is routinely applied, strict criteria for the selection of patients for thyroidectomy must be used. It should be recognized that a well differentiated thyroid cancer may occasionally decrease in size[5]. Unless resolution of the lesion is complete, carcinoma cannot be ruled out with certainty. With the increasing use of needle aspiration biopsy and diagnosis of benign thyroid disease, thyroid suppression may be of value for therapeutic reasons or to prevent further enlargement or the development of new nodules. In most patients, 120 mg of dessicated thyroid, or 0.15 mg of sodium levothyroxin, suppresses TSH and causes no symptoms of thyroid hormone excess. Patients treated by thyroid suppression for 'benign' thyroid disease should be carefully reviewed at regular intervals by a physician experienced in evaluating thyroid glands.

Other diagnostic studies

Currently there is only one serum immunoassay specific for the diagnosis of thyroid carcinoma. With a few exceptions, usually clinically obvious, an elevated serum calcitonin level is diagnostic of medullary carcinoma. Although this test is extremely valuable in screening at-risk MEN IIa and IIb family members for possible thyroid carcinoma, its use for everyone with a thyroid nodule is impractical and wasteful. Sporadic medullary carcinoma of the thyroid accounts for fewer than 4% of all thyroid malignancies. A serum calcitonin level should be obtained whenever a needle biopsy is diagnostic or suspicious of medullary carcinoma.

Serum thyroglobulin is another assay frequently used. Elevated levels may occur, however, in patients with both benign and malignant thyroid lesions. The test is not specific enough to be useful in selection of patients for operation. Serum thyroglobulin levels may be helpful in detecting residual or recurrent thyroid carcinoma after total thyroidectomy, however.

Antithyroid antibiodies are useful in the overall evaluation of patients with suspected Hashimoto's disease. The presence of a discrete nodule in association with Hashimoto's disease, however, does not preclude the diagnosis of an associated thyroid carcinoma. In the context of this discussion an elevation of thyroid antibody levels is of no clinical significance.

THE OPERATIVE TREATMENT OF THE SOLITARY THYROID NODULE

Total extracapsular lobectomy and isthmusectomy is the procedure of choice when a decision has been made to surgically remove a suspicious thyroid nodule[20]. The entire lobe, with the isthmus, is submitted for frozen section pathological examination. When a nodule is located in the isthmus, it is excised with a margin of normal thyroid tissue on both sides for the biopsy. In performing total lobectomy, both parathyroid glands are carefully preserved with their blood supply by either dissecting them from the surface of the thyroid gland or completely avoiding them if they are not in the immediate proximity of the thyroid capsule. This is done anticipating that total thyroidectomy may be necessary if either the frozen or permanent histological sections confirm the presence of thyroid carcinoma. Total lobectomy offers the best opportunity for accurate histological diagnosis and is associated with the lowest complication rate when the need for reoperation is considered. In our last 800 consecutive cases in which total unilateral lobectomy was performed for benign or malignant nodules suspected of being cancer, no permanent recurrent laryngeal nerve palsies have occurred. We are firmly convinced that a total lobectomy is safer than a partial lobectomy followed by resection of the lobe after delayed diagnosis of malignancy. Reoperation to complete a lobectomy after an interval of several days or weeks is associated with a greater risk to both the recurrent laryngeal nerve and the parathyroids on the ipsilateral side. Furthermore, the possibility of implanting carcinoma cells is increased by subtotal lobectomy. Although there is controversy as to whether a total lobectomy and isthmusectomy or a total thyroidectomy is the best definitive operation for a unilateral papillary carcinoma, a subtotal lobectomy is universally considered an inadequate operation[15, 20]. A definitive cancer operation can be accomplished with one procedure in 80% of cases when a skilled thyroid pathologist is available for frozen section interpretation. Therefore it is critical that a frozen section diagnosis be determined so that a definitive operation may be selected whenever open surgical biopsy of a thyroid nodule is performed. A lobectomy or biopsy should not be done without the aid of a competent pathologist who is familiar with the histopathology of thyroid lesions on frozen sections. As confidence is gained in the interpretation of needle biopsies obtained preoperatively, it is likely that the need for intraoperative pathological consultation will decrease. The surgeon may then determine preoperatively what definitive thyroid operation is required, perhaps modified by the gross findings at operation.

CONCLUSIONS

The purpose of this chapter has been to outline in some detail the process of selecting patients with thyroid nodules for exploration when thyroid carcinoma is suspected. It has been shown that by selective use of the diagnostic techniques reviewed, in addition to important clinical considerations (including the age and sex of the patient, characteristics of the nodule, presence or absence of lymphadenopathy or recurrent laryngeal nerve palsy, and history of radiation exposure), many exploratory thyroid operations can be avoided. The surgical patients with solitary thyroid nodules seen at the University of Michigan Hospital between 1966 and 1972 were reviewed 10 years ago[6]. The incidence of malignancy in 202 patients with clinically solitary thyroid nodules undergoing surgery was 28.7%. Patients less than 40 years of age had a 35.7% incidence of malignancy. It was concluded that at that time no sufficiently specific diagnostic studies were available to differentiate benign from malignant lesions. It was also concluded that most patients under the age of 40 years with solitary thyroid nodules should have an exploration with a minimal delay, regardless of sex. The highest incidence of carcinoma was found in patients under 20 years of age and in patients older than 60 years of age with new nodules. Our experience of the last few years, during which needle biopsy has been increasingly used, has led us to the conclusion that the single most important diagnostic aid, in addition to careful clinical evaluation, is the needle biopsy. The incidence of thyroid carcinoma in solitary nodules surgically explored at the University Hospital during the past 5 years is approximately 50%. This does not imply that the incidence of thyroid cancer in solitary nodules has increased. We interpret this to mean that the ability to select patients for operation has improved considerably during the last decade.

References

1 BLUM, M. and ROTHSCHILD, M. Improved nonoperation diagnosis of the solitary 'cold' thyroid nodule. *Journal of the American Medical Association*, **243**, 242–245 (1980)

2 BROOKS, J. R. The solitary thyroid nodule. *American Journal of Surgery*, **125**, 477–482 (1973)

3 ESSELSTYN, C. B. and CRILE, C. Jr Needle aspiration and needle biopsy of the thyroid. *World Journal of Surgery*, **2**, 321–329 (1978)

4 HAMBURGER, J. I., MILLER, J. M. and KINI, S. R. *Clinical Pathology of Thyroid Nodules: Handbook and Atlas*. Private publication (1979)

5 HILL, L. D. and BEEBE, H. G. Thyroid suppression. *Archives of Surgery*, **108**, 403–408 (1974)

6 HOFFMAN, G. L., THOMPSON, N. W. and HEFFRON, C. The solitary thyroid nodule: a reassessment. *Archives of Surgery*, **105**, 379–385 (1972)

7 LIECHTY, R. D. and ZIMMERMAN, D. Solitary thyroid nodules. *Archives of Surgery*, **112**, 59–61 (1977)

8 LÖWHAGEN, T., GRANBERG, P. O., LUNDELL, G. Aspiration biopsy cytology (ABC) in nodules of the thyroid gland suspected to be malignant. *Surgical Clinics of North America*, **59**, 3–18 (1979)

9 LÖWHAGEN, T., WILLEM, J. S., LUNDELL, G. Aspiration biopsy cytology in diagnosis of thyroid cancer. *World Journal of Surgery*, **5**, 61–73 (1981)

10 MILLER, J. M. Needle biopsy of the thyroid: methods and recommendations. *Thyroid Today*, **1**, 1–5 (1982)

11 MILLER, J. M., KINI, S. R., REBUCK, J. *Controversies in Clinical Thyroidology*. New York, Springer-Verlag (1981)

12 MILLER, J. M., HAMBURGER, J. I. and SINI, S. Diagnosis of thyroid nodules. *Journal of the American Medical Association*, **241**, 481–484 (1979)
13 NEWSOME, H. H. and FRATKIN, M. J. Thyroid nodules: selecting patients and operations. *Journal of Clinical Surgery*, **1**, 15–21 (1982)
14 OKERLUND, M. D., SOMMER, J., GRELL, T. Clinical importance of the 'indeterminate' nodule in thyroid imaging: the commonest cause of the 'false negative' thyroid imaging study. *Journal of Nuclear Medicine*, **21**, 31 (1980)
15 PERZIK, S. L. *Surgery in Thyroid Disease: The Place of Total Thyroidectomy*. New York, Stratton Intercontinental (1976)
16 ROSEN, I. B., WALFISH, P. G. and MISKEN, M. The ultra sound of thyroid masses. *Surgical Clinics of North America*, **59**, 19–33 (1979)
17 RYO, U. Y., ARNOLD, J., COLMAN, M., ARNOLD, M., FAUUS, M., FROHMAN, L., SCHNEIDER, A., STACHURA, M. and PINSKY, S. Thyroid scintigram sensitivity with sodium pertechnetate ^{99}Tc and gamma camera with phosphate collimator. *Journal of the American Medical Association*, **235**, 1235–1238 (1978)
18 SILVERBURY, E. Cancer statistics. *Cancer*, **30**, 23–38 (1980)
19 THOMAS, C. G., Jr, BUCKWALTER, J. A., STAAB, E. V. and KERR, C. Y. Evaluation of dominant thyroid masses. *Annals of Surgery*, **183**, 463–469 (1976)
20 THOMPSON, N. W., NISHIYAMA, R. H. and HARNESS, J. K. Thyroid carcinoma: current controversies. *Current Problems in Surgery*, **15**, 1–67 (1978)
21 VANDER, J. B., GASTON, E. A. and DAWBER, T. R. The significance of non-toxic thyroid nodules: final report of a 15-year study on the incidence of thyroid malignancy. *Annals of Internal Medicine*, **69**, 537–554 (1968)
22 WONG, C., VICKERY, A. L., Jr and MALOOF, F. Needle biopsy of the thyroid gland. *Surgery, Gynecology and Obstetrics*, **143**, 365–368 (1976)

3
Transplantation of the parathyroid glands

Mikael E. Romanus, John R. Farndon and
Samuel A. Wells, Jr

INTRODUCTION

The clinical importance of the parathyroid glands was appreciated early in the 1900s, 20 years after Sandstrom[45] had discovered the organs and 10 years after Gley[21] had demonstrated their importance in the maintenance of a stable serum calcium level. It was recognized that the carpal spasm, laryngeal stridor and circumoral tingling which often developed after extensive thyroid surgery were due to iatrogenic damage of the parathyroid glands. Halsted[25] realized the seriousness of these complications and initiated the first animal experiments on parathyroid transplantation.

The successful autotransplantation of parathyroid glands has been clearly demonstrated in both laboratory animals[14, 29, 49, 52] and man[1, 20, 26, 55]. Survival of allografted parathyroid tissue has also been demonstrated in the immunosuppressed host[23, 53, 55]. Function of the transplanted parathyroid has been proved by its ability, as the only source of parathyroid hormone (PTH), to maintain the grafted host in a normocalcemic state. Also, graft function has been demonstrated by a high concentration of PTH in the grafted tissue or its venous effluent.

During the last decade it has become clear that autotransplantation of parathyroid tissue is a valuable technique in certain clinical situations:

Primary parathyroid hyperplasia
Secondary parathyroid hyperplasia
Re-exploration for persistent or recurrent hyperparathyroidism
Total thyroidectomy for carcinoma

Parathyroid allotransplantation is indicated in cases of failure of medical management in the aparathyroid patient and in DiGeorge's syndrome.

During the last 8 years we have performed parathyroid autotransplants in 160 patients and our clinical experience forms the basis of this report.

CLINICAL INDICATIONS

Autotransplantation at initial surgery

Primary parathyroid hyperplasia

Less than 15% of patients with primary hyperparathyroidism have enlargement of four or more[3] glands (parathyroid hyperplasia)[40,61]. In contrast to those with a single enlarged parathyroid gland, patients with hyperparathyroidism due to parathyroid hyperplasia are difficult to manage. The surgical procedure most commonly advocated for patients with primary hyperplasia is 3½-gland parathyroidectomy. Castleman and Cope[10] reported that 55% of their patients with water clear cell hyperplasia (WCCH) developed persistent or recurrent hyperparathyroidism 1 to 10 years postoperatively, and Romanus et al.[40] found that 15% of patients with WCCH developed postoperative hypercalcemia. Chief cell hyperplasia, the common form of generalized parathyroid enlargement, may occur alone or in association with familial endocrinopathies: multiple endocrine neoplasia type I (MEN I), multiple endocrine neoplasia type IIa (MEN IIa) or familial hypocalciuric hypercalcemic hyperparathyroidism (FHHH). In reviewing the literature, Clark, Way and Hunt[13] found recurrent postoperative hypercalcemia in 33% of 22 patients undergoing surgery for familial hyperparathyroidism. Lamers and Froeling[31] reported recurrent hypercalcemia postoperatively in 5 (38%) of 13 patients with MEN I. Of the 12 patients with MEN I reported by Prinz et al.[37], 5 (42%) became normocalcemic, 3 (25%) became hypocalcemic and 4 (33%) developed persistent or recurrent hypercalcemia following subtotal parathyroidectomy. Marx et al.[33] reported that 6 (86%) of 7 patients with FHHH remained hypercalcemic and 1 became aparathyroid after parathyroid surgery.

Because of such poor results in patients with four gland hyperparathyroidism treated by subtotal parathyroidectomy, we suggested a technique where all parathyroids are removed from the neck and pieces from one gland are autotransplanted to the forearm[56].

The mass of hyperfunctioning parathyroid tissue is markedly reduced by this procedure, and should graft-dependent hypercalcemia later develop, a portion of the transplanted tissue could be removed under local anesthesia. In patients having 3½-gland parathyroidectomy, a repeat neck exploration under general anesthesia would be required to correct the recurrent hypercalcemia.

We have performed this procedure in 21 patients undergoing their first operation for hyperparathyroidism due to generalized hyperplasia (Table 3.1). Of these, 11 had familial hyperparathyroidism associated with either MEN I (5 patients), MEN IIa (3 patients) or FHHH (3 patients), and 10 had non-familial parathyroid hyperplasia. Immediately postoperatively, 20 of the 21 patients developed hypocalcemia and most were placed on oral vitamin D and calcium therapy. After termination of therapy (less than 2 months) the 20 patients became normocalcemic. In one patient (5%) with MEN I, prolonged replacement therapy with vitamin D and calcium was required to maintain normocalcemia, despite a functioning parathyroid graft (as demonstrated by a high concentration of PTH in the venous

Table 3.1 Autotransplantation of parathyroid tissue in 160 patients

	Time of autotransplantation		
Diagnosis	Initial surgery	Reoperation	Deferred (cryopreserved tissue)
Primary hyperparathyroidism			
Hyperplasia			
Non-familial	10	6	4
MEN I, MEN IIa	8	2	2
FHHH	3	1	0
Adenoma	0	0	3
Secondary hyperparathyroidism	58	5	2
Normal parathyroid tissue (in conjunction with thyroid surgery)			
1–3 glands	40	0	0
4 glands	16	0	0
Total	135	14	11

Table 3.2 Hyperparathyroidism and hypoparathyroidism following parathyroid autotransplantation in 104 patients

	Time of autotransplantation								
	Initial surgery			Reoperation			Deferred (cryopreserved tissue)		
	Hyper	Hypo	Normo	Hyper	Hypo	Normo	Hyper	Hypo	Normo
Primary hyperplasia									
Non-familial	3/10*	–	7/10	3/6	–	3/6	–	–	4/4
Familial									
MEN I, MEN IIa	4/8	1/8	3/8	–	–	2/2	–	1/2	1/2
FHHH	3/3	–	–	1/1	–	–	–	–	–
Adenoma	–	–	–	–	–	–	–	1/3	2/3
Secondary hyperplasia	2/58	–	56/58	1/5	–	4/5	1/2	–	1/2

* One of these patients had persistent hyperparathyroidism, all others recurrent hyperparathyroidism (increased serum calcium concentration at least 5 months after surgery).
Hyper = hyperparathyroidism; hypo = hypoparathyroidism; normo = normoparathyroidism.

effluent of the grafted compared to the non-grafted arm). In one patient (5%) with non-familial hyperparathyroidism, persistent hypercalcemia was evident in the immediate postoperative period (presumably indicative of a supernumerary parathyroid gland).

Two (20%) of the 10 patients with non-familial hyperparathyroidism have developed recurrent hypercalcemia after parathyroidectomy and autotransplantation, and 7 (64%) of the 11 patients with familial hyperparathyroidism developed recurrent hypercalcemia 5–56 months after surgery (*Table 3.2*). We have resected a portion of the transplanted parathyroid tissue in 4 of the 7 patients with recurrent graft-dependent hyperparathyroidism (*see later in this chapter*) and all 4 are currently normocalcemic[60].

Secondary hyperparathyroidism

Patients with chronic renal failure and renal osteodystrophy are candidates for parathyroidectomy. Indications for surgical intervention are medically intractable bone disease (pain/fractures), pruritus and extra-osseous calcification[8, 34, 48]. There have been two proposed operations: total parathyroidectomy[35] and 3½-gland resection[20, 62]. Neither procedure has given optimal results. In our clinic we have elected to perform total parathyroidectomy with heterotopic autotransplantation of a portion of the resected parathyroid tissue[55]. As *Table 3.1* shows, 58 patients with secondary hyperparathyroidism due to renal osteodystrophy underwent total parathyroidectomy and autotransplantation at initial surgery.

After a mean period of 20 months, 26 (87%) of 30 patients evaluated had a higher concentration of PTH in the venous effluent of the grafted arm compared to the non-grafted arm. The 4 patients who did not have a high PTH level in blood from the grafted arm were, however, normocalcemic without vitamin D or calcium replacement therapy.

Postoperatively, about 80% of patients experienced symptomatic improvement such as lessening of bone pain and pruritus. In 10% there was no improvement in symptoms and in 10% the symptoms worsened.

Because of the severity of the bone disease, postoperative hypocalcemia is prolonged and replacement therapy with vitamin D and oral calcium may be required for 6–9 months.

Early in the series we performed biopsies of the grafts in 10 patients; the parathyroid architecture was consistent with parathyroid hyperplasia. Secretory granules were demonstrated by electron microscopy[55].

In 10 patients parathyroid autografts were performed either before (8) or after (2) renal allografts[18]. Two children (aged 9 and 14) showed markedly increased growth and bone healing after parathyroidectomy and autotransplantation.

Tertiary hyperparathyroidism

Persistent hyperparathyroidism (tertiary hyperparathyroidism) after successful renal transplantation in patients with renal osteodystrophy occurs in approximately 20% of patients[20] and is usually managed by subtotal parathyroidectomy. We have had 2 patients with chronic renal failure who developed tertiary hyperparathyroidism 3 and 14 months after renal allotransplantation. One patient developed severe bone pain following the kidney graft and the symptoms were dramatically relieved by parathyroidectomy and transplant[18].

Carcinoma of the thyroid (normal parathyroid)

Occasionally the vascular supply to one or more parathyroid glands has to be sacrificed or is inadvertently compromised during total or near-total thyroidectomy for carcinoma or other thyroid diseases. An incidence of permanent hypocalcemia as high as 30–40% has been reported in patients undergoing total thyroidectomy[19, 50].

If the vascular supply to any parathyroid gland is compromised or the gland cannot be left *in situ*, it has been proposed that it be sliced into slivers (*see later*) and autografted, if normal, to the adjacent sternocleidomastoid muscle or, if hyperfunctional, to the forearm[12, 30, 32, 36, 39, 43, 55].

In 56 of our 186 patients treated by total thyroidectomy for carcinoma, one or more parathyroid glands were autotransplanted because they could not be preserved *in situ* (*see Table 3.1*). In 16 patients four macroscopically normal parathyroid glands were resected and immediately transplanted. No replacement therapy was necessary in 8 patients, while the other 8 required vitamin D and calcium for a mean period of 1.5 months. All 16 patients are currently normocalcemic without supplementary therapy.

If the parathyroid glands are normal they should be grafted to the sternocleidomastoid muscle, as it is unlikely that they will subsequently become hyperfunctional. If the parathyroid glands are enlarged, however, and there is evidence of hyperparathyroidism they should be autografted to a heterotopic site such as the brachioradialis muscle of the non-dominant forearm. Should subsequent graft-dependent hypercalcemia develop it could be managed by resecting a portion of the parathyroid graft under local anesthesia.

Transplantation at reoperation

Most patients (65–75%) undergoing surgery for primary hyperparathyroidism are found to have a single enlarged gland[7, 40, 61], the removal of which almost always results in a cure[7, 13, 15, 40, 46].

Occasionally, however, an enlarged gland cannot be found at the primary exploration and the patient remains hyperparathyroid. If an insufficient amount of tissue has been removed in a patient with generalized four-gland parathyroid hyperplasia, a similar dilemma is encountered. Most patients with persistent or recurrent hyperparathyroidism require re-exploration of the neck and it is of foremost importance to identify and resect the hyperfunctioning parathyroid gland(s). During reoperation, however, the removal of an enlarged parathyroid gland may cure the hyperparathyroidism, yet render the patient aparathyroid. The reported incidence of hypoparathyroidism in patients re-explored for recurrent hyperparathyroidism ranges from 25% to 30%[2, 5, 15]. This complication can be prevented by parathyroid autotransplantation. If, after reviewing previous operative notes and pathological materials, the surgeon is sure that three or more parathyroid glands have been removed, then an enlarged gland identified at re-exploration may be resected and autografted immediately during a single procedure[17, 58]. If, however, it is not clear that the identified enlarged gland(s) represents the only remaining parathyroid tissue, or if it is suspected that no other parathyroid tissue remains in the neck, the gland should be resected and cryopreserved. Unfortunately the operative note describing previous surgery may be incomplete or there may be a discrepancy between the operative note and the pathology report[5, 47]. If at the end of the re-exploration there is any doubt about the existence of other parathyroid tissue in the neck, the resected tissue should be cryopreserved and autotransplanted later when it becomes evident that the patient has been rendered aparathyroid.

In 9 patients with primary hyperparathyroidism and previously failed operations (*see Table 3.1*) we performed immediate parathyroid autografts when it was clear that the identified enlarged parathyroid gland at reoperation was either the fourth (8 patients) or the fifth (1 patient) gland. Of the 6 patients with non-familial parathyroid hyperplasia 3 developed graft-dependent recurrent hyperparathyroidism (*see Table 3.2*) and of the 3 patients with familial parathyroid disease 1 (with FHHH) developed graft-dependent hypercalcemia postoperatively (serum calcium 11.6 mg/dl or 2.9 mmol/l). None of the 9 patients developed hypocalcemia and 8 had at least 2.5 times higher PTH levels in the venous effluent of the grafted arm compared to levels in the non-grafted arm.

Deferred autotransplantation

Various investigators have shown in experimental animals that parathyroid tissue can retain function after several months of cryopreservation[29, 42, 49, 54]. Since the first report of clinically successful cryopreservation and deferred autotransplantation in 1977[57], approximately 15 cases have been recorded[6, 34, 51, 60].

The technique of parathyroid cryopreservation will be used most often in patients with persistent or recurrent hyperparathyroidism who are undergoing repeat neck exploration, as previously described. In patients treated by total parathyroidectomy and autotransplantation for parathyroid hyperplasia, parathyroid tissue may also be cryopreserved in case the grafted tissue becomes infected.

From December 1978 to August 1981 we cryopreserved tissue from 17 patients undergoing repeat neck exploration. As previously reported[60], 6 patients were rendered aparathyroid and required autotransplantation. In 5 (83%) the parathyroid grafts functioned and the patients became normocalcemic (1 patient is intermittently hypercalcemic). Since the initial report, 5 additional patients have had neck exploration and parathyroidectomy followed by parathyroid cryopreservation and deferred autotransplantation within 2.2 months. In the 11 patients a single large gland, believed to be either an adenoma (5 patients) or a hyperplastic gland (6 patients), was found at surgery. Currently 10 of the 11 patients grafted with cryopreserved tissue have measurable serum PTH levels; however, 4 still require supplementary vitamin D and/or calcium therapy. Two patients had their grafts performed less than 5 months ago. Patients receiving no medication at present required replacement therapy for a mean of 7 months following autotransplantation of cryopreserved tissue.

Parathyroid allotransplantation

Success with parathyroid allotransplantation without immunosuppression has been reported in rodents[14, 41]. In other species, parathyroid allotransplantation has only been achieved in the immunosuppressed host[53]. Parathyroid tissue has been incubated in tissue culture media in an attempt to diminish antigenicity and increase graft survival. The results, however, have not been encouraging[22, 28, 38].

Patients with iatrogenic hypoparathyroidism who are poorly controlled medically are candidates for parathyroid allotransplantation. Such patients are uncommon; furthermore, the side-effects of immunosuppressive therapy are appreciable and usually constitute a greater risk than chronically administered vitamin D and calcium. A previously reported patient[58] with renal osteodystrophy underwent total parathyroidectomy. He later received a renal allograft from his father. Although the transplanted kidney functioned, the patient became hypocalcemic and could not be managed satisfactorily with vitamin D and calcium replacement. Subsequently, under local anesthesia, he received a parathyroid allograft (from the renal donor). Function of the transplanted parathyroid tissue was confirmed by biochemical and histological examination. After 2½ years the patient experienced a late immunological rejection of both renal and parathyroid allografts. He now requires vitamin D and calcium replacement therapy and there is no biochemical evidence of parathyroid graft function.

DiGeorge's syndrome (congenital deficiency of the thymus and parathyroid glands; pharyngeal pouch derivatives[3]) is also an indication for allografting parathyroid tissue. Theoretically, patients could be grafted without immunosuppression, but no well documented successful cases have been reported.

Two infants in our series with complete DiGeorge's syndrome received parathyroid allografts intramuscularly. Both children were severely hypoxic secondary to cardiovascular defects and they died before parathyroid graft function could be assessed.

TECHNIQUE

Transplantation at the time of total parathyroidectomy

The parathyroid glands are resected and, after frozen-section confirmation, immediately placed in chilled sterile saline or tissue culture media (e.g. Waymouth's or RPMI 1640). The lower temperature not only decreases metabolism but also makes the tissue firmer. The parathyroids are then sliced into slivers $1 \times 1 \times 3$ mm in size. Using microsurgical instruments, each sliver of parathyroid tissue is carefully placed into an intramuscular pocket (volar portion of the brachioradialis muscle of the forearm or the sternocleidomastoid muscle). About 15 to 20 pieces are implanted. Care is taken not to induce hemorrhage, and each implantation site is closed with a non-absorbable marking suture, which not only keeps the parathyroid piece from being extruded but also aids in locating the embedded tissue. Should graft-dependent hyperparathyroidism subsequently develop, a portion of the graft could easily be removed under local anesthesia. We have elected to resect half of the implanted parathyroid tissue. Furthermore, graft function can be monitored by measuring plasma levels of parathyroid hormone in the antecubital venous effluent draining the graft bed and comparing them to levels in the antecubital vein of the non-grafted arm. If normal parathyroid tissue is to be transplanted, as in patients undergoing extensive exploration for thyroid carcinoma, the sternocleidomastoid muscle is a preferred transplant site since it is readily accessible in the surgical field and there is a remote likelihood that the parathyroid tissue will hyperfunction and require graft reduction.

Deferred parathyroid autotransplantation

Technique of cryopreservation

The removed parathyroid tissue is immediately placed into sterile saline or tissue culture media. Tissue from the smallest gland is sliced into 30–50 slivers ($1 \times 1 \times 3$ mm) in the same fashion as if they were to be immediately transplanted. The slivers are then put into 3-ml glass vials, 10 pieces in each, together with 1–1.5 ml solution containing 10% dimethylsulfoxide (DMSO), 10% autologous serum and 80% tissue culture media. Since DMSO is toxic at room temperature the freezing process should start immediately after the slivers are immersed in the freezing media. The use of DMSO in the freezing media gives a higher yield of viable tissue in the cryopreservation process. The vials are placed in a freezing chamber (Linde BF-4/6 biological freezing system, Linde Division, Union Carbide, Indianapolis, Indiana, USA) and the freezer is programmed to provide a decrease of 1 °C per min to −60 to −80 °C. The vials are then stored at −190 °C in the vapor phase of a liquid nitrogen freezer (LR 1000 nitrogen storage freezer, Linde Division, Union Carbide).

In preparing the parathyroid slivers at the time of deferred transplantation, they are rapidly thawed in a 37 °C water bath until the last crystals are barely visible. Using a sterile technique, the tissue is washed three times in tissue culture media. The parathyroid pieces are then brought on ice to the operating suite and grafted by the previously described microsurgical technique.

POSTOPERATIVE MANAGEMENT

Immediate postoperative period

Following parathyroidectomy and autotransplantation the serum calcium concentration will fall. The grafted parathyroid tissue does not function immediately; therefore substitution therapy is almost always needed. In 31 (97%) of our 32 patients with primary parathyroid hyperplasia the serum calcium level dropped to 7 ± 0.5 mg/dl (1.75 ± 0.125 mmol/l) within 3 to 10 days. In 6 of these the fall was gradual and no supplemental calcium or vitamin D was required. Each of the 6 patients currently has a serum calcium concentration ranging between 8.3 and 10.0 mg/dl (2.18 and 2.5 mmol/l). The other 25 patients needed initial replacement therapy with glubionate calcium 350 mg four times a day and dihydrotachysterol 0.625 mg/day for a mean of 1.5 ± 2.2 months (range 1–10 months). When the serum calcium level rose to 8 mg/dl (2 mmol/l) the patients were discharged on oral calcium but with a reduced dose of dihydrotachysterol (0.125 mg/day). After approximately 6 weeks the dihydrotachysterol was discontinued, and if the serum calcium concentration remained normal the oral calcium was terminated 2 weeks later. The demonstration of a high concentration of parathyroid hormone in antecubital vein blood of the grafted compared to the non-grafted arm further confirmed graft function. Only 1 (3%) of the 32 patients was considered to have a failed graft. In spite of a high concentration of PTH in the vein draining the grafted arm, this patient required chronic vitamin D and oral calcium replacement therapy. The patient had had a total gastrectomy for the Zollinger-Ellison syndrome and the presumed decreased calcium absorption perhaps accounted in part for his hypocalcemia.

In 11 patients in whom deferred autografting of cryopreserved tissue was performed the mean serum calcium nadir was 6.6 mg/dl (1.65 mmol/l), with a range of 5.5–7.5 mg/dl (1.38–1.88 mmol/l). Intravenous supplementation with calcium gluconate in addition to the oral vitamin D and calcium therapy was given in 10 patients. Substitution therapy was instituted at the time of parathyroidectomy and continued until after transplantation of the frozen tissue for a mean of 8 months (range 1.5–26 months; for 8 patients currently on no replacement therapy). Supplementation is still required in 2 patients even though there is biochemical evidence of graft function. In 1 patient there is no biochemical evidence of graft function (possibly due to an error in the cryopreservation technique).

Graft-dependent hyperparathyroidism

If there is no drop in the serum calcium concentration after presumed total parathyroidectomy and autotransplantation or if the serum calcium level increases to preoperative levels within a few days of surgery, one must suspect residual hyperfunctioning parathyroid tissue in the neck (a supernumerary parathyroid gland rather than graft-dependent hyperparathyroidism).

That recurrent hyperparathyroidism will develop in a certain percentage of patients who have had total parathyroidectomy and autotransplantation is to be expected[24,59], since the transplanted tissue is hyperfunctional and does not assume a normal character when relocated[4]. Anticipating this problem we chose the forearm as an accessible transplant site. The indications for removal of a portion of grafted parathyroid tissue are (1) a serum calcium level above 11 mg/dl (2.75 mmol/l) or (2) a serum calcium level of 10.5 mg/dl (2.63 mmol/l) associated with hypercalciuria (more than 400 mg calcium/24-hour urine).

In our series of patients with primary hyperparathyroidism and autotransplantation (done both at initial and secondary operations) 30% developed recurrent graft-dependent hyperparathyroidism. The recurrence rate was significantly higher (8 of 15; 53%) in patients with familial hyperparathyroidism (MEN I, MEN II or FHHH) than in those with non-familial hyperparathyroidism (5 of 17; 29%). Graft resection was performed in 5 patients and 4 became normocalcemic (1 is intermittently normocalcemic and mildly hypercalcemic). This high incidence of recurrent hyperparathyroidism in patients with familial disease has also been documented by others[31, 33, 37].

Patients undergoing total parathyroidectomy and autotransplantation for renal osteodystrophy frequently do not develop hypercalcemia as a result of graft hyperfunction. Partial graft resection is indicated if the patient develops recurrent secondary hyperparathyroidism manifested by bone pain or fractures, pruritus or extra-osseous metastatic calcification. In our series of 65 patients with renal osteodystrophy treated by parathyroidectomy and transplantation, 2 required subsequent partial graft removal. Resolution of the recurrent osteodystrophy resulted. A third patient had his entire parathyroid graft removed because of calciphylaxis characterized by calcification of peripheral arteries endangering circulation to extremities[59]. However, only temporary symptomatic improvement was achieved following graft reduction.

Persistent hypoparathyroidism

Fortunately our experience with persistent hypoparathyroidism is limited. A few patients have required calcium and/or vitamin D substitution therapy for several months and up to 2 years but have eventually been able to maintain a normal serum calcium concentration without medication. Two patients (one with MEN I, the other with MEN II) developed hypoparathyroidism and required continuous replacement therapy. In one patient the failed graft was due to an error in the technique of cryopreservation. In the other patient a high concentration of PTH was detected in the venous effluent of the graft, but he still required replacement therapy to remain normocalcemic.

Latent hypoparathyroidism

The question of latent hypoparathyroidism after autotransplantation of parathyroid tissue has been addressed by Salander and Tisell[44]. They found that 38% of normocalcemic patients who were solely dependent on transplanted parathyroid tissue became hypocalcemic (without symptoms) if subjected for a week to a low calcium diet in combination with an oral cellulose phosphate suspension taken with meals. It is important to realize that transplanted patients receiving parathyroid autografts may not have a normal reserve capacity of parathyroid tissue and during extreme situations may become hypocalcemic. The same could be said for patients with parathyroid hyperplasia who have had their parathyroid mass reduced by subtotal parathyroidectomy.

DISCUSSION

Surgery is the treatment of choice for patients with primary hyperparathyroidism and advanced secondary hyperparathyroidism. Recently it has been suggested that pharmacological agents (propranolol and cimetidine) effect parathyroid hormone secretion in patients with renal osteodystrophy[9, 27]; however, the role of these agents in the treatment of hyperparathyroidism is not clear. The primary surgical therapy for patients with hyperparathyroidism due to single-gland disease is extirpation of the enlarged gland with verification that the three remaining parathyroids are normal. Patients with generalized parathyroid enlargement are much more difficult to manage. Before this disease entity was widely recognized, surgeons often did not appreciate at operation that there was generalized parathyroid involvement, and patients frequently developed postoperative hypercalcemia when an insufficient amount of tissue was resected. It has further become evident that within the primary hyperplasia group there is a marked difference between patients with non-familial and those with familial parathyroid hyperplasia. In the latter there is a marked tendency for the residual parathyroid to hyperfunction and cause recurrent hyperparathyroidism.

The accepted therapy for patients with four-gland hyperplasia, primary or secondary, has been radical subtotal 3½-gland parathyroidectomy. The results with this method have not been entirely satisfactory, with an incidence of postoperative hypercalcemia as high as 55% being reported in an early series[10]. More recent reports demonstrate hypocalcemia in 5–15% and hypercalcemia in 11–13%[11, 16] of patients. Patients with familial hyperparathyroidism have a substantially higher risk of encountering persistent or recurrent hyperparathyroidism postoperatively (22–85%), and will require subsequent repeat neck exploration[13, 31, 33, 37].

We have proposed an alternative surgical treatment: total parathyroidectomy and heterotopic autotransplantation[55]. Concerned voices regarding the efficacy and reliability of this method were raised. It has also been questioned whether the results of 3½-gland resection have been poor enough to demand consideration of an alternative method. It was feared that many patients would experience prolonged hypocalcemia after parathyroid transplantation and that graft failure would frequently occur. It was also felt that should a supernumerary gland be present its diagnosis would be delayed and confused by a functioning parathyroid graft. Our data show that these concerns were unwarranted.

Immediate parathyroid grafting is successful in virtually all patients and the incidence of graft failure is very low. Only in 2 patients of 106 (both primary and secondary hyperparathyroidism) did the graft fail to render the patient normocalcemic, and in 1 of the 2 despite high levels of PTH in the venous effluent of the parathyroid graft bed. We have had no patients with late graft failure, such as the 3 patients with secondary hyperparathyroidism reported by Mozes *et al.*[34].

On the contrary, our experience is that with time there appears to be an increase in the parathyroid hormone level measured in the graft venous effluent[60]. In a third of patients with primary hyperparathyroidism graft-dependent hypercalcemia develops. In our series recurrent hypercalcemia has occurred in all patients with familial hypocalciuric hypercalcemic hyperparathyroidism. To 'titrate' the exact amount of parathyroid tissue needed in a patient, a portion of the autografted tissue could be resected. It may take more than one graft reduction to achieve normocalcemia, but this seems preferable to repeated neck explorations.

Patients with secondary hyperparathyroidism treated by total parathyroidectomy and autotransplantation have done well, and approximately 80% have had symptomatic improvement. Three patients needed their grafts reduced because of recurrent hyperparathyroidism (2) or calciphylaxis.

The patients in whom parathyroid autotransplantation has proved particularly useful have been those undergoing reoperation for persistent or recurrent hyperparathyroidism. The 9 re-explored patients with primary disease would have been rendered aparathyroid if the pathological tissue found had been resected but not autotransplanted. The method of cryopreserving parathyroid tissue allows the surgeon to delay autotransplantation. The postoperative course will show if the patient is aparathyroid and therefore in need of a parathyroid graft. The optimal length of the observation period between resection and transplantation of the cryopreserved tissue is controversial. Mean observation time between resection and transplantation for our 11 patients was 2.2 months. Although we have grafted patients successfully with parathyroid tissue frozen for as long as 8.5 months it has been documented that in animals tissue can be favorably grafted after 9 months of cryopreservation and in humans after 18 months[6].

The technique of parathyroid autotransplantation, with or without cryopreservation, increases the surgeon's versatility in managing patients with primary or secondary hyperparathyroidism. Our results and those of others suggest that it may provide the optimal treatment modality in patients with familial hyperparathyroidism and in patients subjected to repeat neck exploration due to persistent or recurrent hyperparathyroidism.

References

1 ALVERYD, A., El-ZAWAHRY, M. D., HERLITZ, P. and NORDENSTAM, H. Primary hyperplasia of the parathyroids: report on the management of eight cases. *Acta Chirurgica Scandinavica*, **141**, 24–30 (1975)

2 BEAZLEY, R. M., COSTA, J. and KETCHAM, A. S. Reoperative parathyroid surgery. *American Journal of Surgery*, **130**, 427–429 (1975)

3 BOYD, J. D. Development of the thyroid and parathyroid glands and the thymus. *Annals of the Royal College of Surgeons of England*, **7**, 455–471 (1950)

4 BRENNAN, M. F., BROWN, E. M., MARX, S. J., SPIEGEL, A. M., BROADUS, A. E., DOPPMAN, J. L., WEBBER, B., PATH, F. F. and AURBACH, G. D. Recurrent hyperparathyroidism from an autotransplanted parathyroid adenoma. *New England Journal of Medicine*, **299**, 1057–1059 (1978)

5 BRENNAN, M. D., DOPPMAN, J. L., MARX, S. J., SPIEGEL, A. M., BROWN, E. M. and AURBACH, G. D. Reoperative parathyroid surgery for persistent hyperparathyroidism. *Surgery*, **83**, 669–674 (1978)

6 BRENNAN, M. F., BROWN, E. M., SPIEGEL, A. M., MARX, S. J., DOPPMAN, J. L., JONES, D. C. and AURBACH, G. D. Autotransplantation of cryopreserved parathyroid tissue in man. *Annals of Surgery*, **189**, 139–142 (1979)

7 BRUINING, H. A., VAN HOUTEN, H., JUTTMANN, J. R., LAMBERTS, S. W. J. and BIRKENHAGER, J. C. Results of operative treatment of 615 patients with primary hyperparathyroidism. *World Journal of Surgery*, **5**, 85–90 (1981)

8 BURNETT, H. F., THOMPSON, B. W. and BARBOUR, G. L. Parathyroid autotransplantation. *Archives of Surgery*, **112**, 373–379 (1977)

9 CARO, J. F., BESARAB, A., BURKE, J. F. and GLENNON, J. A. A possible role for propranolol in the treatment of renal osteodystrophy. *Lancet*, **2**, 451–454 (1978)

10 CASTLEMAN, B. and COPE, O. Primary parathyroid hypertrophy and hyperplasia. *Bulletin of the Hospital for Joint Diseases*, **12**, 368–378 (1951)

11 CASTLEMAN, B., SCHANTZ, A. and ROTH, S. I. Parathyroid hyperplasia in primary hyperparathyroidism. *Cancer*, **38**, 1668–1675 (1976)

12 CATELL, R. B. Parathyroid transplantation: a report of autografts of parathyroid glands removed during thyroidectomy. *American Journal of Surgery*, **7**, 4–8 (1929)

13 CLARK, O. M., WAY, L. W. and HUNT, T. K. Recurrent hyperparathyroidism. *Annals of Surgery*, **184**, 391–399 (1976)

14 DIB-KURI, A., REVILLA, A. and CHAVEZ-PEON, F. Successful rat parathyroid allograft and xenografts to the testis without immunosuppression. *Transplantation Proceedings*, **7**, 753–756 (1975)

15 EDIS, A. J., SHEEDY, P. F., BEAHRS, O. H. and VAN HEERDEN, J. A. Results of reoperation for hyperparathyroidism with evaluation of preoperative localization studies. *Surgery*, **84**, 384–391 (1978)

16 EDIS, A. J., VAN HEERDEN, J. A. and SCHOLZ, D. A. Results of subtotal parathyroidectomy for primary chief cell hyperplasia. *Surgery*, **86**, 462–466 (1979)

17 EDIS, A. J., LINOS, D. A. and KAO, P. C. Parathyroid autotransplantation at the time of reoperation for persistent hyperparathyroidism. *Surgery*, **88**, 588–592 (1980)

18 FARNDON, J. R., MARTINEZ, S., DALE, J. K., DILLEY, W. G., GUNNELLS, J. C. and WELLS, S. A. Total parathyroidectomy and heterotopic autotransplantation with renal transplantation in the management of renal osteodystrophy. (Unpublished observation)

19 GANN, D. S. and PAONE, J. F. Delayed hypocalcemia after thyroidectomy for Graves' disease is prevented by parathyroid autotransplantation. *Annals of Surgery*, **190**, 508–512 (1979)

20 GEIS, W. P., POPOVTZER, M. D., CORMAN, J. L., HALGRIMSON, C. G., GROTH, C. G. and STARZL, T. E. The diagnosis and treatment of hyperparathyroidism after renal homotransplantation. *Surgery, Gynecology and Obstetrics*, **137**, 997–1010 (1973)

21 GLEY, M. E. Sur les effets de l'extipation du corps thyroide. Sur les fonctions de la gland thyroide chez le lapin et chez le chien. *Comptes Rendues Hebdomadaires Societé de Biologie*, **43**, 551–554, 843–847 (1891)

22 GOUGH, I. R. and FINNIMORE, M. Transplantation of organ cultured rat parathyroids. *Australian and New Zealand Journal of Surgery*, **49**, 716–720 (1979)

23 GROTH, C. G., POPOVTZER, M., HAMMOND, W. S., CASCARDO, S., IWATSUKI, S., HALGRIMSON, C. G. and STARZL, T. E. Survival of a homologous parathyroid implant in an immunosuppressed patient. *Lancet*, **1**, 1082–1084 (1973)

24 HAASE, G. M., LUCE, J. M., LOCK, J. P., HAMMOND, W. S. and PENN, I. Hyperparathyroidism following parathyroid autotransplantation. *Surgery*, **86**, 694–697 (1979)

25 HALSTED, W. S. Auto and isotransplantation in dogs of parathyroid glandules. *Journal of Experimental Medicine*, **11**, 175–199 (1909)

26 HICKEY, R. C. and SAMAAN, N. A. Human parathyroid autotransplantation. *Archives of Surgery*, **110**, 892–895 (1975)

27 JACOB, A. I., LANIER, D., CANTERBURY, J. and BOURGOIGNIE, J. J. Reduction by cimetidine of serum parathyroid hormone levels in uremic patients. *New England Journal of Medicine*, **302**, 671–674 (1980)

28 JORDAN, G. L., ERICKSON, E., GORDON, W. B. and ROSE, R. G. The treatment of hypoparathyroidism by parathyroid transplantation. *Surgery*, **52**, 134–143 (1962)

29 KAPUR, M. M., MEHTA, S. N., MOULIK, B. K. and SANG, V. K. Parathyroid preservation and transplantation. *Indian Journal of Medical Research*, **64**, 1793–1798 (1976)

30 LAHEY, F. The transplantation of parathyroids in partial thyroidectomy. *Surgery, Gynecology and Obstetrics*, **42**, 508–509 (1926)

31 LAMERS, C. B. H. W. and FROELING, P. G. A. M. Clinical significance of hyperparathyroidism in familial multiple endocrine adenomatosis type I (MEA I). *American Journal of Medicine*, **66**, 422–424 (1979)

32 LUNDSTROM, B., ANDERBERG, B. and GILLGUIST, J. Clinical experience of parathyroid autotransplantation. *Acta Chirurgica Scandinavica*, **144**, 451–453 (1978)

33 MARX, S. J., SPIEGEL, A. M. and BROWN, E. M. Family studies in patients with primary parathyroid hyperplasia. *American Journal of Medicine*, **62**, 698–706 (1977)

34 MOZES, M. F., SOPER, W. D., JONASSON, O. and LANG, G. R. Total parathyroidectomy and autotransplantation in secondary hyperparathyroidism. *Archives of Surgery*, **115**, 378–384 (1980)

35 OGG, C. S. Total parathyroidectomy in treatment of secondary (renal) hyperparathyroidism. *British Medical Journal*, **4**, 331–334 (1967)

36 PALOYAN, E., LAWRENCE, A. M., BROOKS, M. H. and PICKLEMAN, J. R. Total thyroidectomy and parathyroid autotransplantation for radiation associated thyroid cancer. *Surgery*, **80**, 70–76 (1976)

37 PRINZ, R. A., GAMVROS, O. I., SELLU, D. and LYNN, J. A. Subtotal parathyroidectomy for primary chief cell hyperplasia of the multiple endocrine neoplasia type I syndrome. *Annals of Surgery*, **193**, 26–29 (1981)

38 RAAF, J. H., FARR, H. W., MYERS, W. P. L. and GOOD, R. A. Transplantation of fresh and cultured parathyroid glands in the rat. *American Journal of Surgery*, **128**, 478–483 (1974)

39 RAAF, J. M., SAMAAN, N. and HICKEY, R. C. Autografts of normal and hyperplastic human parathyroid: experience in eleven patients, with immunoassay monitoring of function in seven. *World Journal of Surgery*, **4**, 209–221 (1980)

40 ROMANUS, R., HEIMANN, P., NILSSON, O. and HANSSON, G. Surgical treatment of hyperparathyroidism. *Progress in Surgery*, **12**, 22–76 (1973)

41 RUSSELL, P. S. and GITTES, R. F. Parathyroid transplants in rats. *Journal of Experimental Medicine*, **109**, 571–578 (1959)

42 RUSSELL, P. S., WOOD, M. L. and GITTES, R. F. Preservation of living tissue in the frozen state. A study using parathyroid tissue. *Journal of Surgical Research*, **1**, 23–31 (1961)

43 SALANDER, H. and TISELL, L.-E. Incidence of hypoparathyroidism after radical surgery for thyroid carcinoma and autotransplantation of parathyroid glands. *American Journal of Surgery*, **134**, 358–362 (1977)

44 SALANDER, H. and TISELL, L. E. Latent hypoparathyroidism in patients with autotransplanted parathyroid glands. *American Journal of Surgery*, **139**, 385–388 (1980)

45 SANDSTROM, I. Om en ny kortel hos menniskan och atskilliga daggdjur. *Upsala Lakareforenings Forhandlingar*, **15**, 441–472 (1879–1880)

46 SATAVA, R. M., BEAHRS, O. H. and SCHOLZ, D. A. Success rate of cervical exploration for hyperparathyroidism. *Archives of Surgery*, **110**, 625–628 (1975)

47 SAXE, A. W. and BRENNAN, M. F. Strategy and technique of reoperative parathyroid surgery. *Surgery*, **89**, 417–423 (1981)

48 SIVULA, A., KUHLBACK, B., KOCK, B., KAHRI, A., WALLENIUS, M. and EDGREN, J. Parathyroidectomy in chronic renal failure. *Acta Chirurgica Scandinavica*, **145**, 19–25 (1979)

49 SONODA, T., OHKAWA, T., TAKEUCHI, M. and YACHIKU, S. Successful parathyroid preservation: experimental study. *Surgery*, **64**, 791–796 (1968)

50 TOLLEFSEN, H. R. and DeCOSSE, J. J. Papillary carcinoma of the thyroid. *American Journal of Surgery*, **106**, 728–734 (1963)

51 WAGNER, P. K., ROTHMUND, M., KUMMERLE, F., KESSLER, F. J., GABBERT, M. and KRAUSE, U. Autotransplantation von kälte konserviertem menschlichem Nebenschilddrüsengewebe. *Deutsch Medizinische Wochenschrift*, **106**, 363–367 (1981)

52 WELLS, S. A., BURDICK, J. F., KETCHAM, A. S., CHRISTIANSEN, C., ABE, M. and SHERWOOD, L. Transplantation of the parathyroid glands in dogs. *Transplantation*, **15**, 179–182 (1973)

53 WELLS, S. A., BURDICK, J. F., HATTLER, B. G., CHRISTIANSEN, C., PETTIGREW, H. M. ABE, M. and SHERWOOD, L. M. The allografted parathyroid gland. Evaluation of function in the immunosuppressed host. *Annals of Surgery*, **180**, 805–813 (1974)

54 WELLS, S. A. and CHRISTIANSEN, C. The transplanted parathyroid gland: evaluation of cryopreservation and other environmental factors which affect its function. *Surgery*, **75**, 49–55 (1974)

55 WELLS, S. A., GUNNELS, J. C., SHELBURNE, J. D., SCHNEIDER, A. B. and SHERWOOD, L. M. Transplantation of the parathyroid glands in man: clinical indications and results. *Surgery*, **78**, 34–44 (1975)

56 WELLS, S. A., ELLIS, G. J., GUNNELLS, J. C., SCHNEIDER, A. B. and SHERWOOD, L. M. Parathyroid autotransplantation in primary parathyroid hyperplasia. *New England Journal of Medicine*, **295**, 57–62 (1976)

57 WELLS, S. A., GUNNELLS, J. C., GUTMAN, R. A., SHELBURNE, J. D., SCHNEIDER, A. B. and SHERWOOD, L. M. The successful transplantation of frozen parathyroid tissue in man. *Surgery*, **81**, 86–90 (1977)

58 WELLS, S. A., STIRMAN, J. A., BOLMAN, R. M. and GUNNELLS, J. C. Transplantation of the parathyroid glands. Clinical and experimental results. *Surgical Clinics of North America*, **58**, 391–402 (1978)

59 WELLS, S. A. Hypercalcemia following parathyroid transplantation. *Surgery*, **86**, 775–776 (1979)

60 WELLS, S. A., FARNDON, J. R., DALE, J. K., LEIGHT, G. S. and DILLEY, W. G. Long-term evaluation of patients with primary parathyroid hyperplasia managed by total parathyroidectomy and heterotopic autotransplantation. *Annals of Surgery*, **192**, 451–456 (1980)

61 WELLS, S. A., LEIGHT, G. S. and ROSS, A. J. Primary hyperparathyroidism. *Current Problems in Surgery*, **17,** 397–463 (1980)
62 WILSON, R. E., HAMPERS, C. L., BERNSTEIN, D. S., JOHNSON, J. W. and MERRILL, J. P. Subtotal parathyroidectomy in chronic renal failure. *Annals of Surgery*, **174,** 640–652 (1971)

4
Reoperation for suspected hyperparathyroidism
Murray F. Brennan and Samuel A. Wells

INTRODUCTION

The patient with hypercalcemia following a prior cervical or mediastinal exploration for hypercalcemia thought to be due to primary or secondary hyperparathyroidism is a major challenge for the surgeon. The problems of reoperation are well illustrated by the first successful parathyroidectomy by Dr Mandl. The patient, Albert Jahne, born 12 March 1886, had severe bony changes of hyperparathyroidism and sustained a fracture of the left femur in December 1914. On 30 July 1925 a left inferior parathyroid 'adenoma' measuring 2.5 × 1.2 cm was removed. Marked improvement was noted postoperatively; however, by June 1932 his symptoms had recurred. He had a re-exploration of the neck on 18 October 1932, and a subtotal resection of the thyroid revealed two 'normal' parathyroid glands. The patient did not improve following this re-exploration and died with uremia on 26 February 1932. No parathyroid tissue was found at autopsy[1,16].

The prevalence of persistent and recurrent hyperparathyroidism following an initial operation was summarized in 1976 by Clark, Way and Hunt[6]. As the distinction between persistence and recurrence has been applied loosely in the literature, true figures are difficult to obtain. The true prevalence of recurrent disease is extremely small. Using rigorous criteria for recurrence, and excluding patients with parathyroid carcinoma, Mueller[19] saw no recurrent disease in 348 patients managed personally. However, there were 16 patients (5%) with persistent disease[19]. The same has been true in our own experience, where persistent hyperparathyroidism was present in 116 (92%) of 125 patients undergoing reoperation. Data from the first 106 of these patients have recently been reported by Brennan et al[5]. A summary of the experience from the literature is given in *Table 4.1*. It can be seen that in single institutions the persistence or recurrence rate is 5 or 6%[17,24]. In smaller series, however, it may reach 20%. In most referral institutions, the proportion of patients with first operations for hyperparathyroidism who will require reoperation varies from 7%[15] to 16%[24]. In very unusual circumstances, such as in a referral institution interested predominantly in patients with persistent

Table 4.1 Incidence of recurrent and persistent hyperparathyroidism following initial parathyroid surgery

Reference	Year	Number of patients	Persistence	Recurrence	Both	(%)	Comment
8	1975	178	–	–	15	(8)	
6	1976	3788	0	51	51	(1)	Literature review
6	1976	242	0	1	1	(0.04)	Non-familial; single series
6	1976	21	0	7	7	(33)	Familial disease
15	1976	110	–	–	20	(18)	
24	1977	712	–	–	112	(16)	Includes referrals
24	1977	637	–	–	37	(6)	Single hospital series
11	1978	714	–	–	51	(7)	Includes referrals
17	1980	500	25	0	25	(5)	Single hospital series

The dashes indicate no data available

Table 4.2 Prevalence of recurrent or persistent hypercalcemia following reoperation

Reference	Year	Number of patients	Persistence or recurrence (%)
6	1976	28	11 (40)
24	1977	112	10 (9)
11	1978	51	8 (16)
5	1982	106	15 (14, 5*)

* Excluding parathyroid carcinoma and patients subsequently shown not to have primary hyperparathyroidism.

hypercalcemia, the number of reoperations can approximate the number of primary explorations[5].

The persistence or recurrence rate in patients undergoing a second or subsequent re-exploration (*Table 4.2*) is, of course, much higher. This may vary from 40% in patients with predominantly familial disease to 10–20% when all cases of persistent hypercalcemia are included[5,6].

DECISIONS REQUIRED IN PATIENTS WITH PERSISTENT AND RECURRENT HYPERCALCEMIA

When presented with a patient with persistent hypercalcemia following prior parathyroid exploration, a number of decisions need to be made in logical sequence. We believe that the most important decisions are (1) the confirmation of the diagnosis, (2) whether or not the disease is familial, and (3) whether or not the patient's symptoms warrant the risks of reoperation. We use the following clinical and biochemical tests to confirm or exclude the diagnosis of hyperparathyroidism.

(1) Clinical
    (a) Signs and symptoms
    (b) Family history
    (c) Associated diseases
    (d) Presence of malignancy

(2) Laboratory
    (a) Blood: calcium, phosphorus, alkaline phosphatase, chloride, peripheral and selective parathyroid hormone (PTH), bicarbonate, magnesium, blood urea nitrogen (BUN), creatinine, albumin
    (b) Urine: calcium, cyclic AMP, creatinine
    (c) X-ray: bone, plain abdomen (intravenous pyelogram)

A careful examination of the family history will determine whether single or multiple gland disease is likely. Patients with a family history of mild hyperparathyroidism unassociated with renal or skeletal disease who have undergone unsuccessful surgery should raise the suspicion of familial hypercalcemic hypocalciuria (FHH)[18]. The FHH syndrome has been shown to be present in 9% of patients referred with persistent hypercalcemia[18]. As operation less than total parathyroidectomy or total parathyroidectomy with autotransplantation will not help these patients, and total parathyroidectomy should not be recommended, this diagnosis must be suspected. Central to the diagnosis of FHH is the presence of low urinary calcium and a calcium-to-creatinine clearance ratio of less than 0.01.

Patients who are referred with persistent hypercalcemia following previous surgery will have a higher incidence of multiple gland disease than those presenting for operation for the first time. In a recent experience, 37% of patients who came to reoperation had multiple gland disease rather than a single adenoma[5]. The factors that would lead one to suspect multiple gland disease are: previous abnormal hyperfunctional tissue removed; a family history of hypercalcemia or multiple endocrine neoplasia; associated disease of pituitary, thyroid, adrenal or endocrine pancreas; renal failure; or physical features suggestive of multiple endocrine neoplasia type II B. Particular effort should be made to diagnose a familial hyperparathyroid syndrome or multiple endocrine neoplasia syndrome. The diagnoses in 125 patients undergoing reoperation at the National Institutes of Health (NIH) between August 1975 and July 1981 are listed in *Table 4.3*. Diagnoses were confirmed, in some cases, following unsuccessful reoperation.

The determination of how much normal and abnormal tissue has been removed previously is difficult; operative notes are often not consistent with pathological reports. However, careful attention paid to the preceding surgeon's note can give clues in the subsequent identification of where the missing gland may be.

An important problem is the identification of the need for reoperation. We have based this on the severity of the disease once the diagnosis has been confirmed.

Table 4.3 Diagnoses of patients undergoing reoperation for persistent or recurrent hypercalcemia at the National Institutes of Health between August 1975 and July 1981

	Persistent	Recurrent	Both
Single adenoma	67	2	69
Primary hyperplasia	19	3	22
Familial hyperplasia	2	1	3
Multiple endocrine neoplasia			
Type I	10	1	11
Type II	3	0	3
Familial hypocalciuric hypercalcemia	2	0	2
Secondary hyperplasia	4	0	4
Parathyroid carcinoma	4	1	5
Other	6	0	6
Total	117	8	125

Table 4.4 Distribution of symptoms in 125 patients undergoing reoperation at the National Institutes of Health between August 1975 and July 1981

	Persistent %	Recurrent %	Both %
Nephrolithiasis	51	88	53
Bone disease	27	50	29
Gastrointestinal symptoms	18	0	17
Muscle weakness	18	38	19
Psychiatric symptoms	8	0	8

Mild asymptomatic hypercalcemia, even when due to established primary hyperparathyroidism, is rarely an indication for a second operation. Similarly, if the patient has severe underlying disease which is likely to make an operation additionally hazardous the risk must be balanced against the benefit.

Patients who present with persistent or recurrent hyperparathyroidism can be expected to have severe and disabling disease. One feature not commonly appreciated is the profound proximal muscle weakness that can make ambulation a major problem. Severe bone disease and nephrolithiasis continue to be the most prevalent symptoms (*Table 4.4*) in patients referred for reoperation.

LOCALIZATION STUDIES

Once the diagnosis has been established and the indications for reoperation confirmed, localization studies should be considered. In centers where invasive localization can be performed with minimal risk or morbidity all patients with disease severe enough to warrant reoperation should be candidates for localization. In centers where invasive localization is not readily available, non-invasive studies should be performed and, if negative, one should consider patient referral. Localization studies available for the identification of parathyroid tissue are listed below:

Preoperative
Minimally invasive
  Barium swallow
  Neck massage, PTH and urinary cyclic AMP
  Ultrasound
  Thyroid scan
  Selenomethionine scan
  Computed assisted double isotope scanning
  Computed tomography

Invasive
  Selective venous sampling for PTH
  Selective arteriography
  Arterial injection of selenomethionine Se75
  Needle aspiration

Intraoperative
  Methylene blue
  O-Toluidine blue
  Urinary cyclic AMP

If the first operation was performed by a highly experienced parathyroid surgeon, then the likelihood of success by a relatively inexperienced surgeon is very low in a patient who has no preoperative localization. If the first operation was performed by a relatively inexperienced surgeon, then the likelihood of success by an experienced surgeon is high, even without the use of invasive studies[11]. The minimally invasive studies cover a wide range. We have previously suggested that the cine-esophagram is of no value in patients who undergo reoperation[2]. This suggestion has been confirmed by a study of 51 esophagrams obtained from 106 patients with persistent hyperparathyroidism. There was a positive yield of less than 4%. Neck massage with concomitant determination of peripheral venous parathyroid hormone (PTH) and urinary cyclic AMP is of little value[21]. Ultrasound in patients for reoperation has also not been helpful. Ultrasonography is best performed with a high-resolution, high-frequency real time small parts scanner[12]. While larger glands have been visualized with lower frequency, static B-mode scanners[10], the experience in patients who have had a prior operation is disappointing.

We use a thyroid scan to assist interpretation of the more invasive study of selective arteriography. The selenomethionine scan has generally been non-specific although it has been suggested that the combination of a double isotope scan using iodine-125 and selenomethionine Se75 is more specific[13]. In one report of 36 patients, 30 adequate computed double isotope scans were obtained, and 16 of these (53%) provided localization: 14 were positive at the time of exploration, with 10 of them less than 1.5 g in weight[13]. While these are most impressive figures, subsequent follow-up studies have not been forthcoming, and we are unaware of other studies investigating the use of this method prior to reoperation. Intra-arterial injection of selenomethionine Se75 has been employed following thyroid uptake block by pretreatment with thyroxine[23], but is non-specific and rarely helpful.

Computed tomography may be particularly valuable for the detection of mediastinal glands. Scan thickness needs to be 1 cm or less with contiguous or overlapping slices and should extend from the low neck to several centimeters below the carina. Routine scans are performed without intravenous contrast material although intravenous bolus injection of contrast may improve the definition of some glands[14].

We have examined particularly the more invasive studies prior to reoperation. It has always been our approach to employ selective arteriography prior to selective venous sampling. This gives a better identification of the venous drainage of selected areas, which may be confirmed by careful selective venous sampling. If samples from selective venous sampling show high levels of PTH in areas not adequately studied by arteriography, a second arteriographic approach via the axillary route can occasionally be performed[4].

Venous sampling for PTH is performed to obtain selective samples from all thyroid, vertebral and thymic veins. Although the large vessels of the neck and mediastinum are sampled, they are rarely of help in specific localization. Our recent results are documented in *Table 4.5*.

Table 4.5 Results of arteriographic (AG) and venographic (VG) localization studies in 125 reoperations

	Number of patients	Percent
AG and VG both correct	35	28
Either AG or VG correct	78	62
Neither AG nor VG correct	47	38
AG correct	58	46
VG correct	54	43

Theoretically, needle aspiration of a palpable mass in the neck can give a positive diagnosis either by histopathological examination or by the determination of high levels of PTH in the aspirated sample. Again, except in rare cases such as those with large parathyroid cysts, this is not of practical importance.

Intraoperative localization tests during reoperation are of minimal value. The use of methylene blue as a 5 mg/kg dose diluted in 500 ml of saline which has been emphasized in the unoperative case has not helped us in the reoperative situation[9]. The period of staining by methylene blue is short and the glands must be able to be visualized before the stain can be identified. Other thiazide dyes, such as

O-toluidine blue, have proved too toxic for clinical use. We have employed the intraoperative assessment of urinary cyclic AMP excretion as a localization indicator and to confirm the adequacy of extirpation[22]. On occasion an unexpected high rise in urinary cyclic AMP at the time of massage of what is thought to be a thyroid lobe may redirect attention to an area of inadequate exploration. With rapid γ-flow radioimmunoassay, urinary cyclic AMP values can be available to the surgeon within 30 min of sampling.

OPERATIVE CONSIDERATIONS

Our technique and strategy have recently been described[20]. The majority of glands will be found in the neck even in the reoperative situation. Mediastinal glands as the source of the hyperparathyroidism are naturally more common following previous unsuccessful surgery. In a recent experience at the NIH with 125 reoperations, there were 8 patients (6%) who had mediastinal exploration and 21 (17%) who had both cervical and mediastinal exploration, i.e. almost one quarter underwent mediastinal exploration.

RESULTS OF REOPERATION

Persistence or recurrence can be expected in between 8 and 30% of patients undergoing reoperation. A recent evaluation (*Table 4.6*) confirmed that hypercalcemia remained in 15 of 106 patients undergoing reoperation[5]. Of added importance, however, is the fact that in 7 patients the diagnosis of hyperparathyroidism

Table 4.6 Results of reoperation for primary hyperparathyroidism in 106 patients*

	Number of patients	Percent
Hypercalcemia	15	14
Probable FHH	4	
Not primary HPTH	3	
Parathyroid carcinoma	3	
MEN I	2	
Primary HPTH	2	
Familial HPTH	1	
Hypocalcemia	55	52
Eucalcemia	36	34

* Data from Brennan *et al.*[5]
FHH = familial hypocalciuric hypercalcemia; HPTH = hyperparathyroidism; MEN I = multiple endocrine neoplasia type I.

was in doubt: 4 presumptively had the FHH syndrome and 3 were clearly not hyperparathyroid. The remaining 8 patients who had persistence included 3 with carcinoma and 5 with unequivocal hyperparathyroidism. Again, of the latter 5 patients only 2 had uncomplicated presumed primary hyperparathyroidism. The other 3 had a familial variety. In addition, 55 (52%) had hypocalcemia following reoperation and required calcium and vitamin D at the time of discharge from the hospital. This very high prevalence of hypocalcemia reflects the severity of the associated bone disease and the high risk of hypoparathyroidism following multiple operations. It should be emphasized, however, that the majority of patients leaving hospital on vitamin D and calcium can be slowly weaned from these supplements so that less than one-third will be candidates for autografting at 6 months.

AUTOTRANSPLANTATION

As already mentioned, the possibility exists that the parathyroid gland resected during reoperation of a patient with hyperparathyroidism may be the only functioning tissue remaining. The surgeon, therefore, should have a plan to obviate rendering the patient aparathyroid. An adequate search for parathyroid tissue cannot be performed in a scarred field, and the only means of gauging the parathyroid tissue reserve is to read the previous surgeon's operative notes and to examine histological slides of the resected tissue. Operative notes, unfortunately, often do not accurately portray the number of glands remaining and their character. Histological preparations of resected or biopsied parathyroid tissue provide a more accurate index of the number of parathyroid glands indentified, but one cannot totally depend on these because a parathyroid gland may have been damaged by handling or may have had its vascular supply compromised during the operation. Also, supernumerary parathyroid tissue may be present in a small percentage of patients.

Parathyroid autotransplantation provides a mechanism for markedly reducing the likelihood of aparathyroidism in patients being re-explored for hyperparathyroidism. One must be very careful in employing this technique because the indiscriminant autografting of hyperfunctioning parathyroid tissue may result in a situation where parathyroid tissue remains in the neck and at the transplant site as well. The management of such patients if postoperative hypercalcemia develops is difficult and requires two or more operations.

Theoretically this problem can be avoided by tissue cryopreservation. If in a reoperative patient with hyperparathyroidism an enlarged parathyroid gland is identified, but it is not clear how many other parathyroid glands remain, the resected tissue can be cryopreserved[3, 25] and the patient observed. If it becomes obvious after lengthy replacement therapy that the patient cannot be weaned from calcium and vitamin D then the autologous parathyroid tissue can be thawed and grafted. Currently there is some controversy regarding the time of optimal replacement therapy, and the exact role of autotransplantation in the reoperative situation is still undergoing critical evaluation. Whether to deliberately attempt complete parathyroidectomy and immediate autografting or to reserve autografting until permanent hypoparathyroidism is documented is a matter of debate[3, 25, 26]. The problem is additionally compounded by the fact that not all cryopreserved grafts function sufficiently to allow the patient to be taken off vitamin D and calcium support within one year.

Delayed autografting in this group is one possible approach because of the difficulty of being certain that the patient is aparathyroid. If the patient does not have familial disease and a fourth gland is being removed, immediate autografting may be wiser.

Complications of reoperative surgery are very real[7]. Although mortality is low, the morbidity after reoperation in this severely ill population can be high (*Table 4.7*).

Table 4.7 Complications of reoperation in 125 patients

	Number of patients
Death within 30 days of operation (candida endocarditis; sepsis; immunodeficiency)	2
Wound hematoma	3
Horner's syndrome	1
Temporary nerve injury	6
Temporary tracheostomy	2
Pneumothorax	1
Pulmonary embolism	1

SUMMARY AND CONCLUSIONS

Reoperative parathyroid surgery continues to be a major intellectual and technical challenge. As physicians and surgeons become more experienced, one can hope that the first operation will be more successful and errors of diagnosis avoided. With judicious use of localization studies and appropriate selection of patients who need reoperation, a successful outcome in more than 90% of patients undergoing reoperation can be anticipated.

References

1 BARR, D. P. and BULGER, H. A. The clinical syndrome of hyperparathyroidism. *American Journal of the Medical Sciences*, **1979,** 449 (1930)

2 BRENNAN, M. F., DOPPMAN, J. L., MARX, S. J., SPIEGEL, A. M., BROWN, E. M. and AURBACH, G. D. Reoperative parathyroid surgery for persistent hyperparathyroidism. *Surgery*, **83,** 669 (1978)

3 BRENNAN, M. F., BROWN, E. M., SPIEGEL, A. M., MARX, S. J., DOPPMAN, J. L., JONES, D. C. and AURBACH, G. D. Autotransplantation of cryopreserved parathyroid tissue in man. *Annals of Surgery*, **189,** 139 (1979)

4 BRENNAN, M. F., DOPPMAN, J. L., KRUDY, A. G., MARX, S. J., SPIEGEL, A. M. and AURBACH, G. D. Assessment of techniques for reoperative parathyroid gland localization in patients undergoing reoperation for hyperparathyroidism. *Surgery,* **91,** 6–11 (1982)

5 BRENNAN, M. F., MARX, S. J., DOPPMAN, J. L., COSTA, J., SAXE, A., SPIEGEL, A., KRUDY, A. and AURBACH, G. D. Results of reoperation for persistent and recurrent hyperparathyroidism. *Annals of Surgery*, **194**, 671–676 (1981)

6 CLARK, O. H., WAY, L. W. and HUNT, T. K. Recurrent hyperparathyroidism. *Annals of Surgery*, **184**, 391 (1976)

7 DOPPMAN, J. L., BRENNAN, M. F., KOEHLER, J. O. and MARX, S. J. Computed tomography for parathyroid localization. *Journal of Computer Assisted Tomography*, **1**, 30 (1977)

8 DUBOST, C. Hyperparathyroidie. Les Réinterventions. *Journal de Chirurgie (Paris)*, **110**, 179 (1975)

9 DUDLEY, N. F. Methylene blue for rapid identification of the parathyroid sonography: a useful aid to preoperative localization. *British Medical Journal*, **3**, 680–681 (1971)

10 DUFFY, P., PICKER, R. H., DUFFIELD, S., REEVE, T. and HEWLETT, S. Parathyroid sonography: a useful aid to preoperative localization. *Journal of Clinical Ultrasound*, **8**, 113 (1980)

11 EDIS, A. J., SHEEDY, P. F., BEAHRS, O. H. and VAN HEERDEN, J. A. Results of reoperation for hyperparathyroidism with evaluation of preoperative localization studies. *Surgery*, **84**, 384 (1978)

12 EDIS, A. J. and EVANS, T. C. High resolution, real time ultrasonography in the preoperative localization of parathyroid tumors. *New England Journal of Medicine*, **301**, 532 (1979)

13 ELL, P. J., POKROPEK, A. T. and BRITTON, K. E. Localization of parathyroid adenomas by computer assisted parathyroid scanning. *British Journal of Surgery*, **62**, 553 (1975)

14 KRUDY, A. G., DOPPMAN, J. L., BRENNAN, M. F., MARX, S. J., SPIEGEL, A. M. and AURBACH, G. D. The detection of mediastinal parathyroid glands by computed tomography and angiography. Analysis of 17 proven cases. *Radiology*, **140**, 739–744 (1981)

15 LIVESAY, J. J. and MULDER, D. G. Recurrent hyperparathyroidism. *Archives of Surgery*, **111**, 688 (1976)

16 MANDL, F. Hyperparathyroidism. *Surgery*, **21**, 394 (1947)

17 MARTIN, J. K., VAN HEERDEN, J. A., EDIS, A. J. and DAHLIN, D. C. Persistent post-operative hyperparathyroidism. *Surgery, Gynecology and Obstetrics*, **151**, 764 (1980)

18 MARX, S. J., STOCK, J. L., ATTIE, M. F., DOWNS, R. W., GARDNER, D. G. and BROWN, E. M. Familial hypocalciuric hypercalcemia: recognition among patients referred after unsuccessful parathyroid exploration. *Annals of Internal Medicine*, **92**, 351 (1980)

19 MUELLER, H. True recurrence of hyperparathyroidism: proposed criteria of recurrence. *British Journal of Surgery*, **62**, 556 (1975)

20 SAXE, A. W. and BRENNAN, M. F. Strategy and technique of reoperative parathyroid surgery. *Surgery*, **89**, 417 (1981)

21 SPIEGEL, A. M., DOPPMAN, J. L., MARX, S. J., BRENNAN, M. F., BROWN, E. M., DOWNS, R. W. et al. Preoperative localization of abnormal parathyroids: neck massage versus arteriography and selective venous sampling. *Annals of Internal Medicine*, **89**, 935 (1978)

22 SPIEGEL, A. M., EASTMAN, S. T., ATTIE, M. F., DOWNS, R. W., LEVINE, M. A., MARX, S. J. et al. Utility of rapid measurement of intraoperative urinary cyclic AMP excretion in guiding surgery for primary hyperparathyroidism. *New England Journal of Medicine*, **303**, 1457 (1980)

23 STOCK, J. L., KRUDY, A., DOPPMAN, J. L., JONES, A. E., BRENNAN, M. F., ATTIE, M. F. et al. Parathyroid scanning after intra-arterial injections of [^{75}Se] selenomethionine. *Journal of Clinical Endocrinology and Metabolism*, **52**, 835 (1981)

24 WANG, C. A. Parathyroid re-exploration. *Annals of Surgery*, **186**, 140 (1977)

25 WELLS, S. A. and CHRISTIANSEN, C. The transplanted parathyroid gland: evaluation of cryopreservation and other environment factors which affect its function. *Surgery*, **75**, 49 (1974)

26 WELLS, S. A., GUNNELLS, J. C., LESLIE, J. B., SCHNEIDER, A. B., SHERWOOD, L. M. and GUTMAN, R. A. Transplantation of the parathyroid glands in man. *Transplant Proceedings*, **9**, 241 (1977)

Editors' commentary on Chapter 4

These experienced authors have reviewed very thoroughly the problems associated with recurrent and persistent hypercalcemia following an initial exploration. They have emphasized the importance of an absolutely confirmed diagnosis and the presence of symptomatic hyperparathyroidism before embarking upon a second, more hazardous re-exploration. They point out the need for and limitations of localization studies. Their experience with selective arteriography has been extensive and they advocate this procedure, although it correctly localized the disease in only 46% of their cases. It should be emphasized that they have been associated with a highly skilled angiographer who has had no major complications arising from those studies. A significant incidence of major neurological complications (2%) has, however, been reported from a number of other hospitals and this fact, in association with a relatively high false negative rate, has caused many clinicians to use this test only on rare occasions. The Ann Arbor Group have used selective arteriography less frequently than any of the localization studies noted but have found it very useful in several difficult cases. We would agree entirely with the authors that angiography and selective venous sampling should be done only in centers where there is an interested and experienced angiographer available. In contrast to the authors, we have found ultrasound of the neck to be of some value in the reoperative cases. We have used it to evaluate the thyroid gland for the presence of an intrathyroidal parathyroid adenoma that has been overlooked. In two cases it has been specifically helpful in identifying the missing adenoma before a second operation was undertaken. We, like the authors, have found that the operative notes or map of the initial findings, in conjunction with the pathological report and a discussion with the original surgeon, are very important in leading to a successful reoperation. In our experience the missing adenoma has been found during cervical re-exploration in nearly all referred cases from outside hospitals. Because of this, we no longer do invasive localization studies in any of these patients unless four proven parathyroid glands have been identified at the original operation. In all but one of our own cases requiring reoperation a missing adenoma has been found at mediastinal exploration, usually after one or more invasive localizing studies had been performed. Selective venous parathyroid hormone levels have been of some help but are not in themselves reliable in specifically localizing an adenoma. A high level tends to regionalize or lateralize the source of parathyroid hormone and confirms the diagnosis. The authors have presented a well balanced discussion of the indications for parathyroid transplantation after reoperations. They emphasize that autografting should be selective and for the most part delayed, using cryopreservation. We would agree entirely with their recommendations as we have found that only a small percentage of patients become permanently hypoparathyroid after reoperation, but the risk is always present.

5
The role of adrenalectomy in the management of Cushing's syndrome
R. B. Welbourn and K. J. Manolas

HISTORY

Before adrenalectomy became available for the treatment of Cushing's syndrome, half the patients died from the disease within 5 years of the first symptom[71]. Adrenalectomy was a hazardous procedure until the discovery of cortisone and its use as replacement therapy during and after operation. This transformed the situation so that the disease could be treated effectively and reliably for the first time. In 1951 Priestley *et al.*[73] from the Mayo Clinic reported their remarkable early results in 29 patients, in 1955 Cope and Raker[14] from Boston followed, and the operation was soon adopted generally[2].

At that time it was appreciated that excessive production of cortisol by the adrenal cortex was the immediate cause of the clinical and metabolic features of the syndrome, but the underlying causes and their relative incidence had not been defined in large series of patients (*Figure 5.1*). Diagnosis depended on clinical assessment and measurement of non-specific adrenal steroids in the urine. Cortisol itself and ACTH could not be measured routinely, and no methods had been devised to test the dependence or independence of the adrenals on the pituitary. Pituitary tumours, which had been described by Cushing[16] in all but two of his cases, could not be recognized in life unless they were large enough to increase the size of the sella turcica as a whole, and this was seen on X-rays in only about 15% of patients[1]. Adrenal carcinomas could usually be recognized, but adenomas were rarely distinguishable from hyperplastic glands except at operation. The ectopic ACTH syndrome had not been described.

Bilateral adrenalectomy was used for the treatment of patients with bilateral adrenal hyperplasia with or without evidence of a large pituitary tumour. During the past 30 years many hundreds of patients have been treated, and the immediate and long-term results in adults[63, 81, 92] and children[59] have been studied and reported in detail.

At first most surgeons removed one or both glands subtotally (by analogy with subtotal thyroidectomy) in the hope that normal adrenal function would be

53

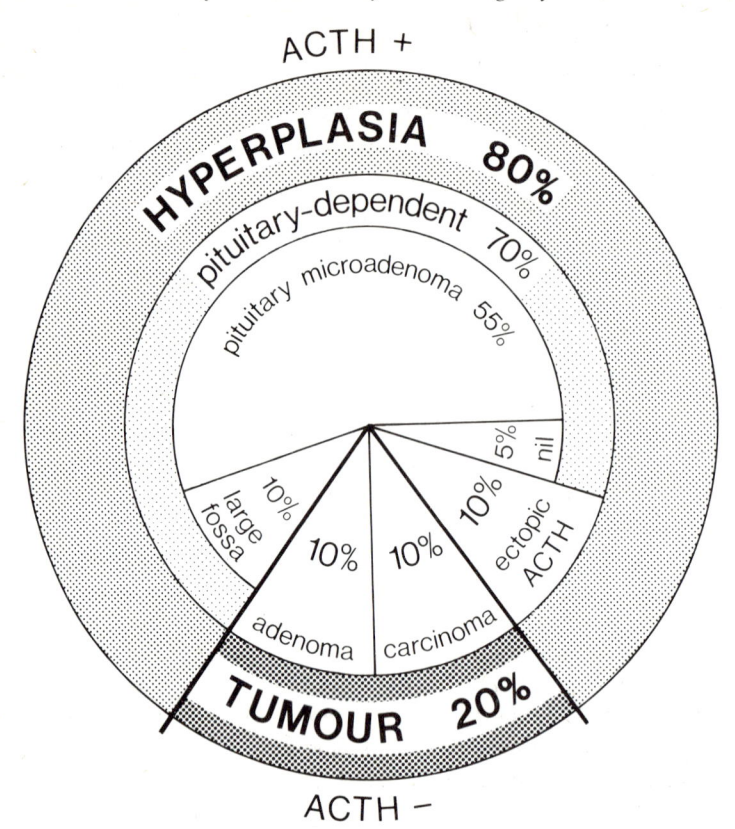

Figure 5.1 Causal lesions in Cushing's syndrome (percentages are approximate). 'ACTH +' indicates that excess of ACTH causes adrenal hyperplasia. 'ACTH −' means that an adrenal tumour inhibits the production of ACTH by the pituitary. (From Welbourn[91], courtesy of the Editor and Publishers, *British Journal of Surgery*)

restored and that steroids would not be required after the early postoperative period. About 10% of those undergoing operation and 30% of those who survive 10 years remain in remission without requiring replacement therapy. In the majority the remnants either fail to function adequately, necessitating replacement therapy, or enlarge so that the syndrome recurs[92]. For these reasons total bilateral adrenalectomy with permanent replacement therapy has become the usual standard practice.

Steroid replacement, properly controlled by the doctor and reliably taken by the patient, is literally vital, and death from adrenocortical insufficiency is a constant hazard. However, provided that the patient and his or her relatives understand this, problems are infrequent and death is very rare[61].

RESULTS OF ADRENALECTOMY

The operative mortality is about 2–5%[36,92], pulmonary embolism being a common cause of death[6,83]. Remission follows rapidly in the great majority who survive[92].

In the first few days and weeks the blood pressure falls, but remains labile, and the skin often peels, particularly at the hair margins, until remission is complete. The electrolyte balance returns to normal, and diabetes usually remits if it is mild, but tends to persist if it is severe. During the next few weeks and months the appearance, shape, strength, energy, mental state and sexual function all return towards normal. The cardiovascular system improves in most patients, but deteriorates in a few, who may suffer fatal cerebrovascular or cardiovascular accidents within the first year after operation. Later the blood pressure returns almost to normal in most patients and the cardiovascular system reaches a stable state. The bones regain their protein matrices but do not recalcify (except in children). Deformities become stable and the bones no longer fracture. Hirsutism diminishes but does not disappear completely. Cutaneous striae become pale. Growth is restored in children but lost height is rarely regained. Renal stones, if treated effectively, do not reform. Fertility is restored.

While in the first year after adrenalectomy the main hazard is a vascular accident, later the major complication is the continued growth of a pituitary tumour. The growth may, in part, be accelerated by removal of the inhibiting effect of a high concentration of cortisol in the blood. The sella turcica enlarges, the plasma ACTH level rises and, as a result, Addisonian pigmentation appears. This condition, known as Nelson's syndrome[66], usually develops within 2 to 3 years, but may not do so until much later[63]. Eventually it may affect 30% or more of patients, both adults[13, 64] and children[34]. In the first author's personal series (*see Table 5.2*) about 50% of patients developed pathological pigmentation. Several methods, both surgical and radiotherapeutic, may be used successfully to treat the established syndrome, but some of the pituitary tumours are locally invasive and incurable[92].

A few patients can be weaned off replacement therapy after apparent total bilateral adrenalectomy and remain well, while in a very few the syndrome either persists or recurs[3, 10]. While the adrenals may not have been removed completely in some of these patients, experienced surgeons are confident that they were in others. Ectopic adrenocortical tissue has been found in some 30% of all people at autopsy[26], and it seems likely that this may hypertrophy in the same way as the adrenal remnant after subtotal adrenalectomy.

In all, about two-thirds of the patients who undergo adrenalectomy remain alive and in remission for 5 to 15 years after operation and one half are alive after 20 years[63, 92] (*Figure 5.2*). These are the standards with which other, newer methods of treatment must be compared.

Adrenocortical tumours causing Cushing's syndrome are nearly always unilateral and have been treated by surgical excision for many years. Cortisone rendered these operations safe also. Malignant tumours cannot always be removed, owing to local invasion. When they can be excised, the syndrome usually remits rapidly, but the tumour frequently recurs locally and metastasizes to the lungs, the skeleton and elsewhere. The syndrome then commonly recurs also, and even after treatment with mitotane, which is occasionally effective, most patients die within 5 years[37, 38, 46, 60].

Benign adenomas are quite different. The operative morbidity and mortality are negligible, nearly all patients are weaned off replacement therapy, and a very high

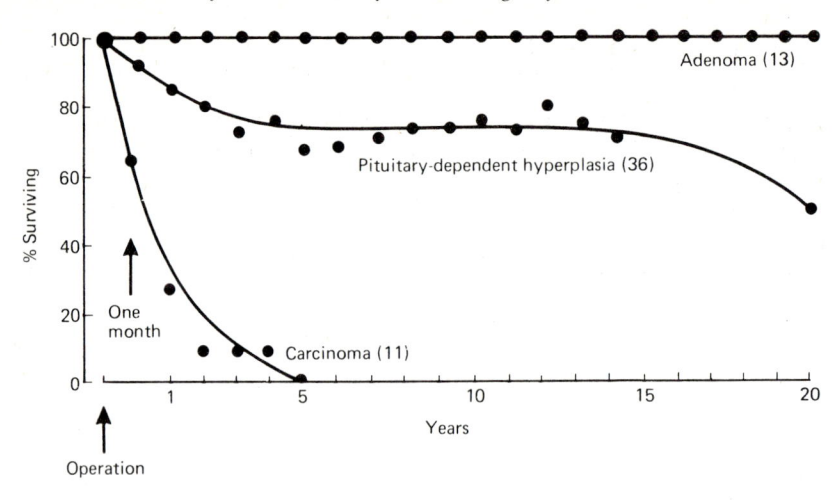

Figure 5.2 Survival after adrenalectomy for Cushing's syndrome (numbers of patients in parentheses). (From Welbourn[91], courtesy of the Editor and Publishers, *British Journal of Surgery*)

proportion remain alive and well for many years[69]. In one series of 13 patients[91] all were alive and in remission, the first 7 having survived more than 10 years after operation (*see Figure 5.2*). In a series of 25 patients, which included these 13, all but one, who was lost to follow-up, were alive between 1 and 25 years after[23].

Pituitary tumours

Before the advent of cortisone, surgical hypophysectomy was hazardous and was usually postponed for as long as possible. In Cushing's syndrome the transcranial approach was used and the operation was limited to removal by suction of the adenoma, thought to be accessible just beneath the diaphragma sellae[43]. At first, after the introduction of cortisone, patients with obvious pituitary tumours were treated initially by adrenalectomy and were subjected to craniotomy later only if the pituitary tumour caused local complications or pigmentation[77].

Within a few years, however, the situation changed. Cortisone rendered operations on the pituitary safer, like those on the adrenals, and surgeons developed expertise in hypophysectomy from employing it in the treatment of large numbers of women with advanced breast cancer. As a result, patients with Cushing's syndrome, whose sellae were large, came to be treated initially by hypophysectomy, usually followed by radiotherapy, either external or internal[20]. Adrenalectomy was reserved for those who failed to respond or in whom the syndrome recurred owing to incomplete removal or invasiveness of the tumour[92]. In general, unless the tumour is invasive, the results are good.

CUSHING'S SYNDROME TODAY

During the past 30 years, knowledge about Cushing's syndrome has increased very greatly. The main causative lesions and their *approximate* relative proportions are now known[21] (*Table 5.1*).

Table 5.1 Causative lesions of Cushing's syndrome

Lesion	Relative proportion*	
Bilateral adrenal hyperplasia due to ACTH excess		80%
Pituitary tumour	65%	
Hypothalamic/pituitary hyperfunction without tumour	5%	
Paraendocrine tumour	10%	
Unilateral adrenocortical tumour		20%
Adenoma	10%	
Carcinoma	10%	

* All percentages are approximate.

Bilateral adrenal hyperplasia[67] is frequently associated with micronodules up to 2 or 3 mm in diameter. In about 10 to 20% of patients the nodules are larger and may reach a size of 2.5 cm. This condition is known as nodular hyperplasia and is generally ACTH-dependent. Adrenal tumours secrete autonomously, inhibit the production of ACTH, and cause atrophy of the non-tumorous parts of the glands. However, one patient has been described in whom an autonomous macronodule or adenoma, 4 cm in diameter, coexisted with bilateral ACTH-dependent hyperplasia[80].

Cushing's syndrome can be diagnosed with precision by measurement of cortisol in the blood and urine, and ACTH in the blood. The dependence of hyperplastic adrenal glands on the pituitary can be assessed particularly by the dexamethasone and metyrapone tests[24].

In the past, some 85% of pituitary tumours have not been detected by conventional X-rays, which include measurement of sellar area and volume[1]. Cushing's syndrome is now usually diagnosed at an earlier stage than formerly, so that even more escape detection by these means. Diagnostic procedures are, however, improving and the more extensively patients are investigated radiologically, the more frequently pituitary tumours are diagnosed with confidence without resort to needle biopsy or operation (*see later*). Angiography, computed tomographic (CT) scanning, use of the water-soluble contrast medium metrizamide combined with conventional radiology or with CT scanning[19,30], and thin-section (hypocycloidal) tomography have all contributed. The last is perhaps the most sensitive, and lateral tomograms, taken at 2 mm intervals, often reveal evidence of tumours not detected by conventional X-rays[76].

Paraendocrine tumours, namely extrapituitary tumours which secrete ACTH and cause the ectopic ACTH syndrome[58], may often be diagnosed with confidence[39], and benign ones amenable to operation can sometimes be identified.

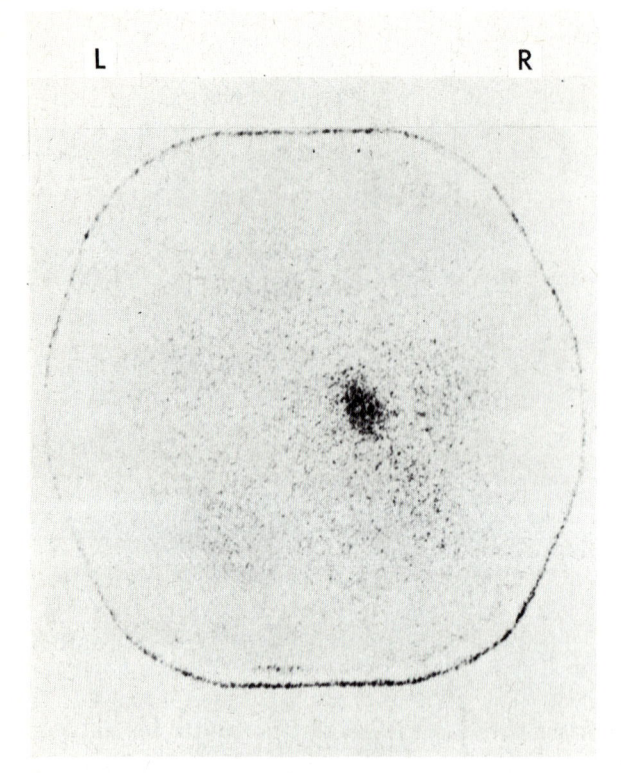

Figure 5.3 Patient with Cushing's syndrome due to right adrenal adenoma. Posterior view of upper abdomen 14 days after intravenous injection of selenium-75 norcholesterol (Scintadren, Amersham International) 250 μCi (10 MBq) showing uptake in right suprarenal area. (Courtesy of Dr J. P. Lavender)

Thirty years ago there was no reliable technique for the localization of adrenal tumours. Now the number available is almost embarrassing[41, 85, 88]. They include angiography, selective venous sampling, ultrasonography, and radiocholesterol (*Figure 5.3*) and CT scanning (*Figure 5.4*). The last two particularly, alone or in combination, allow the localization of benign and malignant tumours with great accuracy. Adrenal venography should be avoided because it frequently ruptures the gland and results in haematoma formation around it. This renders subsequent operations unnecessarily difficult.

ALTERNATIVES TO ADRENALECTOMY

While this knowledge has been accumulating, many alternative therapeutic procedures have been introduced, particularly for the treatment of Cushing's syndrome due to pituitary-dependent adrenal hyperplasia, when no large pituitary tumour is apparent. No prospective controlled trials comparing different procedures have been reported. The methods include drug therapy, radiotherapy and surgical operations. They have been used alone and in various combinations.

Alternatives to adrenalectomy 59

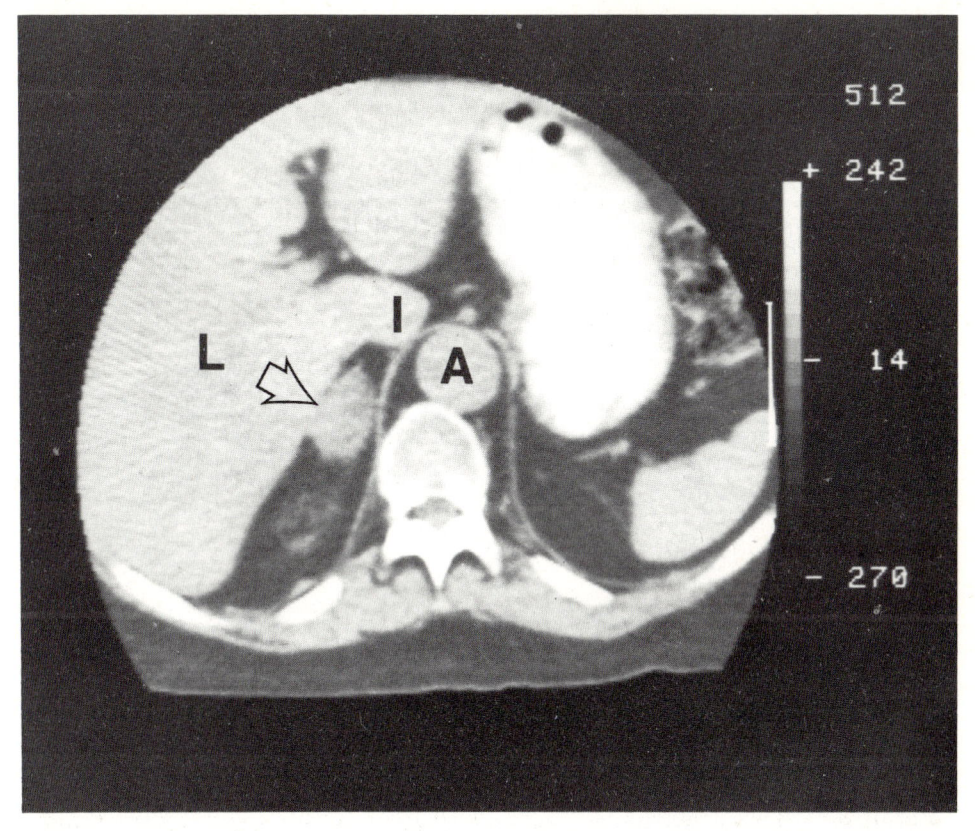

Figure 5.4 Same patient as in *Figure 5.3*. Computed tomography (CT) scan, showing tumour (arrow) medial to the liver (L) and posterolateral to the inferior vena cava (I). The right crus of the diaphragm and aorta (A) are medial to the tumour. (Courtesy of Dr G. Bydder)

Drug therapy

Drug therapy requires close supervision by clinical assessment and by frequent measurement of plasma cortisol levels, and the dosages need to be adjusted from time to time according to the circumstances. When effective, drugs do not cause remission as rapidly as surgical operations.

Metyrapone

Metyrapone inhibits selectively, and to a varying degree, the conversion of 11-deoxycortisol (compound S) to cortisol and was the first agent to receive extensive trial. Unlike cortisol, compound S does not inhibit the secretion of ACTH by the pituitary. Hence, when ACTH is of pituitary origin, its concentration in the plasma rises, but it does not do so when it is secreted by an ectopic tumour[42].

Metyrapone, in doses of 0.5 to 4 g per day, causes remission within weeks or months in most patients with Cushing's syndrome, whatever the underlying lesion. Long-term therapy is very expensive and is liable to unpleasant complications, particularly nausea and vomiting, skin rashes and, in women, hirsutism and acne. It has been found to be most effective as an adjunct to other forms of therapy, particularly external irradiation of the pituitary[42], and in the preparation of patients for adrenalectomy or hypophysectomy[68].

Aminoglutethimide

Aminoglutethimide, which inhibits the conversion of cholesterol to pregnenolone, a step common to the biosynthesis of all adrenal steroids, has been found less effective[94] and also to cause sedation and other undesirable side-effects. A combination of metyrapone and aminoglutethimide may be better than either alone as an adjunct to more definitive forms of therapy[11].

Trilostane

Trilostane blocks the conversion of pregnenolone to progesterone and inhibits the synthesis of cortisol and aldosterone without interfering with gonadal function. Preliminary reports suggest that it may be effective in the same circumstances as the two previous drugs. However, it may also cause unpleasant complications[49].

Mitotane

Mitotane (*o'p*-DDD) causes necrosis of the normal or hyperplastic zona fasciculata and zona reticularis and also of adrenal tumours. It is of most value in the treatment of carcinomas[38] but has also been employed in the management of pituitary-dependent Cushing's syndrome[7]. It has toxic side-effects, particularly nausea, but in one large series good long-term results were reported in over 80% of patients[60].

Centrally acting drugs

These drugs, including the dopamine agonist *bromocryptine*[52] and the serotonin antagonist *cyproheptadine*[27,50], have proved effective in some hands but not in others[18] and have not been used widely.

Radiotherapy

All forms of irradiation are more effective in patients whose fossae are of normal size on conventional X-rays than in those in whom they are enlarged. Radiotherapy, though perhaps safer, does not, when effective, cause such rapid remission as adrenalectomy or surgical excision of a pituitary tumour.

External irradiation

External irradiation of the pituitary with *photons* from conventional sources has been in use for many years. Indeed, some patients responded well before the advent of cortisone and safe adrenalectomy[84]. In recent years, therapy from a cobalt source or a linear accelerator has been used extensively, and a dose of 4500 to 5000 rad over one month is effective in about 30 to 40% of patients in most series[29]. Higher success rates have been reported[69,81], especially in patients with milder forms of the disease. Because remission ensues very slowly, patients usually need to be controlled with adjuvant drugs, particularly metyrapone. The syndrome recurs in some, and, while the method is usually safe, various complications have been reported[62]. Children appear to respond better than adults, and excellent results, without impairment of pituitary function, have been reported[44].

A new technique, known as 'closed stereotactic radiosurgery', allows a small area of the pituitary to be irradiated intensively while the rest is spared[75]. Now that many small tumours can be located precisely, the results of external irradiation are likely to improve[65,86].

External irradiation with *protons* (α-particles) from a synchrocyclotron has been pioneered by Lawrence[57] at Berkeley and by Kjellberg[48] in Boston. It allows a very large dose (about 7000 rad) to be delivered accurately to the tumour or to the centre of the pituitary in one short session. Irradiation of the brain and the periphery of the gland is much less than with photon therapy. Results are satisfactory, at least in the short term, in nearly 90% of patients[48,57], most of whom do not require replacement therapy.

Interstitial irradiation

Interstitial irradiation of the pituitary with radon seeds at craniotomy was pioneered by Pattison of Newcastle in 1938 with encouraging results in two patients[70]. Twenty years later Fraser and Joplin[8] at Hammersmith started to develop the technique of interstitial irradiation, at first with gold-198 and later with yttrium-90 inserted under radiological control via a cannula introduced through the nose or beside it. The technique has now been perfected and, at Hammersmith, provides the best form of irradiation for patients without large tumours[8]. In patients with normal-sized glands the results are similar to those of bilateral adrenalectomy, at least for 10 years or so. Approximately 30 to 40% require replacement therapy with thyroxine or steroids[45] (personal communication). The further growth of small pituitary tumours is prevented. As with external irradiation, results are less satisfactory in patients with enlarged pituitary fossae. Interstitial irradiation may be used safely and effectively in children[9] and interferes little with pituitary function. Only 1 of the last 9 children treated required replacement therapy[8]. Other workers have attempted the same procedure, but have been far less successful, and no comparable results have been reported.

Surgical removal of pituitary adenomas

For many years a transsphenoidal approach for the decompression of pituitary tumours has been used as an alternative to the transcranial route. In experienced hands this is a less traumatic procedure. In the late 1960s it received new impetus from the adoption of the operating microscope for pituitary surgery, and surgeons started to *remove* adenomas by this route. Even quite large ones, extending up to 1 cm above the diaphragm, can be excised satisfactorily. The technique was developed mainly by James[40] of Bristol, an ENT surgeon, and Hardy[31] of Montreal, a neurosurgeon. At first it was employed mainly by ENT surgeons, but later other neurosurgeons, especially Guiot[28] in France and Kjellberg and Kliman[47] in the USA, came to use it also.

The results are usually good, and remission follows rapidly. The few who fail to respond, presumably because of incomplete removal, are still treated by adrenalectomy, which cures the Cushing's syndrome. In some of these the residual pituitary tumour lies dormant and the patients remain in good health for years. In others, as in some patients with Nelson's syndrome, the tumour is invasive and rapidly fatal[92].

Pituitary microsurgery

When *small* tumours (less than 10 mm) are detected by radiographic methods, an increasing number of surgeons are now removing them by microsurgical techniques, using the transsphenoidal route[33, 78, 89]. Moreover, microsurgical exploration of the pituitary fossa by the same route, without special preoperative methods for the detection of a tumour, is being practised in some centres[5, 51]. Tumours are found in a high proportion of cases and are enucleated, the rest of the gland being left undisturbed. In a small proportion no adenoma is found and the gland is removed totally. In these cases a minute tumour or generalized hyperplasia may be found histologically[79, 87]. Preliminary reports indicate that in *experienced* hands the mortality and complication rates are very low and that nearly 80% of patients, on the average, undergo rapid and satisfactory remission. The range is about 50% (6/11)[55] to 100% (16/16)[89]. The largest series so far reported contain less than 40 patients each[4, 22]. All patients require replacement therapy immediately, but most become independent of it after a few months.

There are several possible causes of failure. (1) The dura mater may be involved microscopically by adenomas which are frankly invasive[82], so that some of the tumour may be left behind at operation and enlarge later. (2) Only one of multiple microadenomas present may be recognized and removed at operation[54]. (3) Small, clinically silent pituitary adenomas have been found at autopsy in over 20% of people. Some such tumours may be found in patients with Cushing's syndrome and be removed without clinical benefit[15].

It should be emphasized that, although the early results of microsurgical removal of adenomas in small series are encouraging, very few results beyond 5 years have

DEVELOPMENT OF ADRENALECTOMY

been reported and the incidence of recurrence is not yet known. No complete comparisons can therefore be made with adrenalectomy or with other well-established methods of treatment[93].

DEVELOPMENT OF ADRENALECTOMY

During the time that these alternative therapeutic measures have been evolving, adrenalectomy itself has developed and undergone refinements. While controlled prospective trials have not been undertaken, it seems clear that the operative morbidity has been reduced. Four measures are probably responsible, but their relative importance is uncertain:

(1) Preoperative preparation with drugs, especially metyrapone, induces partial remission within a few weeks in most patients, so that they come to operation in a much better state than previously and the immediate postoperative period is smoother.
(2) The recognition that patients with Cushing's syndrome are greatly at risk from deep venous thrombosis and pulmonary embolism has led to the routine use of measures to prevent these complications. They include intermittent pneumatic compression of the legs, low dose heparin, and intravenous dextran. There is some evidence that the last of these may be of benefit in adrenalectomy for Cushing's syndrome[17].
(3) Wound dehiscence and infection were previously common and serious complications. They can now be almost eliminated by the preoperative preparation described, and by the use of vitamin A[35] and appropriate prophylactic antibiotics[25,72] over the period of operation.
(4) Formerly most operations were undertaken by the lateral or anterior (transabdominal) approach. Both these are major and potentially complicated undertakings in patients with Cushing's syndrome, although they are still indicated in some circumstances. The anterior route, in particular, often resulted in subphrenic abscess[92]. Most surgeons now employ the posterior route for the removal of hyperplastic glands and adenomas[90]. It is much less traumatic and allows a rapid convalescence.

Although these procedures have, to unknown and probably different degrees, reduced the immediate postoperative morbidity, there is little evidence that they have influenced the operative *mortality*. In the author's own series (*see Table 5.2*) of adrenalectomies for benign adrenal disease (hyperplasia or adenoma), 3 of 77 patients (4%) failed to leave hospital alive. In retrospect, only one patient, an Italian who had been bedridden for a long time, might have been saved. Pituitary implantation with yttrium-90 was attempted, but abandoned because c.s.f. leaked through the cannula. Adrenalectomy was uneventful until 10 weeks later when, during mobilization, the patient died from a massive pulmonary embolus. Further analysis shows that 3 of 56 patients (5%) died in the years 1953 to 1974 and that none of 21 (0%) have died since. The difference is not significant, but it may indicate a trend. During the same period, 4 of 10 patients (40%) died soon after exploration of adrenal carcinoma. In 3 of these the tumour could not be resected.

The incidence of Nelson's syndrome in patients with pituitary-dependent disease may be reduced by external pituitary irradiation at about the time of adrenalectomy[69] but the evidence is inconclusive[64].

A variant of this regime has been proposed, namely *unilateral* adrenalectomy followed by pituitary irradiation for both adults[53] and children[56]. Half the patients respond well and do not need replacement therapy. However, the other half relapse and require total adrenalectomy.

Some surgeons have removed both glands completely, grafting small fragments of them into a superficial muscle so that, if the syndrome persists or recurs, they can remove them progressively until normal function is restored. This practice has rarely been successful in the past, but recent attempts by Hardy[32] in the USA and by others[74] have been more encouraging, and the technique should, perhaps, receive further attention.

Most paraendocrine tumours secreting ACTH are highly malignant and cause acute Cushing's syndrome only as a terminal event. Some, however, especially carcinoids of the bronchus or elsewhere, are less aggressive or entirely benign. If the primary tumour can be recognized initially, it may be removed, causing remission without the need for adrenalectomy and replacement therapy, as in 2 patients in the Hammersmith series[16a] (*see later*). If no primary tumour can be found, adrenalectomy causes excellent remission, as in 5 of these cases. In one a benign tumour revealed itself later, and was then removed.

SELECTION OF TREATMENT

Most physicians and surgeons would agree with Orth and Liddle[69] that the ideal form of treatment for patients with Cushing's syndrome would:

(1) reduce the secretion of cortisol to normal
(2) eradicate any tumour threatening health
(3) avoid permanent endocrine deficiency and
(4) avoid permanent dependence on medicines

They would probably add that it would also be free from iatrogenic morbidity and mortality.

These principles underlie the conclusions which follow. In the absence of objective controlled trials, they reflect subjective judgements of the available evidence.

The outcome of treatment in any individual patient depends partly on the nature of the causative lesion and partly on the method of treatment provided. At one extreme, an adrenal adenoma or a benign paraendocrine tumour, removed surgically, provides the best possible result. At the other, an adrenal carcinoma, an invasive pituitary tumour or a malignant paraendocrine tumour, however treated, carries a bad prognosis. Intermediate are patients with pituitary-dependent adrenal hyperplasia with benign pituitary tumours or hyperplasia.

Drug therapy, especially with metyrapone, is very valuable as an adjunct to all surgical and radiotherapeutic measures, but no pharmacological agent has yet been found which is both sufficiently efficacious and free from complications to be generally suitable for long-term definitive therapy of Cushing's syndrome.

No effective alternative to adrenalectomy has been advanced for the treatment of adrenal tumours. Patients with adenomas fare singularly well, and this form of therapy, which has been tested for many years, satisfies the principles of treatment more completely than any other for this or any variety of the syndrome.

Carcinomas have a bad prognosis, whatever methods are used, and surgical excision, combined with chemotherapy in the form of mitotane, is the best that can be provided at present.

Pituitary tumours, which cause generalized enlargement of the fossa, respond best to surgical hypophysectomy combined with radiotherapy, although some are invasive and, at present, incurable.

There are several alternative procedures which may prove as good as, or better than, total bilateral adrenalectomy for the small fossa, pituitary-dependent group of patients. Although other measures may enter the lists seriously in the future, the main contenders at present are:

(1) microsurgical removal of pituitary adenoma
(2) yttrium-90 pituitary implantation
(3) proton therapy

The first is being employed more and more as surgeons become proficient in the technique. The procedure is not as satisfactory as surgical excision of an adrenal adenoma, because there is a greater likelihood of recurrence and perhaps of permanent need for replacement therapy. On the other hand it may prove more effective than total adrenalectomy, not in terms of control of the syndrome but in providing freedom from the almost invariable necessity of permanent replacement therapy and from the development of Nelson's syndrome.

Facilities for the other two measures are available in very few centres, but they fulfil the first two and the last criteria very well in the hands of those who practise them. Their success in relation to the third and fourth criteria (avoidance of endocrine deficiency and dependence on medicines) is only moderate. The *availability* of a therapeutic measure therefore plays a large part in determining which is most appropriate in any one centre.

Personal series

It is instructive to analyze the indications for adrenal exploration and (except in the case of unresectable adrenal carcinoma) adrenalectomy in the author's own practice in the years 1953 to 1981 (*Table 5.2*). The findings reflect changing policies, the availability and efficacy of different therapeutic methods, and improving diagnostic procedures.

Table 5.2 Indications for adrenal exploration in 95 patients with Cushing's syndrome*

	Number of patients	
	Belfast (1953–1963)	Hammersmith (1963–1981)
A Pituitary-dependent adrenal hyperplasia suspected		
(1) Bilateral adrenalectomy treatment of choice if fossa of normal size	21 (adenoma found in 2)	11 (last in 1976)
(2) Pituitary implant impossible for technical reasons	–	4
(3) Pituitary implant failed to control syndrome	–	8 (last in 1976)
(4) Hypophysectomy failed to control syndrome	1	1
(5) Implant and hypophysectomy failed to control syndrome	–	3 (last in 1969)
(6) Child or adolescent	–	2
B Pituitary-independent adrenal hyperplasia suspected		
(1) Ectopic ACTH syndrome proved or probable	0	7
(2) Ectopic ACTH syndrome possible	0	3
C Adrenal tumour suspected		
(1) Adenoma	0	16 (none found in 3)
(2) Carcinoma	4	6
Total adrenal explorations	26	61
D No adrenal exploration; surgical hypophysectomy	1	3
E No operation on adrenals or pituitary	2	2
Total (no adrenal exploration)	3	5

* Personal series, R. B. Welbourn. The 14 patients treated by D. A. D. Montgomery and T. L. Kennedy in Belfast from 1963–1967 which were included in the series of Welbourn, Montgomery and Kennedy[92] have here been excluded, and 49 patients treated at Hammersmith since 1968 have been added.

From 1953 to 1963 all patients in Northern Ireland (whose population was 1.5 million) suspected of having Cushing's syndrome were referred to D. A. D. Montgomery and the author[2, 63, 92] in Belfast. Bilateral adrenalectomy was regarded as the treatment of choice for patients with apparently pituitary-dependent adrenal hyperplasia but a normal-sized fossa, and 21 patients were operated on for this reason[92] (A1; Table 5.2). Two of them were found at operation to have adenomas, and these were removed. During the same period 2 patients presented with enlarged pituitary fossae and were treated by transcranial hypophysectomy. One patient (D) was cured, but the other (A4) had an invasive tumour and required adrenalectomy subsequently.

At Hammersmith (1963–1981) patients from many countries were referred, some directly and some via the endocrinologists. The author's patients were therefore highly selected. He, and some endocrinologists (particularly C. L. Cope) and surgeons who referred patients adopted the same policy in relation to adrenalectomy as that practised in Belfast. In the same hospital, however, Fraser and Joplin were developing the technique of interstitial irradiation and employed this in most of their patients[8]. Consequently only 11 patients underwent bilateral adrenalectomy *as the first treatment of choice* (A1), the last in 1976. Four patients were treated by adrenalectomy because a pituitary implant was not possible for technical reasons (A2). One of these had an empty sella, one had such severe osteoporosis that the sella was invisible on X-rays, and two suffered leakage, one of blood and one of c.s.f., when the cannula entered the gland.

Pituitary implantation did not always control the syndrome in the early years, and 8 patients required subsequent adrenalectomy (A3), the last in 1976. One patient in whom hypophysectomy had failed to control the syndrome (A4) and three in whom both interstitial irradiation *and* hypophysectomy had failed (A5) underwent adrenalectomy. (During this same period three other patients about whom the author was consulted underwent surgical hypophysectomy as the first form of treatment (D)).

Six children or adolescents (below the age of 18) underwent adrenalectomy, the first four because it was regarded as the treatment of choice for *all* patients of this type (A1), the last two (in 1976 and 1977) because of the fear that any therapy directed at the pituitary might prevent normal growth and sexual development (A6).

In 10 patients investigation suggested that the adrenals were independent of pituitary control (B1 and B2), and adrenalectomy was employed for this reason. Seven of them definitely or probably had paraendocrine tumours causing the ectopic ACTH syndrome.

While in Belfast two adrenal adenomas which had not been recognized previously were found at operation, at Hammersmith 3 of 16 patients suspected of having such tumours were found to have bilateral hyperplasia. The last of these presented in 1976. Two of them were subjected to total adrenalectomy (C1), and the third had one macronodular hyperplastic gland removed and was later treated successfully by yttrium implantation.

Four adrenal carcinomas were diagnosed correctly and operated on in Belfast and six at Hammersmith (C2).

It is interesting to note that 1976 was the last year in which adrenalectomy was used as the treatment of choice for pituitary-dependent Cushing's syndrome in an adult, the last in which adrenalectomy was performed for a failed pituitary implant, and the last in which a preoperative false positive diagnosis of adrenal adenoma was made. The next year, 1977, was the last in which adrenalectomy was preferred to pituitary implantation in an adolescent.

Four patients were neither irradiated nor treated by operations on the adrenals or the pituitary (E). One refused operation and underwent spontaneous remission; the other three suffered from the ectopic ACTH syndrome. One, with an oat-cell bronchial carcinoma, died and two (as already mentioned) had carcinoid tumours excised without need for adrenalectomy.

Indications for adrenalectomy

In the light of these principles, facts and arguments it seems reasonable to draw the following conclusions about the role of adrenalectomy in the treatment of patients suffering from Cushing's syndrome:

(1) Adrenal tumours, benign or malignant, are best treated by surgical excision when it is possible.
(2) Adrenal hyperplasia or nodular hyperplasia which is apparently independent of pituitary control may be treated by total adrenalectomy with relief of the Cushing syndrome. Many such patients have paraendocrine tumours secreting ACTH. If a primary tumour is identified and can be removed completely, adrenalectomy is *not* required. If it eludes detection, or is growing slowly and cannot be excised, total adrenalectomy provides rapid symptomatic relief. When the tumour cannot be found initially, it should be sought at regular intervals thereafter. When it cannot be eradicated, radiotherapy or chemotherapy may be of benefit.
(3) Surgical or radiotherapeutic measures to remove or destroy a pituitary adenoma (small or large) may be impractical for technical reasons. In such cases total adrenalectomy is the best alternative.
(4) Similar measures may fail to control the Cushing syndrome. Adrenalectomy is then required.
(5) In many centres specialized neurosurgical and radiotherapeutic facilities are not available. Adrenalectomy is an entirely satisfactory alternative and should probably be followed by conventional external irradiation of the pituitary.
(6) Children and adolescents require special consideration. While as recently as 1977 therapy to the pituitary was regarded as possibly hazardous, it is now clear that external radiotherapy[44] or interstitial irradiation[9] provides excellent results in this age group. It would seem reasonable therefore, in patients below the age of 18, to try the effect of metyrapone and interstitial irradiation at Hammersmith, or external irradiation elsewhere. If these facilities are not available, or if they fail, total adrenalectomy would appear to be the treatment of choice. Pituitary microsurgical procedures do not appear to have been used.

OPERATIVE APPROACH

The operative approach[90] to the adrenals influences the ease with which adrenalectomy may be accomplished and also the postoperative morbidity. The authors employ three different approaches – posterior, anterior and lateral – and each is ideal in certain circumstances.

The *posterior route* is usually best for the removal of bilateral hyperplastic glands and of small adenomas (up to 2 or 3 cm in diameter). The patient is placed face down, the 12th rib is resected on one or both sides, and one or both adrenals are removed. The postoperative course is usually remarkably smooth and free from pain. If, as rarely happens today, the wounds become infected, they drain downhill and heal rapidly.

An *anterior abdominal* incision is convenient when the patient is suspected of having a paraendocrine, ACTH-secreting tumour. The primary lesion may be found, for instance, in the pancreas or, as in one patient in the Hammersmith series, in the appendix. Secondary deposits may be found in the liver, biopsies may be taken and the adrenals can be removed. Unless the patient is obese, a midline epigastric incision is suitable. Otherwise a 'roof-top' or double 'Kocher' type of incision gives the best access.

The *lateral approach* provides the best access to large tumours, to adrenals which have been operated on previously, and in any circumstances when difficulty is expected. On the left an extrapleural incision through the bed of the 11th rib provides the best access, and on the right a transthoracic exploration through the bed of the 10th rib is most satisfactory.

In *children* a lateral incision through the bed of the 11th rib on each side provides good access. For bilateral adrenalectomy the child may be turned from one side to the other during operation. Even in teenagers both the posterior and anterior approaches may not provide adequate access.

CONCLUSION

It must be emphasized again that no controlled trials have been reported, comparing adrenalectomy with other methods of treatment for any type of Cushing's syndrome. It is therefore difficult to reach firm conclusions. However, it is clear that different forms of therapy are appropriate in different circumstances and that these should be regarded as complementary. For example, adrenalectomy is effective when procedures designed to remove or destroy the pituitary fail. Conversely, hypophysectomy or pituitary irradiation is indicated when Nelson's syndrome develops or on the rare occasions when Cushing's syndrome recurs after bilateral adrenalectomy.

Adrenalectomy under cortisone cover was the first reliably effective form of treatment of Cushing's syndrome. It remains a valuable therapeutic measure in many circumstances.

References

1 ANONYMOUS. New drug treatment for Cushing's disease. *Lancet*, **Dec. 6**, 1135–1136 (1975)

2 BECK, R. N., MONTGOMERY, D. A. D. and WELBOURN, R. B. Cushing's syndrome: six cases treated surgically. *Lancet*, **1**, 1140–1144 (1954)

3 BERGAN, A., HAUGEN, H. N. and FLATMARK, A. Recurrent and persistent Cushing's syndrome after assumed total bilateral adrenalectomy. *Acta Chirurgica Scandinavica*, **144**, 13–15 (1978)

4 BIGOS, S. T., SOMMA, M., RASIO, E., EASTMAN, R. C., LANTHIER, A., and JOHNSTON, H. H. Cushing's disease: management by transphenoidal pituitary microsurgery. *Journal of Clinical Endocrinology and Metabolism*, **50**, 348–354 (1980)

5 BIGOS, S. T., ROBERT, F., PELLETIER, G. and HARDY, J. Cure of Cushing's disease by transsphenoidal removal of a microadenoma from a pituitary gland despite a radiographically normal sella turcica. *Journal of Clinical Endocrinology and Metabolism*, **45**, 1251–1260 (1977)

6 BLICHERT-TOFT, M., BAGERSKOV, A., LOCKWOOD, K. and HASNER, E. Cushing's syndrome: surgical management and postoperative complications. *Surgery, Gynecology and Obstetrics*, **131**, 261–265 (1972)

7 BRICAIRE, H. and LUTON, J. P. Douze ans de traitement médical de la maladie de Cushing. Usage prolongé de l'*o'p*-DDD dans quarante-six cas. *Nouvelle Press Médicale*, **6**, 325–329 (1976)

8 BURKE, C. W., DOYLE, F. H., JOPLIN, G. F., ARNOT, R. N., MACERLEAN, D. P. and FRASER, R. T. Cushing's disease: treatment by pituitary implantation of radioactive gold or yttrium seeds. *Quarterly Journal of Medicine*, **168**, 693–714 (1973)

9 CASSAR, J., DOYLE, F. H., MASHITER, K. and JOPLIN, G. F. Treatment of Cushing's disease in juveniles with interstitial pituitary irradiation. *Clinical Endocrinology*, **11**, 313–321 (1979)

10 CHALMERS, R. A., MASHITER, K. and JOPLIN, G. F. Residual adrenocortical function after bilateral 'total' adrenalectomy for Cushing's disease. *Lancet*, **2**, 1196–1199 (1981)

11 CHILD, D. F., BURKE, C. W., BURLEY, D. M., REES, L. H. and FRASER, T. R. Drug control of Cushing's syndrome. *Acta Endocrinologica*, **82**, 330–341 (1976)

13 COHEN, K. L., NOTH, R. H. and PECHINSKI, T. Incidence of pituitary tumors following adrenalectomy. A long-term follow-up study of patients treated for Cushing's disease. *Archives of Internal Medicine*, **138**, 575–579 (1978)

14 COPE, O. and RAKER, J. Cushing's disease: surgical experience in care of 46 cases. *New England Journal of Medicine*, **253**, 165–172 (1955)

15 COSTELLO, R. T. Subclinical adenoma of the pituitary gland. *American Journal of Pathology*, **12**, 205–208 (1936)

16 CUSHING, H. The basophil adenomas of the pituitary body and their clinical manifestations (pituitary basophilism). *Bulletin of the Johns Hopkins Hospital*, **50**, 137–195 (1932)

16a DAVIES, C. J., JOPLIN, G. F. and WELBOURN, R. B. Surgical management of the ectopic ACTH syndrome. *Annals of Surgery*, **196**, 246–258 (1982)

17 DELANEY, J. P., SOLOMKIN, J. S., JACOBSON, M. E. and DOE, R. P. Surgical management of Cushing's syndrome. *Surgery*, **84**, 465–470 (1978)

18 D'ERCOLE, A. J., MORRIS, A. M., UNDERWOOD, L. E. and VAN WYK, J. J. Treatment of Cushing's disease in childhood with cyproheptadine (clinical note). *Journal of Pediatrics*, **90**, 834–835 (1977)

19 DRAYER, B. P., ROSENBAUM, A. E., KENNERDELL, J. S., ROBINSON, A. G., BANK, W. O. and DEEB, Z. L. Computed tomographic diagnosis of suprasellar masses by intrathecal enhancement. *Radiology*, **123**, 339–344 (1977)

20 EDELSTYN, G. A., GLEADHILL, C. A., LYONS, A. R., RODGERS, H. W., TAYLOR, A. R. and WELBOURN, R. B. Hypophysectomy combined with intrasellar irradiation with yttrium-90. *Lancet*, **1**, 462–463 (1958)

21 EDIS, A. J., AYALA, L. A. and EGDAHL, R. H. (Comps.) *Manual of Endocrine Surgery*, p. 152. New York, Springer-Verlag (1975)

22 FAHLBUSCH, R. Surgical treatment of pituitary adenomas. In *The Pituitary*, edited by C. Beardwell and G. L. Robinson. *Clinical Endocrinology*, **1**, pp. 76–105. London, Butterworths (1981)

23 FRANCIS, D., JOHNSTON, I. D. A., KENNEDY, D. L. and WELBOURN, R. B. The diagnosis and management of 29 patients with Cushing's syndrome and/or virilism due to adrenocortical adenoma. (Presented at the Meeting of the Association of Surgeons of Great Britain and Ireland, 1982)

24 FRIESEN, S. R. (Ed.) *Surgical Endocrinology: Clinical Syndromes*, pp. 332–335. Philadelphia, J. B. Lippincott (1978)

25 GALLAND, R. B., SAUNDERS, J. H., MOSLEY, J. G. and DARRELL, J. H. Prevention of wound infection in abdominal operations by preoperative antibiotics or povidone-iodine: a controlled trial. *Lancet*, **2**, 1043–1045 (1977)

26 GRAHAM, L. S. Celiac accessory adrenal glands. *Cancer*, **6**, 149–152 (1953)

27 GRANT, D. B. and ATHERDEN, S. M. Cushing's disease presenting with growth failure: clinical remission during cyproheptadine therapy. *Archives of Disease in Childhood*, **54**, 466–468 (1979)

28 GUIOT, G. Transsphenoidal approach in surgical treatment of pituitary adenomas: general principles and indications in non-functioning adenomas. In *Diagnosis and Treatment of Pituitary Tumors*, edited by R. O. Kohler and G. T. Ross, pp. 159–178. Amsterdam, Excerpta Medica (1973)

29 HALL, R., ANDERSON, J., SMART, G. A. and BESSER, M. (Eds.) *Fundamentals of Clinical Endocrinology*, 3rd Edn. p. 233. Tunbridge Wells, Pitman Medical (1980)

30 HALL, K. and McALLISTER, V. L. Metrizamide cisternography in pituitary and juxta-pituitary lesions. *Radiology*, **134**, 101–108 (1980)

31 HARDY, J. Transsphenoidal microsurgery of the normal and pathological pituitary. *Clinical Neurosurgery*, **16**, 185–216 (1969)

32 HARDY, J. D. Surgical management of Cushing's syndrome with emphasis on adrenal autotransplantation. *Annals of Surgery*, **188**, 290–307 (1978)

33 HARDY, J. Ten years after the recognition of pituitary microadenomas. In *Pituitary Microadenomas*, edited by G. Faglia, M. Giovanelli and R. M. MacLeod, pp. 7–14. London, Academic Press (1980)

34 HOPWOOD, N. J. and KENNY, F. M. Incidence of Nelson's syndrome after adrenalectomy for Cushing's disease in children. *American Journal of Diseases of Children*, **131**, 1353–1356 (1977)

35 HUNT, T. K., EHRLICH, H. P., GARCIA, J. A. and DUNPHY, J. E. Effect of vitamin A on reversing the inhibitory effect of cortisone on healing of open wounds in animals and man. *Annals of Surgery*, **170**, 633–641 (1969)

36 HUNT, T. K. and TYRRELL, B. J. Cushing's syndrome: hypercortisolism. In *Surgical Endocrinology: Clinical Syndromes*, edited by S. R. Friesen, pp. 330–344. Philadelphia, J. B. Lippincott (1978)

37 HUTTER, A. M., Jr and KAYHOE, D. E. Adrenal cortical carcinoma: clinical features of 138 patients and results of treatment with $o'p$–DDD. *American Journal of Medicine*, **41**, 572–580 (1966)

38 HUTTER, A. M., Jr and KAYHOE, D. E. Adrenal cortical carcinoma: results of treatment with $o'p$–DDD in 138 patients. *American Journal of Medicine*, **41**, 581–592 (1966)

39 IMURA, H. Ectopic hormone syndromes. *Clinics in Endocrinology and Metabolism*, **9**, 235–260 (1980)
40 JAMES, A. J. The hypophysis (Semon Lecture, 1965). *Journal of Laryngology and Otology*, **81**, 1283–1307 (1967)
41 JAVADPOUR, N., WOLTERING, E. A. and BRENNAN, M. F. Adrenal neoplasms. *Current Problems in Surgery*, **17**, 1–52 (1980)
42 JEFFCOATE, W. J., REES, L. H., TOMLIN, S., JONES, A. E., EDWARDS, C. R. W. and BESSER, G. M. Metyrapone in long-term management of Cushing's disease. *British Medical Journal*, **2**, 215–217 (1977)
43 JEFFERSON, G. Operations on skull and brain. In *Modern Operative Surgery*, 3rd Edn., edited by G. Grey-Turner, pp. 1226–1228. London, Cassell and Co. (1943)
44 JENNINGS, A. S., LIDDLE, G. W. and ORTH, D. N. Results of treating childhood Cushing's disease with pituitary irradiation. *New England Journal of Medicine*, **297**, 957–962 (1977)
45 JOPLIN, G. F., WHITE, M. C. and MASHITER, K. Treatment of Cushing's disease by interstitial irradiation of the pituitary with yttrium-90 (personal communication)
46 KELLY, W. F., BARNES, A. J., CASSAR, J., WHITE, M., MASHITER, K. and COIZOU, S. Cushing's syndrome due to adrenocortical carcinoma – a comprehensive clinical and biochemical study of patients treated by surgery and chemotherapy. *Acta Endocrinologica*, **91**, 303–318 (1979)
47 KJELLBERG, R. N. and KLIMAN, B. A system for therapy of pituitary tumors. In *Diagnosis and Treatment of Pituitary Tumours*, edited by P. O. Kohler and G. T. Ross, pp. 234–252. Amsterdam, Excerpta Medica (1973)
48 KJELLBERG, R. N. and KLIMAN, B. Bragg peak proton treatment for pituitary-related conditions. *Proceedings of the Royal Society of Medicine*, **67**, 32–33 (1974)
49 KOMANICKY, P., SPARK, R. F. and MELBY, J. C. Treatment of Cushing's syndrome with trilostane (WIN 24,540), an inhibitor of adrenal steroid biosynthesis. *Journal of Clinical Endocrinology and Metabolism*, **47**, 1042–1051 (1978)
50 KRIEGER, D. T., AMOROSA, L. and LINICK, F. Cyproheptadine induced remission of Cushing's disease. *New England Journal of Medicine*, **293**, 893–896 (1975)
51 KUWAYAMA, A., KAGEYAMA, N., NAKANE, T., TAKANOHASHI, M., OKADA, C. and KANIE, N. Treatment of Cushing's disease by transsphenoidal microsurgery. *Neurologica Medico-Chirurgica (Tokyo)*, **18**, 279–285 (1978)
52 LAMBERTS, S. W. J. and BIRKENHAGER, J. C. Effect of bromocriptine in pituitary-dependent Cushing's syndrome. *Journal of Endocrinology*, **70**, 315–316 (1976)
53 LAMBERTS, S. W. J., DeJONG, F. H. and BIRKENHAGER, J. C. Evaluation of a therapeutic regimen in Cushing's disease: the predictability of the result of unilateral adrenalectomy followed by external pituitary irradiation. *Acta Endocrinologica*, **86**, 146–155 (1977)
54 LAMBERTS, S. W. J., STEFANCO, S. Z., DeLANGE, S. A. *et al.* Failure of clinical remission after transsphenoidal removal of a microadenoma in a patient with Cushing's disease: multiple hyperplastic and adenomatous cell nests in surrounding pituitary tissue. *Journal of Clinical Endocrinology and Metabolism*, **50**, 793–795 (1980)
55 LAMBERTS, S. W. J., DeLANGE, S. A., SINGH, R., FERMIN, H., KLIJN, J. G. M. and DeJONG, F. H. A comparison between the results of transsphenoidal operation and those of

unilateral adrenalectomy followed by external pituitary irradiation. *Netherlands Journal of Medicine*, **23,** 193–199 (1980)

56 LANDAU, B., LEIBA, S., KAUFMAN, H., SERVADIO, C. and WAINRACH, B. Unilateral adrenalectomy and pituitary irradiation in the treatment of ACTH-dependent Cushing's disease in children and adolescents. *Clinical Endocrinology (Oxford)*, **9,** 221–226 (1978)

57 LAWRENCE, J. H., TOBIAS, C. A., LINFOOT, J. A., BORN, J. L. and CHONG, C. Y. Heavy-particle therapy in acromegaly and Cushing's disease. *Journal of the American Medical Assocation*, **235,** 2307–2310 (1976)

58 LIDDLE, G. W., ISLAND, D. P. and MEADOR, C. K. Normal and abnormal regulation of corticotropin secretion in man. *Recent Progress in Hormone Research*, **18,** 125–166 (1962)

59 McARTHUR, R. G., HAYLES, A. B. and SALASSA, R. M. Childhood Cushing's disease: results of bilateral adrenalectomy. *Journal of Pediatrics*, **59,** 159–165 (1979)

60 MacFARLANE, D. A. Cancer of the adrenal cortex: the natural history, prognosis and treatment in a study of fifty-five cases. *Annals of the Royal College of Surgeons of England*, **23,** 155–186 (1958)

61 MONTGOMERY, D. A. D. and WELBOURN, R. B. (Comps.) *Medical and Surgical Endocrinology*, 1st Edn., pp. 108–110. London, Edward Arnold (1975)

62 MONTGOMERY, D. A. D. and WELBOURN, R. B. *Medical and Surgical Endocrinology*, 1st Edn., pp. 64–65. London, Edward Arnold (1975)

63 MONTGOMERY, D. A. D. and WELBOURN, R. B. Cushing's syndrome: 20 years after adrenalectomy. *British Journal of Surgery*, **65,** 221–223 (1978)

64 MOORE, T. J., DLUHY, R. G., WILLIAMS, G. H. and CAIN, J. P. Nelson's syndrome: frequency, prognosis, and effect of prior pituitary irradiation. *Annals of Internal Medicine*, **85,** 731–734 (1976)

65 NAIDICH, T. P., PINTO, R. S., KUSHNER, M. J. *et al.* Evaluation of sellar and parasellar masses by computed tomography. *Radiology*, **120,** 91–99 (1976)

66 NELSON, D., MEAKIN, J. W., DEALY, J. B., MATSON, D. D., KENDALL, E. and THORN, G. W. ACTH-producing tumor of the pituitary gland. *New England Journal of Medicine*, **259,** 161–164 (1958)

67 NEVILLE, A. M. and SYMINGTON, T. The pathology of the adrenal gland in Cushing's syndrome. *Journal of Pathology and Bacteriology*, **93,** 19–35 (1967)

68 ORTH, D. N. Metyrapone is useful only as an adjunctive therapy in Cushing's disease. *Annals of Internal Medicine*, **89,** 128–130 (1978)

69 ORTH, D. N. and LIDDLE, G. W. Results of treatment in 108 patients with Cushing's syndrome. *New England Journal of Medicine*, **285,** 243–247 (1971)

70 PATTISON, A. R. D. and SWAN, W. G. A. Surgical treatment of pituitary basophilism. *Lancet*, **1,** 1265–1269 (1938)

71 PLOTZ, C. M., KNOWLTON, A. I. and RAGAN, C. The natural history of Cushing's syndrome. *American Journal of Medicine*, **13,** 597–614 (1952)

72 POLK, H. C. and LOPEZ-MAYOR, J. F. Postoperative wound infection: a prospective study of determinant factors and prevention. *Surgery*, **46,** 97–103 (1969)

73 PRIESTLEY, J. T., SPRAGUE, R. G., WALTERS, W. *et al.* Subtotal adrenalectomy for Cushing's syndrome. A preliminary report of 29 cases. *Annals of Surgery*, **134,** 464–475 (1951)

74 PRINZ, R. A., BROOKS, M. H., LAWRENCE, A. M. and PALOYAN, E. Cushing's disease: the role of adrenalectomy and autotransplantation. *Surgical Clinics of North America*, **59**, 159–165 (1979)

75 RAHN, T., THOREN, M., HALL, K. and BACKLUND, E. O. Stereotactic radiosurgery in Cushing's syndrome: acute radiation effects. *Surgical Neurology*, **14**, 85–92 (1980)

76 ROBERTSON, W. D. and NEWTON, T. H. Radiologic assessment of pituitary microadenomas. *American Journal of Roentgenology*, **131**, 489–492 (1978)

77 SALASSA, R. M., KEARNS, T. P., KERNOHAN, J. W., SPRAGUE, R. G. and McCARTY, C. S. Pituitary tumors in patients with Cushing's syndrome. *Journal of Clinical Endocrinology and Metabolism*, **19**, 1523–1539 (1959)

78 SALASSA, R. M., LAWS, E. R., CARPENTER, P. C. and NORTHCUTT, R. C. Transsphenoidal removal of pituitary microadenoma in Cushing's disease. *Mayo Clinic Proceedings*, **53**, 24–28 (1978)

79 SCHNALL, A. M., KOVACS, K., BRODKEY, J. S. and PEARSON, O. H. Pituitary Cushing's disease without adenoma. *Acta Endocrinologica*, **94**, 297–303 (1980)

80 SCHTEINGART, D. E. and TSAO, H. S. Coexistence of pituitary adrenocorticotropin-dependent Cushing's syndrome with a solitary adrenal adenoma. *Journal of Clinical Endocrinology and Metabolism*, **50**, 961–966 (1980)

81 SCOTT, W. H., Jr, LIDDLE, G. W., MULHERIN, J. L., McKENNA, J. J., STROUP, S. L. and RHAMY, R. K. Surgical experience with Cushing's disease. *Annals of Surgery*, **185**, 524–534 (1977)

82 SHAFFI, O. M. and WRIGHTSON, P. Dural invasion by pituitary tumours. *New Zealand Medical Journal*, **81**, 386–390 (1975)

83 SJÖBERG, H. E., BLOMBÄCK, M. and GRANBERG, P. O. Thromboembolic complications, heparin treatment and increase in coagulation factors in Cushing's syndrome. *Acta Medica Scandinavica*, **199**, 95–98 (1976)

84 SOSMAN, M. C. Cushing's disease – pituitary basophilism (Caldwell Lecture, 1947). *American Journal of Roentgenology*, **62**, 1–32 (1949)

85 SUTTON, D. The radiological diagnosis of adrenal tumours. *British Journal of Radiology*, **48**, 237–258 (1975)

86 SYVERTSEN, A., HAUGHTON, V. M., WILLIAMS, A. L. and CUSICK, J. F. The computed tomographic appearance of the normal pituitary gland and pituitary microadenomas. *Radiology*, **133**, 385–391 (1979)

87 TAYLOR, H. C., VELASCO, M. E. and BRODKEY, J. S. Remission of pituitary-dependent Cushing's disease after removal of non-neoplastic pituitary gland. *Archives of Internal Medicine*, **140**, 1366–1368 (1980)

88 THRALL, J. H., FREITAS, J. E. and BEIERWALTERS, W. H. Adrenal scintigraphy. *Seminars in Nuclear Medicine*, **8**, 23–41 (1978)

89 TYRRELL, J. B., BROOKS, R. M., FITZGERALD, P. A., COFOID, P. B., FORSHAM, P. H. and WILSON, C. B. Cushing's disease: selective trans-sphenoidal resection of pituitary microadenomas. *New England Journal of Medicine*, **298**, 753–758 (1978)

90 WELBOURN, R. B. Operations on the adrenal glands. In *Operative Surgery*, edited by C. Rob, R. Smith and H. A. F. Dudley, pp. 403–419. London, Butterworths (1977)

91 WELBOURN, R. B. Some aspects of adrenal surgery. *British Journal of Surgery*, **67**, 723–727 (1980)
92 WELBOURN, R. B., MONTGOMERY, D. A. D. and KENNEDY, T. L. The natural history of treated Cushing's syndrome. *British Journal of Surgery*, **58**, 1–16 (1971)
93 WILSON, C. B., TYRELL, J. B. and FITZGERALD, P. Cushing's disease revisited. *American Journal of Surgery*, **138**, 77–79 (1979)
94 ZACHMANN, N., GITZELMANN, R. P., ZAGALAK, M. and PRADER, A. Effect of aminoglutethimide in urinary cortisol and cortisone metabolites in adolescents with Cushing's syndrome. *Clinical Endocrinology*, **7**, 63–71 (1977)

6
Localization of gastroentero-pancreatic (GEP) tumors

A. I. Vinik, J. Glowniak, B. Glaser, B. Shapiro,
A. Funakoshi, K. Cho, N. W. Thompson
and S. S. Fajans

INTRODUCTION

Tumors of the gastroentero-pancreatic (GEP) axis occur predominantly in the pancreas, and rarely in the duodenum and stomach. Occasionally tumors secreting GEP hormones may even be found in ectopic sites, i.e. in the kidney, ovary, thyroid (G cell), lung (bronchial carcinoid) or adrenal medulla, or they may be apparently confined to a solitary lymph node. When these tumors are small, as they often are, especially if diagnosed early in the course of the disease, localization by angiography[10, 15, 43, 44] may fail. Abdominal ultrasound and computed axial tomography (CAT) have proved of value only in large tumors since the density of the tumors is similar to that of the surrounding normal tissue.

Accurate preoperative localization of islet cell tumors may occasionally be necessary for the appropriate surgical approach and a successful outcome. Most insulinomas are small, ranging from 0.5 to 3.0 cm[10] in diameter, and may not be readily palpable at operation because their consistency is similar to that of normal pancreatic tissue[1,31,36,47]. In these instances it has been the usual practice to perform blind distal pancreatectomy, i.e. without localizing or removing tumor situated in the head of the pancreas. Blind pancreatic resection and unnecessary dissection of the pancreas increase operative morbidity, and may result in incomplete cure or even the need for repeat exploration or total pancreatectomy, with increased morbidity and mortality[1,7,48].

Percutaneous transhepatic portal venous sampling (THVS) for the detection of hormone production has proved valuable for localizing many endocrine tumors. This technique has been applied to gut/pancreatic tumors, but several important problems have arisen and require detailed discussion.

While insulinomas constitute the greatest proportion, tumors secreting gastrin[54], glucagon[17], somatostatin[11, 12, 25, 26, 29, 38, 50], human pancreatic polypeptide (hPP)[28], vasoactive intestinal polypeptide (VIP)[3,46] and thyrocalcitonin[39], and mixed endocrine tumors (MEN)[27], diffuse islet cell adenomatosis[5], hyperplasia and nesidioblastosis[13] have all been described as producing clinical syndromes.

The various hormone-secreting cells are not evenly distributed in islet tissue. Large numbers of cells producing one hormone will be found in some areas and not in others[8, 33, 40]. The peak concentrations of different pancreatic hormones will vary a great deal in venous samples depending on the location of the cells of origin, and thorough knowledge of the variability of the venous drainage of the pancreas and proximal gut is required to allow interpretation of measurements made in the portal venous system in man. For this reason, before embarking on a description of the technique for THVS for the localization of GEP tumors, we will review briefly some of our experience relating to vagaries in venous drainage which could cause confusion.

VENOUS ANATOMY

The portal vein is almost always constant in its topography, and is formed by the confluence of the superior mesenteric and splenic veins posterior to the neck of the pancreas and sweeping towards the porta hepatis. The superior mesenteric vein is formed by the confluence of a right and left trunk. The right trunk usually receives tributaries from the jejunum, ileum and ascending colon, and the left predominantly from the jejunum. The inferior mesenteric vein, which drains the colon, joins the splenic vein within 3 cm of the portal vein in 50% of patients, but may enter more distally. In one third of cases, the inferior mesenteric vein may join the superior mesenteric vein and merge with the splenic vein at the confluence. The left gastric vein, which receives tributaries from the stomach, can end in the last 2 cm of the splenic vein (30%), in the first 1 cm of the portal vein (40%) or, rarely, at the splenoportal confluence[42].

It is important to recognize that the right gastroepiploic vein, which receives tributaries from the stomach, pylorus and first part of the duodenum, constitutes the venous drainage of the normal area of gastrin secretion, namely the antrum and first portion of the duodenum. After following the greater curve of the stomach it enters the anterolateral aspect of the superior mesenteric vein or the proximal portal vein just beyond the confluence. It is invariably joined by the anterior superior pancreatico-duodenal vein, which receives blood from the head of the pancreas, and one or two colic veins. The vessels unite to form the gastrocolic trunk, and hormone levels at this site may thus reflect an origin from either the antrum, duodenum or head of the pancreas. The right gastric vein receives blood from the pylorus, is usually very small, and enters the portal or posterior superior pancreatico-duodenal vein.

The lower anterior part of the head and adjacent duodenum are drained by the anterior inferior pancreatico-duodenal vein, which may enter a jejunal vein or drain directly into the superior mesenteric vein. The posterior portion of the head of the pancreas is drained by two main veins, the posterior superior pancreatico-duodenal vein, which enters the portal vein 1.5–3.0 cm from the confluence, and the posterior inferior pancreatico-duodenal vein, which also receives blood from the duodenum and joins the first jejunal vein or empties directly into the superior mesenteric. Thus, tumors of the head of the pancreas may drain into the proximal portion of the portal vein, the gastrocolic trunk, or the superior mesenteric via the inferior arcade. Tumors of the uncinate process appear to drain via the inferior arcade into the proximal portion of the superior mesenteric vein.

The venous drainage of the neck and body of the pancreas is by a number of small tributaries which enter the splenic vein directly. There are usually about six of these, and tumors in this area are generally detected by raised hormone levels within the splenic veins adjacent to the tumor. However, a transverse inferior pancreatic vein occurs in about 70% of cases; this receives blood from the inferior portion of the body of the pancreas and has a variable termination: the superior mesenteric, inferior mesenteric or splenic vein, and rarely the gastrocolic trunk.

This variable termination of veins must be taken into account when evaluating hormone levels in the venous drainage, since a tumor of the body or tail may cause high hormonal levels in the superior mesenteric, splenic or inferior mesenteric vein. An example of this will be given later. Furthermore, tumors in the distal tail, which normally drain into the splenic vein, may also drain into the gastroepiploic vein, which terminates in the superior mesenteric or portal vein, and lead to erroneous localization.

Lastly, although these major trunks are fairly constant, the tributaries which drain tumors may be inconstant and direct drainage may occur into areas quite different from the expected venous drainage. These complexities emphasize the need for detailed venographic delineation of the portal venous anatomy in every patient. It should also be made clear at the onset that THVS is difficult, time-consuming and expensive and should not be embarked upon without sound biochemical and clinical evidence that oversecretion of a GEP hormone is causing the patient's symptom complex.

PERCUTANEOUS TRANSHEPATIC VENOUS SAMPLING

The feasibility of sampling blood in the venous effluent at the site of the tumor has been demonstrated by several groups by the successful localization of insulinomas[6, 18, 23, 32, 35, 37, 49]. Tumors secreting gastrin[5, 22], glucagon[20] and somatostatin[13], and mixed endocrine tumors[54] have been localized by hormone concentrations in the portal effluent. Aside from tumors, nesidioblastosis hyperplasia, G cell hyperplasia and multiple adenomatosis may be diagnosed by this technique[13, 54]. The method of catheterization will be described briefly.

Catheterization procedure

Before transhepatic portal vein catheterization, the venous phase of the celiac and superior mesenteric angiograms are reviewed to locate and establish the patency of the portal vein. Each subject receives heavy sedation and analgesia with meperidine (Demerol), diazepam (Valium) and chlorpromazine. Under local anesthesia, a 19-gauge Teflon catheter is introduced in the midaxillary line and, with the patient holding his breath, the catheter is advanced in the horizontal plane towards the hepatic hilum. The position of the tip of the catheter in a portal venous radicle is confirmed by the injection of radio-opaque dye. The catheter is then advanced into the portal, splenic and superior mesenteric veins over a curved guide wire. Portograms are obtained with injection of contrast medium into the distal splenic and superior mesenteric veins respectively. Using these portograms to identify sites along the venous drainage (*Figure 6.1*), blood samples are obtained along the superior mesenteric, splenic and portal veins at intervals of 1.5–2.0 cm. Additional samples are obtained from the dorsal pancreatic, gastrocolic, coronary and superior pancreatico-duodenal veins whenever possible. A catheter is also placed in the celiac artery via a percutaneous transfemoral approach, and arterial blood samples are collected simultaneously with many of the venous samples. Another catheter is placed in the hepatic vein via the transfemoral approach and samples are taken simultaneously with each third or fourth venous sample. After the procedure is completed, the transhepatic venous catheter is withdrawn to near the hepatic capsule and the catheter track is filled with one or two pieces of Gelfoam to prevent hemorrhage or leakage of bile.

Blood sampling, storage and assay

Each blood sample (7–8 ml) is immediately divided into two and placed into heparin-coated tubes, one containing aprotinin (Trasylol, Bayer) 1000 KIU/ml whole blood. Both tubes are gently mixed and immediately placed on ice. Plasma is separated in a refrigerated centrifuge within 60 min. All samples are frozen at −20 °C for later assay. Care must be taken to avoid thawing and refreezing of samples before glucagon and somatostatin determinations.

Hormone assays

Insulin[16], gastrin[51], glucagon[41], pancreatic polypeptide[9], somatostatin[53] and motilin are measured by radioimmunoassays.

THE 'NORMAL' HORMONE DISTRIBUTION

The importance of identifying the normal distribution of GEP hormones has been studied in patients with single hormone-producing tumors by measuring the distribution of other GEP hormones which are secreted simultaneously[13, 14].

Clinical details of these patients are given in *Tables 6.1 and 6.2*. Of the 11 patients with organic hyperinsulinism, 9 had single adenomas, 1 (AS) had a macroadenoma and islet hyperplasia, and 1 (AW) had nesidioblastosis. Of the 7 patients with hypergastrinemia, 1 had a sporadic isolated gastrinoma (PA), 1 had G cell hyperfunction (PG), and 5 had MEN I (*Table 6.2*). One patient with carcinoid syndrome (MB) was also studied.

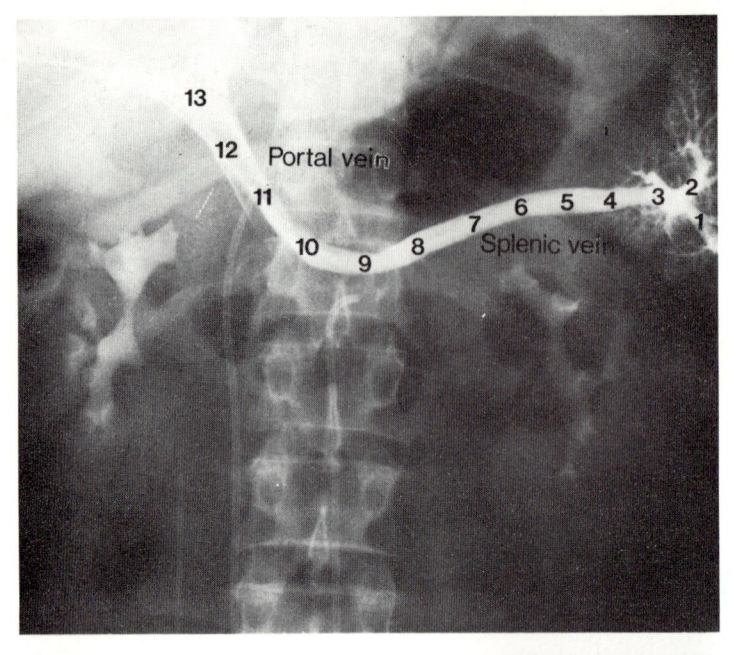

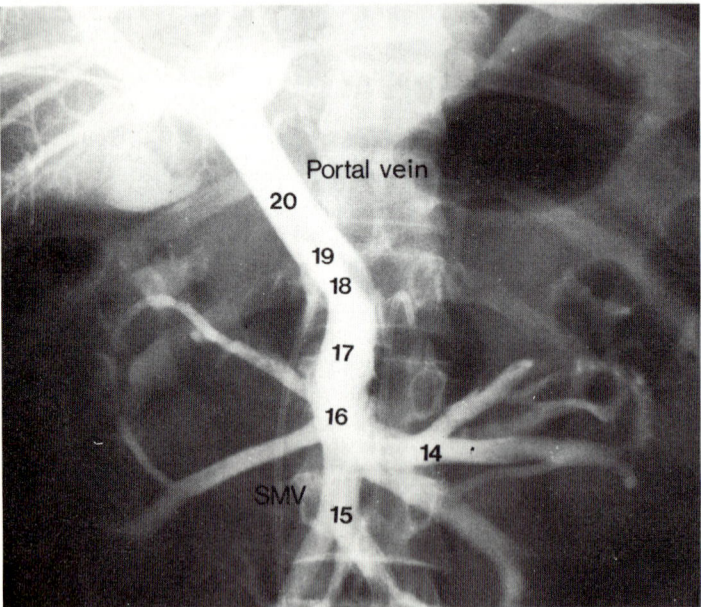

Figure 6.1 Portal venogram obtained during THVS. The catheter is fed through the skin, subcutaneous tissue and liver and then into the portal vein. The numbers indicate sampling sites in the splenic, superior mesenteric (SMV) and portal vein. Further samples for hormone estimations are taken from selected vessels, e.g. gastrocolic trunk, posterior superior pancreatico-duodenal vein and inferior pancreatico-duodenal vein

Table 6.1 Clinical details of 11 patients with organic hyperinsulinism

Patient	Age (years)	Sex	Height (m)	Weight (kg)	Duration of symptoms (years)	Hours to hypoglycemia*	Glucose nadir (mg/dl)	IRI (µU/ml)	I/G†	Fasting proinsulin (%)**	Operative findings††
EV	26	M	1.73	96.3	2.5	16.5	42	22	0.5	62	1
DS	40	F	1.65	80.5	7	15	42	36	0.86	22	1
NH	33	M	1.83	85.0	10	12	41	14	0.34	53	1
RS	21	F	1.60	66.6	1	17.5	39	63	1.66	31	1
AB	60	M	1.78	85.9	2	21	44	30	0.69	44	1
ASa	30	M	1.73	94.9	2	18	41	53	1.29	67	1
AW	20	M	1.60	74.2	19	20.5	40	23	0.58	23	2
AS	58	F	1.68	104.8	1	45	43	17	0.4	31	3
SP	22	F	1.52	46.3	10	66	37	38	1.03	66	1
DT	33	M	1.70	78.3	3	8.5	33	28	0.85	22	1
JS	57	M	1.85	106.6	1	5	37	169	4.56	79	1

Prolonged fast

IRI = Immunoreactive insulin.
* Symptomatic hypoglycemia.
† I/G = insulin (µU/ml)/glucose (mg/dl) (normal level less than 0.3).
** Normal proinsulin: less than 20%.
†† Operative findings: 1 = single adenoma; 2 = nesidioblastosis; 3 = macroadenoma and islet hyperplasia.

Table 6.2 Clinical details of 7 patients with hypergastrinemia

Patient	Age (years)	Sex	Height (m)	Weight (kg)	Duration of symptoms (years)	Basal gastrin (pg/ml)	Maximum response to secretin (pg/ml)	Operative findings
BE*	41	M	1.68	65.2	7	84	189	Pancreatic tumor†; duodenal tumors†
FW*	53	M	1.85	85.9	0.25	150	101	Ductal adenocarcinoma of the pancreas. Islet cell micro- and macroadenomatosis
LS*	49	F	1.47	49.9	7	503	554	Two adenomas in tail of pancreas
PG†	23	M	1.68	57.6	5	336	122	Increased gastric rugal folds with gastritis
JH*	59	F	1.52	60.3	2	1663	1083	Multiple pancreatic adenomas
PA§	49	F	1.57	64.3	6	810	2060	Adenoma in head of the pancreas
PN*	55	F	1.52	79.6	0	520	1650	Two duodenal adenomas

* MEN I.
† G Cell hyperfunction.
§ Isolated sporadic gastrinoma.

The hormone concentrations and portal/systemic arterial gradients of gastrin, glucagon, hPP, somatostatin, VIP and motilin in 5 patients with isolated single insulinomas are given in *Table 6.3*, and those of insulin, glucagon, hPP, somatostatin, VIP and motilin in 5 patients with gastrinoma syndrome in *Table 6.4*.

The highest concentration and a significant gradient of gastrin were found in the gastrocolic trunk, which is compatible with its origin from the gastric antrum. The lack of a significant gradient between the concentrations of gastrin in the pancreatic venous effluent and the systemic circulation supports the observation that there are no gastrin cells in the adult human pancreas and that heptadecapeptide gastrin is not inactivated by passage through the liver[45,52].

A gastrin concentration of more than 300 pg/ml, a gradient of more than 200 pg/ml, and a ratio higher than 3 between the concentration in the gastrocolic trunk and the peripheral concentration suggests a tumor or G cell hyperfunction. A concentration of more than 150 pg/ml and a gradient of more than 50 pg/ml in the portal venous system localizes a tumor. A positive hepatic vein/portal gradient may suggest hepatic metastases and preclude surgical extirpation of tumor.

The mean hPP concentration in the portal vein is 1.3 times greater than that in peripheral veins (*Table 6.3*), indicating hepatic extraction of hPP. The highest level in the portal vein adjacent to the posterior superior pancreatico-duodenal vein is compatible with the localization of PP cells by immunohistochemistry in a separate lobe in the head of the pancreas[8,40]. This particular distribution must be considered when attempting to localize pancreatic polypeptide tumors, since failure to do so

Table 6.3 Hormone concentrations and portal/systemic arterial gradients in patients with single insulinomas*

	Gastrin (pg/ml)	Glucagon (pg/ml)	hPP (pg/ml)	Somatostatin (pg/ml)	VIP (pg/ml)	Motilin (pg/ml)
Splenic vein	82	130	124	108	55	76
V–A	4	47	−1	2	−3	3
Superior mesenteric vein	83	114	96	186	59	93
V–A	−1	25	−6	57	5	21
Portal vein	85	123	164	126	58	81
V–A	5	38	49	2	2	11
Gastrocolic trunk	126	131	144	178	59	84
V–A	46	60	34	55	2	0
Celiac artery	90	94	95	125	58	79
Peripheral vein	76	84	114	126	56	No data
Portal/systemic gradient§	6%	31%†	30%†	2%	3%	14%

* Details of patients EV, DS, NH, RS and AB (*Table 6.1*); for insulin concentrations see *Table 6.5*.
† Significant $P < 0.05$.
§ Portal vein gradient divided by mean portal vein concentration $\times 100\%$.
V–A = Plasma hormone concentration gradient between the vein indicated and the celiac artery (measured simultaneously).

could lead to the mistaken impression of this tumor in the head of the normal pancreas.

The glucagon concentrations are elevated throughout the portal venous system, with positive portal/systemic gradients in the splenic, superior mesenteric and portal veins (*Table 6.3*). The gradient across the liver (about 30%) is compatible with the known hepatic extraction of glucagon[2]. The positive gradients in the superior mesenteric vein and gastrocolic trunk suggest secretion of a 'pancreatic type' glucagon by the stomach and intestine in man[4]. The antiserum used detects the terminal COOH group of glucagon and has negligible cross-reactivity with intestinal glucagon-like immunoreactivity (GLI). It does, however, detect glucagon of varying molecular weight derived from both pancreas and gut.

The highest concentrations of somatostatin are found in the gastrocolic trunk and superior mesenteric veins, suggesting that in man the pancreas does not secrete somatostatin into the portal circulation in the fasting state[13] and that most, if not all, derives from the gut. This corresponds with the tissue content findings in dog and man[34].

VIP concentrations are fairly evenly distributed in the portal venous system (*see Table 6.3*) and are greater in the veins draining the distal gut than in peripheral veins. Since VIP derives predominantly from the colon[30], and probably from neural elements in the gut, these observations are not surprising. Furthermore, since most VIP tumors arise in the pancreas or adrenal medulla, gradients in any of these sites would be significant.

Motilin concentrations are highest in the superior mesenteric vein, indicating the predominantly duodenal origin of this hormone. There appears to be no significant hepatic extraction of motilin. No reports of motilin-secreting tumors have yet been published. The motilin levels (*see Table 6.3*) will be necessary for the interpretation of future studies on the localization of tumors producing these latter two hormones.

The appreciation of gradients across the liver may be important in the diagnosis of metastatic disease since it would be anticipated that the hepatic vein/portal gradient would disappear. In the case of gastrin and motilin, which are not extracted by the liver, higher levels in the hepatic vein than in the portal vein would suggest hepatic metastases.

The insulin concentrations in the gastrinoma patients (*Table 6.4*) suggest an almost even origin from head, body and tail of the pancreas, and a 58% extraction by the liver. A wide range of insulin concentrations is found in the portal venous system and levels can be raised dramatically in obese subjects. Indeed, these can far exceed those found in insulinoma patients if only the absolute levels are considered. A step up at any one site would nonetheless be indicative of a tumor.

An awareness of the effects of catheter placement is necessary when interpreting concentrations of hormones in the portal venous system. Insertion of the catheter tip into small tributaries and occlusion of the vessel lumen can give erroneous values. It is for this reason that we contend that superselective sampling is unnecessary and may even be misleading. Furthermore, multiple sampling at the various sites may be necessary, since variations of 30% or greater may be due to streaming in the portal vein. A catheter with a lateral port rotated through 360 degrees in the same site can give widely differing results. It is not unusual to find

Table 6.4 Hormone concentrations and portal/systemic arterial gradients in patients with gastrinoma syndrome

	Insulin* (μU/ml)	Glucagon* (pg/ml)	hPP* (pg/ml)	Somatostatin† (pg/ml)	Motilin§ (pg/ml)
Splenic vein	156	565	2100	126	253
V–A	112	356	1020	12	−11
Superior mesenteric vein	70	186	1070	136	382
V–A	27	19	92	26	20
Portal vein	113	211	1640	134	366
V–A	66	60	543	23	81
Gastrocolic trunk	89	257	2640	95	258
V–A	48	−19	1640	4	−5
Celiac artery	41	185	1030	117	295
Hepatic vein	86	249	1610	102	347
Portal systemic gradient	58%	28%	33%	17%	22%

* Patients BE, (FW) and PN (*Table 6.2 and 6.6*).
† Patients (BE,FW), JH, PA and PN (*Table 6.2 and 6.6*).
§ Patients JH and PN (*Table 6.2 and 6.6*).
V–A = plasma hormone concentration gradient between the vein indicated and the celiac artery (measured simultaneously).

levels declining during the course of the procedure, possibly due to stress-related factors. Soon after initiation of these studies it became apparent that simultaneous arterial sampling was necessary to avoid differences due to rapid changes of hormone levels being misinterpreted.

THE INSULINOMA SYNDROME

Table 6.5 provides details of tumor site and size and of insulin concentrations in 9 patients with single insulinomas. In 6 of these patients pancreatic angiography, abdominal CAT and ultrasound had failed to localize the tumor. All 9 tumors were localized by the maximum hormone level in the portal venous system. *Figure 6.2* provides two examples of the insulin concentrations measured in tumors of the tail and body of the pancreas.

The maximum insulin concentrations ranged from 64–2600 μU/ml. The mean (±s.e.) insulin concentration of samples drawn simultaneously from the celiac artery was 62 ± 19 μU/ml and that of veins draining the uninvolved pancreas was 58 ± 18 μU/ml. The gradients in tumor site ranged from 39–2547 μU/ml.

Tumors in the head of the pancreas (EV, SP) had high insulin levels in the area of drainage of the superior pancreatico-duodenal vein. Tumors in the uncinate lobe gave high values in the superior mesenteric vein close to the junction with the splenic vein. Tumors in the neck (DS, ASa and RS) drained into the proximal

Table 6.5 Insulin concentrations and gradients in patients with insulin-producing islet cell tumors

Patient	Tumor site	Tumor size (cm)	Maximum insulin level in PVS (µU/ml)	Tumor site — Simultaneous arterial insulin (µU/ml)	Tumor site — P–A gradient (µU/ml)	Level of insulin in PVS (mean ± s.e.) (µU/ml)	Uninvolved area — Simultaneous arterial insulin (mean ± s.e.) (µU/ml)	Uninvolved area — P–A gradient (µU/ml)
EV*	Head	2 × 1	64	25	39	20.1	22	−2
DS*	Neck	0.8 × 1.0	941	43	898	36	44	−8
NH*	Body	1 × 1	690	22	668	37	29	+8†
RS*	Neck	2.5 × 2	240	69	171	55	63	−8
AB*	Tail	2 × 3	292	41	251	30.6	38	−7
ASa*	Neck	1.9 × 1.7	863	80	783	61	69	−8.2
SP	Head	7 × 5	73	21	52	16.5	18	−1.5
DT	Head	2.5 × 2.1	2600	53	2547	65	58	+7†
JS	Head	2.0 × 2.0	1290	204	1086	198	206	−8
Mean (x̄)			784	62	722	58	61	−3.1
s.e.			268	19	262	18	19	2.2

* Abdominal angiogram, CAT and ultrasound negative.
† These patients received glucose during the procedure, which may explain the positive immunoreactive insulin gradient.
PVS = portal venous system; P–A gradient = difference between insulin concentration in PVS and that measured simultaneously in the celiac artery.

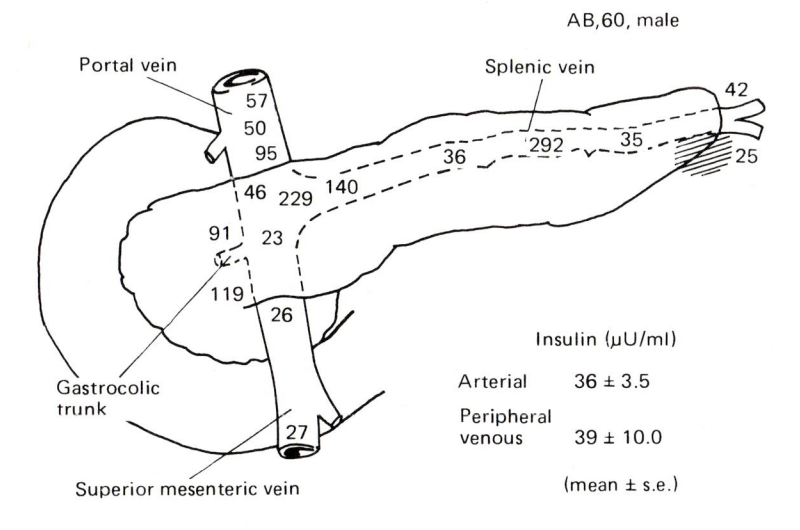

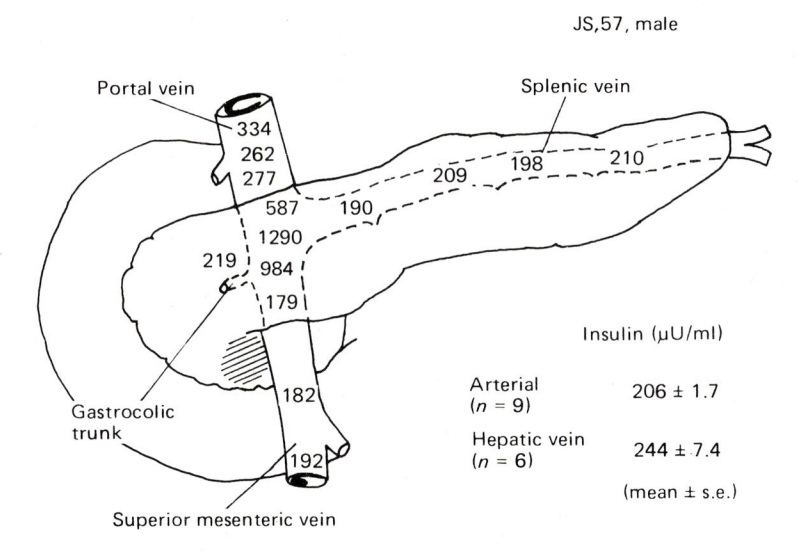

Figure 6.2 Schematic illustration of the sites of tumors and insulin concentrations (mean ± s.e.) in patients with organic hyperinsulinism (*see also Tables 6.1 and 6.5*). The shaded areas indicate tumors, associated with localized insulin elevation. (Modified from Glaser et al.[13])

portal vein or near the confluence of the splenic and portal vein close to the junction of the superior mesenteric and splenic veins. One tumor in the neck of the pancreas was shown to drain directly into the portal vein at surgery (RS). Tumors in the body drained into the splenic vein (NH).

88   Localization of gastroentero-pancreatic (GEP) tumors

AB, 60, male

(a)

AS, 58, female

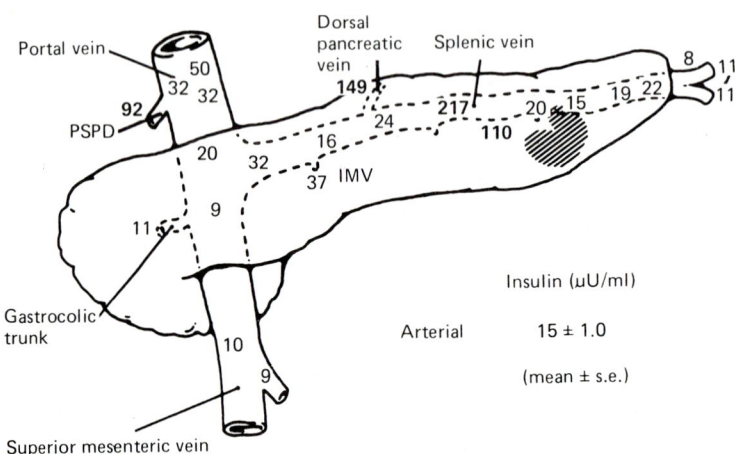

	Insulin (μU/ml)
Arterial	15 ± 1.0
	(mean ± s.e.)

(b)

Figure 6.3 Schematic diagrams of venous drainage patterns which can lead to erroneous localization of a tumor. (*a*) A tumor in the tail of the pancreas draining via the gastroepiploic vein into the superior mesenteric vein (*see also Figure 6.2*). (*b*) A tumor in the tail, with high levels in the dorsal pancreatic and posterior superior pancreatico-duodenal (PSPD) veins, presumably draining via the transverse pancreatic vein(s). IMV = inferior mesenteric vein. (Modified from Glaser *et al.*[13])

Tumors in the tail of the pancreas drain directly into the distal splenic vein (AB), but may give erroneously high values in the gastrocolic trunk because of a venous connection between the tail of the pancreas and the superior mesenteric vein via the gastroepiploic vein (*Figure 6.3*).

ASa, 30, male

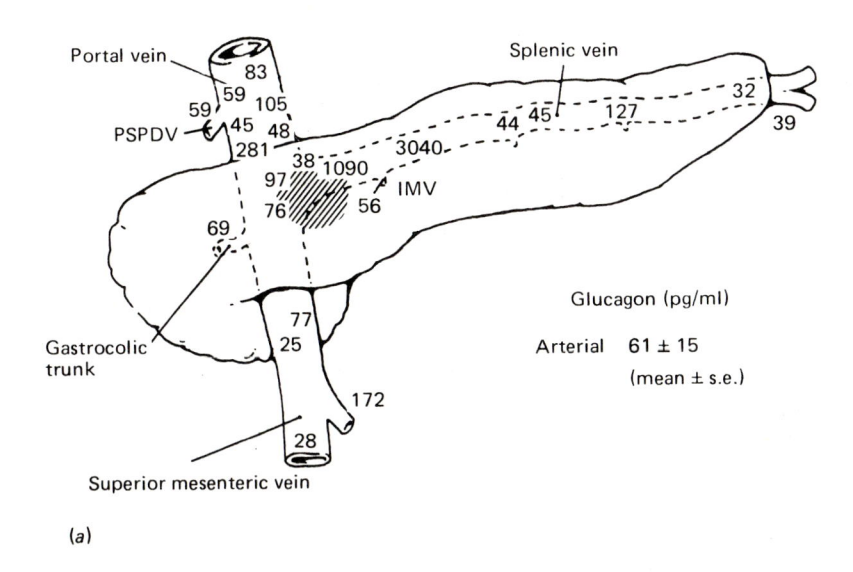

(a)

Glucagon (pg/ml)

Arterial   61 ± 15

(mean ± s.e.)

SP, 22, female

(b)

Somatostatin (pg/ml)

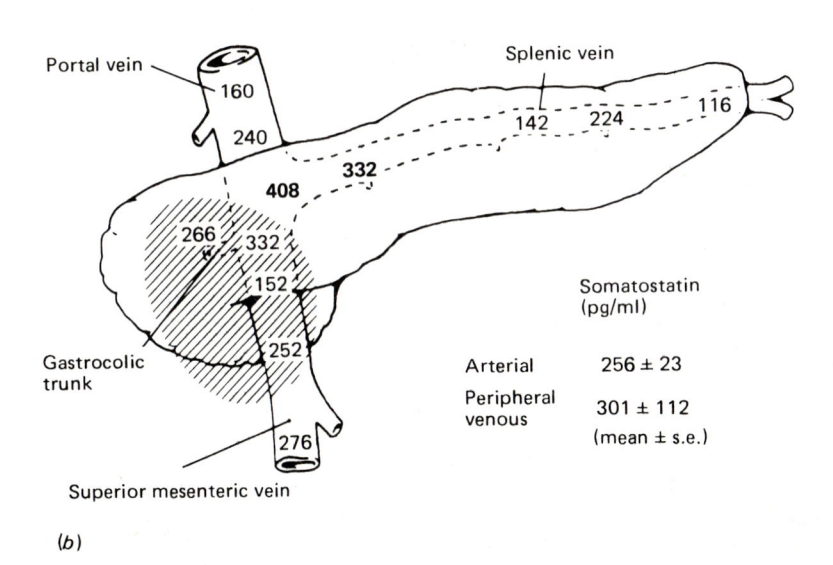

Arterial   256 ± 23

Peripheral venous   301 ± 112

(mean ± s.e.)

Figure 6.4 Illustration of mixed endocrine tumors defined by hormone levels in the portal venous system. (*a*) Glucagon concentrations in a patient with an insulinoma secreting insulin and glucagon. (*b*) Somatostatin concentrations in a patient with an insulinoma secreting insulin and somatostatin. *Next page:* (*c*) Gastrin and (*d*) pancreatic polypeptide (hPP) concentrations in a patient with gastrinomas in the wall of the duodenum and posterior part of head of pancreas and multiple small tumors secreting PP. PSPDV = posterior superior pancreatico-duodenal vein; IMF = inferior mesenteric vein

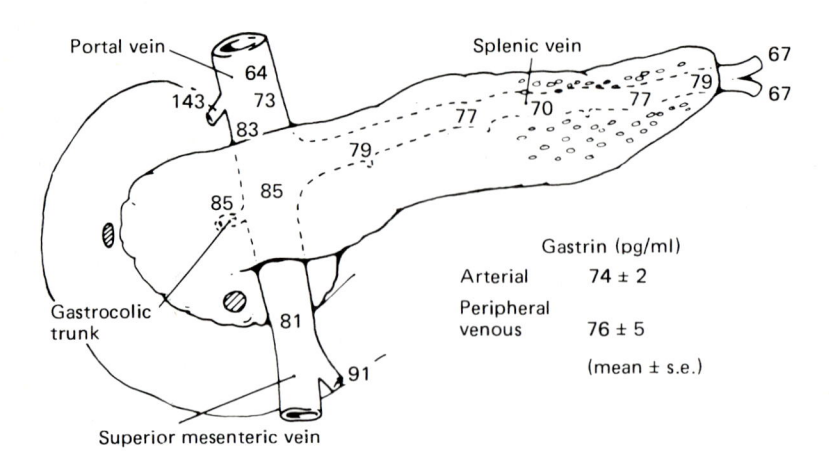

90 *Localization of gastroentero-pancreatic (GEP) tumors*

BE, 41, male

(c)

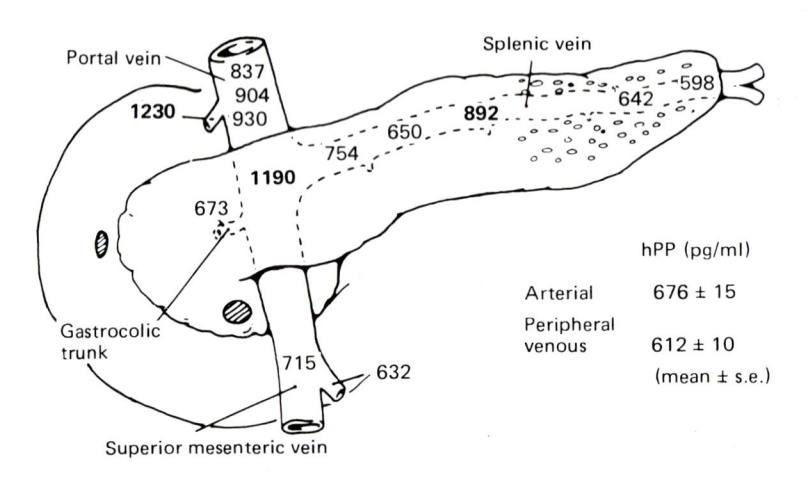

Gastrin (pg/ml)
Arterial   74 ± 2
Peripheral venous   76 ± 5
(mean ± s.e.)

(d)

hPP (pg/ml)
Arterial   676 ± 15
Peripheral venous   612 ± 10
(mean ± s.e.)

Figure 6.4 contd.

DIFFUSE INSULIN HYPERSECRETION

Of the 11 patients with organic hyperinsulinism (*see Table 6.1*) 2 had diffuse elevation of insulin in the portal venous system. In patient AW (*see Figure 6.2*) elevated insulin concentrations were found in the distal and midsplenic veins, the proximal pancreatic vein and the portal vein, suggesting multiple areas of hyperplasia and insulin hypersecretion. A 95% pancreatectomy was performed. The histological diagnosis of nesidioblastosis was made, and confirmed by immunohistochemistry. Patient AS (*see Table 6.1*), who had undergone surgery for removal of a single adenoma of the tail one year before, had an angiographically demonstrable 'recurrence' in the tail. THVS showed elevated insulin concentrations in the midsplenic, inferior mesenteric, posterior superior pancreaticoduodenal and dorsal pancreatic vein (*Figure 6.3b*), which suggests a multicentric process. A distal two-thirds pancreatectomy was carried out at which a single isolated tumor was found, with diffuse islet cell hyperplasia. Since both nesidioblastosis and hyperplasia or multiple adenomatosis give non-homogeneous elevation of insulin levels this cannot be used to differentiate them[13,21]. They can, however, be clearly distinguished from single adenomas, indicating a more radical surgical approach to that in the single adenoma.

MIXED INSULIN/GEP HORMONE TUMORS

Mixed tumors of the GEP axis will usually produce symptoms due to hypersecretion of one of these peptides[54]. Since, in general, insulin has the most dramatic effects, symptoms of hypoglycemia will invariably supersede those of the other hormones except possibly gastrin, as will be seen later. In 2 patients with organic hyperinsulinism, slightly raised portal concentrations of other GEP hormones were found. One (patient ASa) had high glucagon concentrations at the site of the tumor in the neck of the pancreas (*Figure 6.4a*) associated with insulin hypersecretion without the characteristic symptoms of glucagon excess. The other (patient SP) had high somatostatin levels (*Figure 6.4b*) related to a large insulinoma identified by angiography (*see Figure 6.8a*), yet had no symptoms attributable to somatostatin hypersecretion.

THE GASTRIN HYPERSECRETION SYNDROME

Clinical details of these patients have been provided in *Table 6.2*, and the nature of the hypersecretion is given in *Table 6.6*. Of the 7 patients, 5 had MEN I, 1 (patient PA) had an isolated gastrinoma (*Figure 6.5a*), and 1 (PG) had G cell hyperplasia (*Figure 6.5e*). One patient (FW) had hypersecretion of all hormones measured from multiple tumors at different sites in the pancreas (*Figure 6.6*; same patient as in *Figure 6.5d*).

In patient BE the highest concentration of gastrin (143 pg/ml) was found in the posterior superior pancreatico-duodenal vein (*Figure 6.4c*), and two tumors were excised, one in the head of the pancreas and the other in the wall of the duodenum. A distal two-thirds pancreatectomy, performed because of elevated PP concentrations in the splenic vein (*Figure 6.4d*), revealed multiple small pancreatic polypeptide tumors. Ten months postoperatively serum gastrin had risen from 86 to 142 pg/ml, and the response to secretin (rise to 358 pg/ml) was diagnostic of tumor secreting gastrin. Although THVS localized gastrin-secreting tumors, excision of these tumors failed to remove all abnormally secreting tissue.

Table 6.6 Gastrin concentrations and gradients in patients with hypergastrinemic syndromes

Patient	Tumor site	Tumor diameter (cm)	Maximum IG in PVS (pg/ml)	Simultaneous arterial gastrin (pg/ml)	P–A gradient (pg/ml)	Site of maximum IG
BE	Head of pancreas + duodenal wall	0.8, 0.4	143	71	72	Posterior superior pancreatico-duodenal vein
FW	Head of pancreas	0.5	199	125	74	Inferior pancreatico-duodenal vein
LS	Head of pancreas	No data	1107	783	424	Veins draining the head of pancreas
PG	G cell hyperplasia	No data	810	253	557	Gastroepiploic vein
JH	Multiple		1452	1404	48	Pancreatica magna
PA	Head of pancreas	×2.5	5380	2020	3360	Proximal superior mesenteric vein
PN	Two tumors in duodenal wall	0.25, 0.25	945	333	612	Distal gastrocolic trunk
			543	353	190	Proximal superior mesenteric vein

IG = Immunoreactive gastrin; PVS = portal venous system; P = gastrin concentration in PVS; A = simultaneous gastrin concentration in celiac artery.

In patient FW, THVS demonstrated diffuse hypergastrinema, with a raised value in the inferior pancreatico-duodenal vein (*Figure 6.6*). The gastrin hypersecretion was due to gastric outlet obstruction, and the raised value could have come either from the duodenum or from a small gastrinoma associated with a duct adenocarcinoma in the head of the pancreas. Multiple areas of hormone hypersecretion were found at THVS, corresponding with islet cell hyperplasia and macro- and microadenomatosis[54]. The tissue was obtained during a Whipple procedure carried out for the duct carcinoma. Raised gastrin concentrations corresponded with the venous drainage of the tumor, but this proved of no value in the patient's management. The unusual occurrence of an endocrine tumor associated with adenocarcinoma in MEN has been reported[14].

Patients PN, JH and LS are further examples of hypergastrinema in MEN I syndrome. In LS a previous distal two-thirds pancreatectomy identified raised gastrin levels only in relation to the residual tumor in the head of the pancreas. In PN raised values in the distal gastrocolic trunk and the superior mesenteric vein suggested tumor in the wall of the duodenum or head of the pancreas. Two small tumors were excised from the wall of the duodenum. However, 1 month postoperatively serum gastrin concentrations remained elevated, indicating residual hyperfunctioning tumor. Patient JH had diffuse hypergastrinema (*see Figure 6.5c*), indicating tumor besides those identified on angiography (*see Figure 6.8b*) in the body and tail of the pancreas. Multiple tumors were excised which failed to cure the patient.

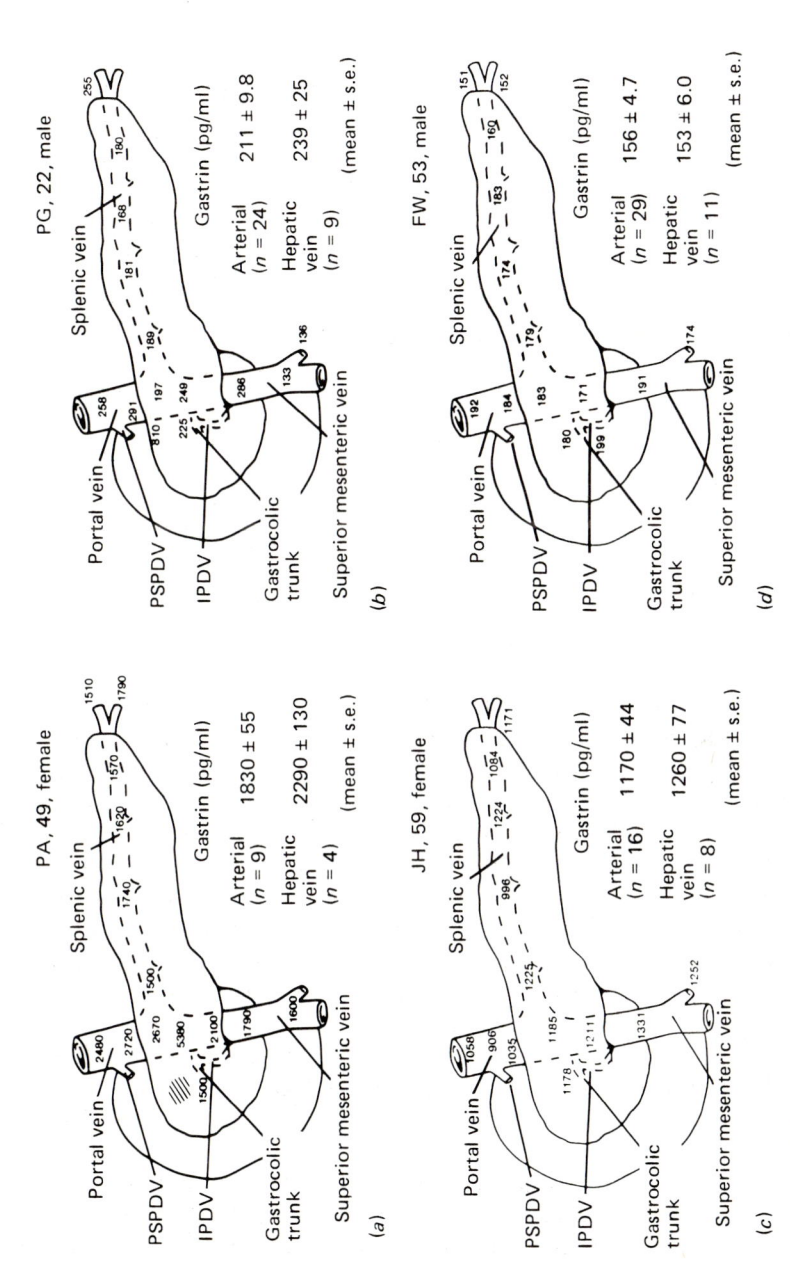

Figure 6.5 Patterns of gastrin concentrations in portal venous system in different conditions. (*a*) A solitary sporadic gastrinoma of the head of the pancreas. (*b*) G cell hyperfunction and high gastrin values in the gastrocolic trunk which drains the antrum. (*c*) This patient had two angiographically demonstrable tumors in the body of the pancreas, but diffuse hypergastrinemia compatible with diffuse disease in MEN. (*d*) A patient with MEN and multiple hormone-secreting tumors and diffusely raised gastrin levels. PSPDV = posterior superior pancreatico-duodenal vein; IPDV = inferior pancreatico-duodenal vein

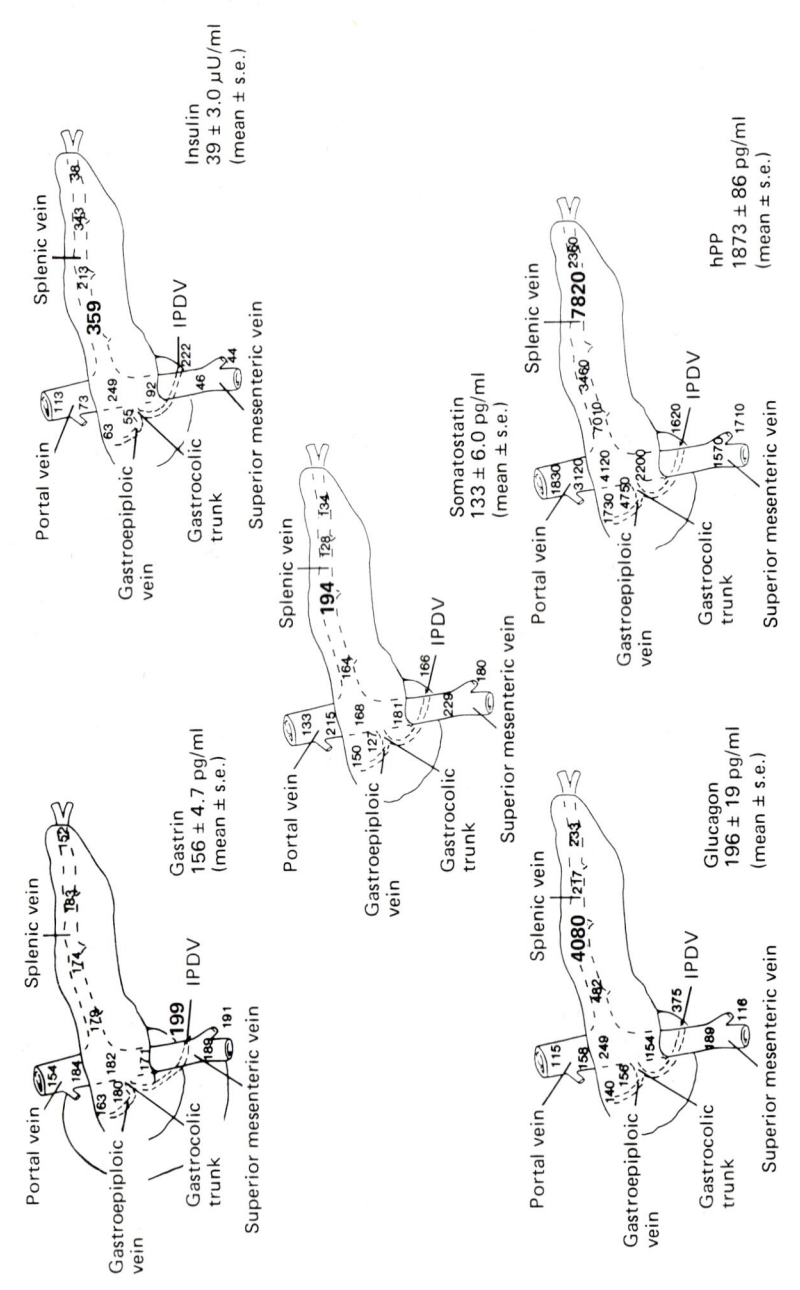

Figure 6.6 Patient FW with MEN I. Diagram showing arterial concentrations of various hormones, with highest concentrations indicating areas of overproduction of these hormones. Histologically these were found to correlate with small adenomas and 'nesidioblastosis' of pancreatic polypeptide cells. IPDV = inferior pancreatico-duodenal vein

In contrast to these patients with MEN I, patient PA (*see Figure 6.5a*) had a single high gastrin value in the high superior mesenteric vein, compatible with a gastrinoma in the head of the pancreas. A single large encapsulated tumor was found in the posterior superior portion of the head of the pancreas. After excision of the tumor, basal gastrin and acid secretion and the response to secretin returned to normal.

Although not essential to the diagnosis, THVS was performed in patient PG (*see Figure 6.5b*), in whom the diagnosis of G cell hyperfunction was made. The highest concentration of gastrin (810 pg/ml) was found in the gastroepiploic vein, suggesting antral origin. After antrectomy and truncal vagotomy, gastrin levels and acid secretion returned to normal, and a normal response to secretin was found.

CARCINOID SYNDROME

Carcinoid tumors which have not metastasized are notoriously difficult to localize.

MB, a white female aged 55, illustrates this problem well. This patient had had flushing of the face and hands, precipitated by alcohol ingestion, for 10 years and frequent (6–7 times a day) soft stools for 6 years. For the last 6 months, intermittent wheezing had accompanied the flushing attacks. She was found to have blue discoloration of the skin and face, no pulmonary hypertension, no hepatomegaly, a diffuse firm irregular goiter and a pelvic mass thought to be ovarian in origin.

Urinary 5-HIAA excretion was increased to 120 mg/day (normal value less than 10 mg/day). Serum calcium concentrations were raised to more than 10.4 mg/dl (2.60 mmol/l), with the C-terminal component of parathyroid hormone of 807 pg-Eq/ml (normal value less than 375 pg-Eq/ml). Thyroxine (T_4) was 4 μg/dl (315 nmol/l) (normal range 4.5–11.5 μg/dl or 362–906 nmol/l) and TSH 29.5 μU/ml (normal range 0–10 μU/ml). Calcitonin was 800 pg/ml (normal value less than 250 pg/ml). Several diagnoses were thus considered, including carcinoid syndrome, hyperparathyroidism, MEN II, medullary carcinoma of the thyroid with carcinoid and hypothyroidism.

A liver/spleen scan was negative. Computed axial tomography of the pelvis revealed a calcified, partially necrotic mass in the pelvis, thought to be a leiomyoma of the uterus. Angiography indicated abnormal vessels arising from the ileocolic artery extending towards the uterus bilaterally, suggesting the presence of a pelvic mass. In November 1980 transhepatic venous catheterization was carried out, with sampling of the superior vena cava, the portal vein, inferior vena cava, and selected pelvic and ovarian veins.

Serotonin concentrations in the various vessels are shown in *Figure 6.7*. Because of the high serotonin concentrations in the left jugular vein, exploration of the neck was carried out. No medullary carcinoma was present. The left lobe of the thyroid and the pyramidal lobe showed features consistent with Hashimoto's thyroiditis. Four-gland parathyroid biopsy was normal. A paratracheal lymph gland was normal. The thymus was excised and an ectopic parathyroid nodule found. Because of these negative findings, exploratory laparotomy was performed and an ovarian carcinoid tumor, 10 × 6 × 8 cm, was removed.

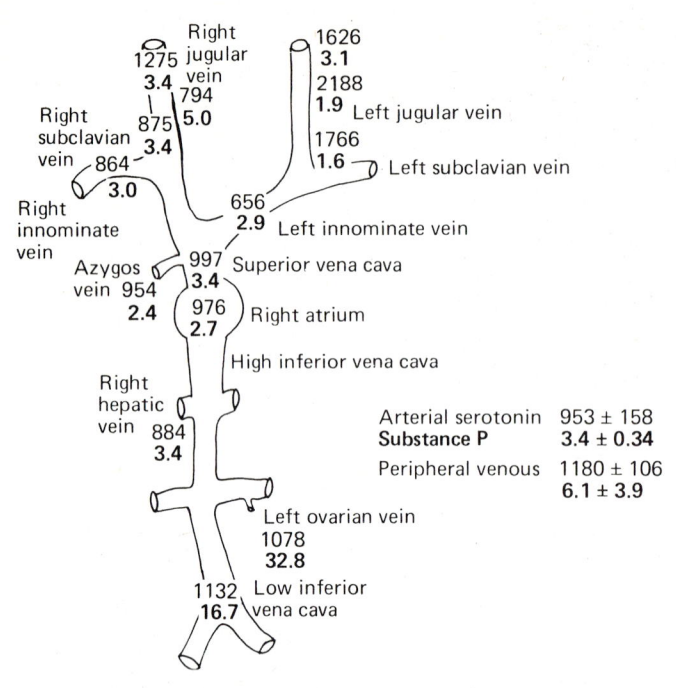

96 Localization of gastroentero-pancreatic (GEP) tumors

```
                Right
         1275  jugular          1626
          3.4   vein            3.1
                 794            2188
  Right        875  5.0         1.9  Left jugular vein
  subclavian   3.4              1766
  vein   864                    1.6   Left subclavian vein
          3.0
  Right              656
  innominate         2.9  Left innominate vein
  vein
         Azygos     997  Superior vena cava
         vein 954   3.4
               2.4  976
                    2.7  Right atrium
                    High inferior vena cava
  Right
  hepatic
  vein   884              Arterial serotonin    953 ± 158
         3.4              Substance P           3.4 ± 0.34
                          Peripheral venous     1180 ± 106
                                                6.1 ± 3.9
                    Left ovarian vein
                    1078
                    32.8
              1132  Low inferior
              16.7  vena cava
```

Figure 6.7 Serotonin and substance P concentrations in a female patient aged 55 with carcinoid syndrome due to a tumor in the left ovary. Raised serotonin levels misdirected us into first exploring the neck, yet substance P levels (shown in bold type) were raised in the vein draining the tumor

Sometime thereafter we received the results of substance P determinations. The concentrations are also shown in *Figure 6.7*. High levels were found in the left ovarian vein and in the low inferior vena cava. Serotonin concentrations at the same sites were similar to those elsewhere and there was no gradient.

It appeared therefore that serotonin concentrations had been misleading and that those of substance P more accurately localized the tumor. Three months postoperatively the patient was well, without flushing or diarrhea. Serotonin, parathyroid hormone, calcitonin and calcium values were all normal.

ANGIOGRAPHY, CAT SCAN AND ULTRASOUND

For many years arteriographic studies have been the most sensitive means of localizing islet cell adenomas, with success rates ranging widely among reported series[1, 31, 44]. Most insulinomas are small, ranging from 0.5–3.1 cm[10], and may not be readily visible because their density is similar to that of normal pancreatic tissue[1, 31, 36, 47]. Angiograms may falsely localize lesions and in unusual cases demonstrate only one tumor when, in fact, multiple adenomas are present[10, 24]. *Figure 6.8a* demonstrates a large tumor in the head of the pancreas in a patient aged 20 with organic hyperinsulinism. A superior mesenteric angiogram showed a

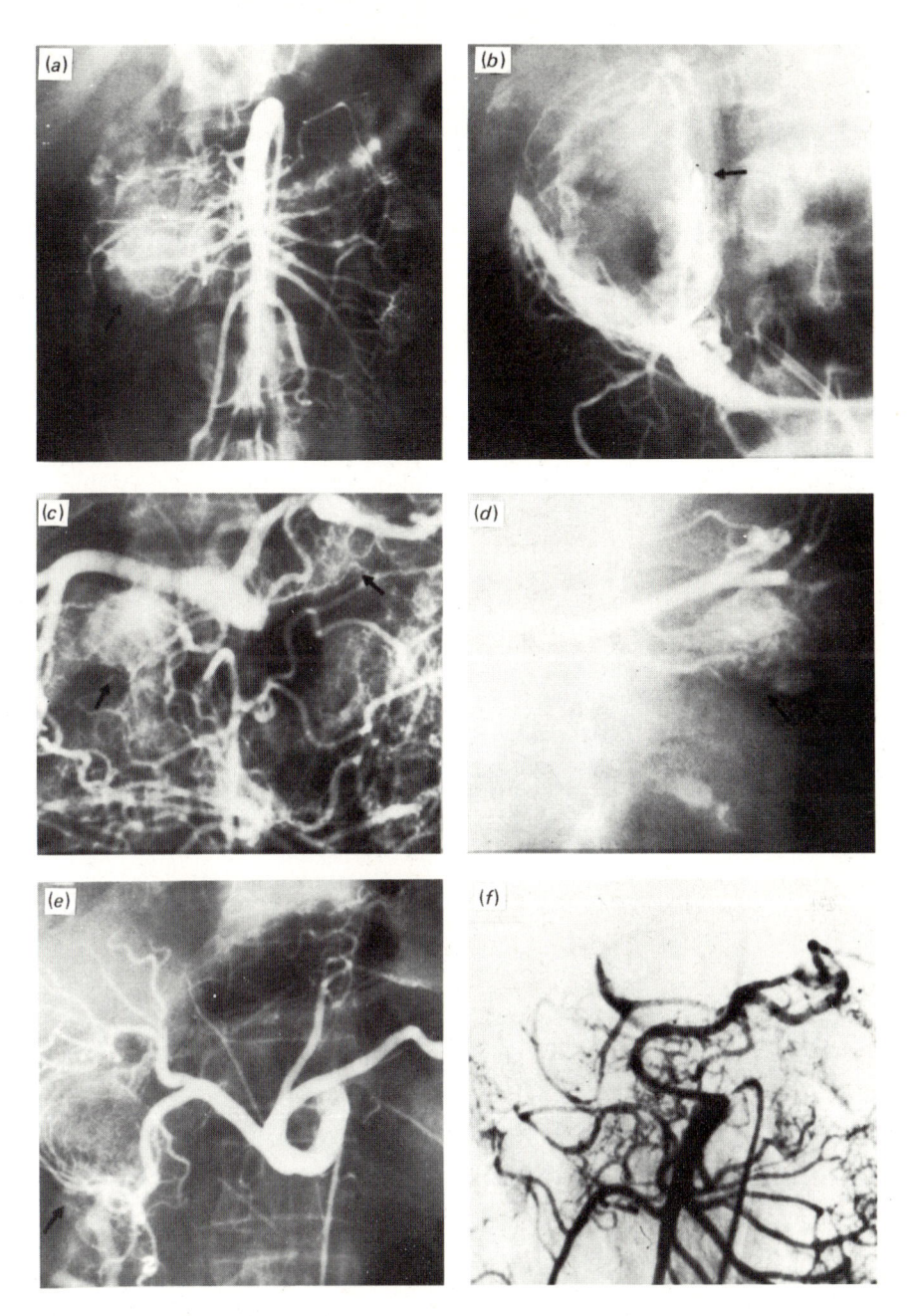

Figure 6.8 Angiographic demonstration of tumors and pseudotumors. (*a*) Insulinoma in head of pancreas. (*b*) Glucagonoma in the body. (*c*) Two gastrinomas. (*d*) False positive spleniculus. (*e*) False positive duodenal bulb. (*f*) Misleading 'tumor' vessels after celiac artery occlusion

large vascular mass in the head of the pancreas supplied by the inferior pancreaticoduodenal artery. THVS showed this to be the only source of insulin. Also shown is the angiogram of a woman aged 58 who had MEN I with peptic ulcer symptoms (*Figure 6.8c*). Two tumors visualized on angiography suggested possible resectability. THVS indicated diffuse origin of gastrin. Excision of the two tumors did not cure the patient. To further illustrate problems that can be encountered in pancreatic angiography, *Figure 6.8* shows false localization of tumors due to (1) an opaque shadow in the area of the duodenal bulb (*Figure 6.8e*) and (2) an apparent tumor which was a spleniculus (*Figure 6.8d*).

In other islet cell tumors, particularly small insulinomas and gastrinomas, we have been singularly unsuccessful, but have had some measure of success with large tumors, as in the case of malignant glucagonomas.

Of the 20 cases studied by the percutaneous transhepatic route we have been able to identify only 2 by computed axial tomography. Ultrasound has been singularly unhelpful in our experience.

Side-effects and morbidity

The most significant side-effects are the pain and discomfort experienced by the patient. However, provided that adequate premedication with analgesics and sedatives is given, as well as occasional supplementation during the procedure, this is well tolerated. In only 1 patient in our experience did mild hemobilia occur, which did not require transfusion. Patients should be kept at rest for at least 6 hours after the procedure. Care must be taken not to oversedate the patient since control of respiration is essential when traversing the liver with the catheter.

SUMMARY

The importance of preoperative localization of islet cell tumors in the surgical management of patients is well established[1,7,48]. Blind pancreatic resection in patients with occult tumors not only increases the operative morbidity but may result in incomplete cure. Angiography, ultrasound and computed axial tomography are only moderately successful in identifying these tumors. THVS may be helpful in localizing tumours under these circumstances. However, a thorough knowledge of the pancreatic venous anatomy is a prerequisite to successful catheterization of the pancreatic veins and interpretation of hormonal measurements made therein. There are a number of pitfalls awaiting the unwary, and false localization may mislead the surgeon in the approach to the tumor. In all our patients the site of insulinomas could be predicted from the site of maximum insulin concentration. In tumors of the head of the pancreas the highest concentrations were found either in the superior mesenteric or in the proximal portal vein.

Tumors in the neck were associated with highest levels in the confluence of splenic and mesenteric veins; uncinate lobe tumors drained into the superior mesenteric vein, and tumors in the body or tail of the pancreas were associated with highest levels of insulin in the splenic vein. When maximum insulin concentrations appear in the superior mesenteric vein it is important to recognize that the tumor may be in one of three locations in the pancreas. In such cases the neck and entire head of the pancreas and uncinate process must be explored carefully and mobilized for palpation. In tumors of the distal body or tail of the pancreas dual drainage may occur by the gastroepiploic and splenic veins, and erroneously high values may be obtained in the superior mesenteric or portal vessels. In such circumstances it is advisable to mobilize the entire tail of the pancreas (in order to reveal a small adenoma often buried deep in the spleen) before mobilizing the head of the pancreas. Multiple elevated hormone concentrations in the portal venous system suggest the diagnosis of hyperplasia, nesidioblastosis or multiple adenomas, but these cannot be distinguished by this procedure. In the case of organic hyperinsulinism it is clear that, in order to prevent hypoglycemia, sufficient pancreatic tissue must be resected to restore circulating insulin levels to normal. In MEN I with hypergastrinemia and peptic ulcer disease it appears to be futile to tackle the pancreas, and the best approach would seem to be medical treatment, with or without total gastrectomy, to treat the gastric acid hypersecretion which is the cause of the symptoms. However, our experience is limited and THVS may well be worthwhile in the hope that in a certain proportion of MEN I patients localized, resectable tumours will be found.

Once the diagnosis has been made, most competent surgeons will be able to determine the site of the lesion at operation and carry out the appropriate surgical procedure. However, to be forewarned of the site of such a lesion gives some degree of comfort, and this is particularly true for tumors in the head, neck and uncinate process of the pancreas. In many instances these tumors are not visualized by angiography, CAT or ultrasound, and may not be palpable at the time of operation. It is therefore easy for the surgeon to carry out a distal two-thirds pancreatectomy, leaving the offending tissue behind. With THVS it has become possible to identify and remove these tumors, yet spare sufficient pancreas to avoid the unnecessary complications of insulin-dependent diabetes and pancreatic steatorrhea. The preoperative assessment of islet cell hyperplasia, multiple adenomas or nesidioblastosis from multiple elevations in hormone concentrations clearly dictates a different approach from that to the single islet cell tumor.

We believe that preoperative portal venous sampling and hormone assays play an important role in the localization of islet cell tumors which are not detectable by conventional diagnostic studies and therefore considered occult. This technique also identifies patients with islet cell hyperfunction but no specific tumor. Furthermore, portal venous sampling may be useful in patients in whom angiography has either falsely localized a lesion or demonstrated only one of several tumors (*see earlier*).

CONCLUSION

We have presented here our experience with 11 patients with organic hyperinsulinism, 7 with hypergastrinema and 1 with carcinoid syndrome in whom percutaneous transhepatic portal and pancreatic vein catheterization was carried out successfully.

This helped to localize tumors, identify multiple tumors, establish the diagnosis of nesidioblastosis or hyperplasia, and identify multiple hormone secretion by the same tumor or multiple tumors within the pancreas. THVS is a safe and reliable procedure and has become an important investigation in the evaluation of patients with angiographically negative functioning islet cell lesions. We believe that the sampling method will play a fairly major role in the localization of adenomas in patients with normal angiographic studies or previously negative surgical explorations. Since no clinical study has managed to distinguish patients with multiple tumors from those with single adenomas or with islet cell hyperplasia or nesidioblastosis, THVS may be the procedure of choice. Portal venous concentrations of a number of hormones have been measured, including gastrin, glucagon, VIP, motilin, somatostatin, insulin and PP, which may prove useful in further studies designed to localize tumors of the GEP axis.

Acknowledgement

Work supported in part by US Public Health Service Grants AM-02244, AM-00888, T32-07245, 5MO1RR-42 and 5-P60-AM20572.

Hormone assays of VIP were kindly provided by Tom Odorisio, MD, University of Ohio, Columbus, Ohio; and of substance P and serotonin by Bernard Jaffee, MD, Downstate Medical Center, Brooklyn, New York.

References

1 ALFIDI, R. J., BHYUN, D. S., CRILE, G. Jr and HAWK, W. Arteriography and hypoglycemia. *Surgery, Gynecology and Obstetrics*, **133,** 447–452 (1971)
2 BLACKARD, W. G., NELSON, N. C. and ANDREWS, S. S. Portal and peripheral vein immunoreactive glucagon concentrations after arginine or glucose infusion. *Diabetes*, **23,** 199–202 (1974)
3 BLOOM, S. R., POLAK, J. M. and PEARSE, A. G. E. Vasoactive intestinal polypeptide and watery diarrhoea syndrome. *Lancet*, **2,** 14–16 (1973)
4 BOTHA, J. L., VINIK, A. I., CHILD, P. T., PAUL, M. and JACKSON, W. P. U. Pancreatic glucagon-like immunoreactivity in a pancreatectomized patient. *Hormone and Metabolic Research*, **9,** 199–205 (1977)
5 BURCHARTH, F., STAGE, J. G., STADIL, F., JENSEN, L. I. and FISCHERMANN, K. Localization of gastrinomas by transhepatic portal catheterization and gastrin assay. *Gastroenterology*, **77,** 444–450 (1979)
6 DOPPMAN, J. L., BRENNAN, M. F., DUNNICK, N. R., KAHN, C. R. and GORDEN, P. The role of pancreatic venous sampling in the localization of occult insulinomas. *Radiology*, **138,** 557–562 (1981)
7 DUNN, E. and STEIN, S. Percutaneous transhepatic pancreatic vein catheterization in localization of insulinomas. *Archives of Surgery*, **116,** 232–233 (1981)
8 ERLANDSEN, S. L., HEGRE, O. D., PARSONS, J. A., McEROY, R. C. and ELDE, R. P. Pancreatic islet cell hormones: distribution of cell types in the islet and the evidence for the presence of somatostatin and gastrin within the D cell. *Journal of Histochemistry and Cytochemistry*, **24,** 883–897 (1976)

9 FLOYD, J. C., Jr, FAJANS, S. S., PEK, S. and CHANCE, R. E. A newly recognized pancreatic polypeptide: plasma levels in health and disease. *Recent Progress in Hormone Research*, **33,** 519–569 (1977)

10 FULTON, R. E., SHEEDY, P. F., McILLRATH, D. C. and FERRIS, D. O. Preoperative angiographic localization of insulin producing tumors of the pancreas. *American Journal of Roentgenology*, **123,** 367–377 (1975)

11 GAHNICHE, J. P., CONLIN, R., DUBOIS, P. M., CHAYVIALLE, J. A., DESCOS, F., PAULIN, C. and GEFFROY, Y. Calcitonin secretion by a pancreatic somatostatinoma. *New England Journal of Medicine*, **299,** 1252 (1978)

12 GANDA, O. P., WEIR, G. C., SOELDNER, J. S., LEGG, M. A., CHICK, W. L., PATEL, Y. C., EBEID, A. M., GABBEY, K. and REICHLIN, S. Somatostatinoma: a somatostatin-containing tumor of the endocrine pancreas. *New England Journal of Medicine*, **296,** 963–967 (1977)

13 GLASER, B., VALTYSSON, G., FAJANS, S. S., VINIK, A. I., CHO, K. and THOMPSON, N. Gastrointestinal/pancreatic hormone concentration in the portal venous system of nine patients with organic hyperinsulinism. *Metabolism*, **30**(10), 1001–1010 (1981)

14 GLOWNIAK, J., SHAPIRO, B., VINIK, A. I., GLASER, B., THOMPSON, N. and CHO, K. Percutaneous transhepatic venous sampling of gastrin. Value in sporadic and familial islet cell tumors and G-cell hyperfunction. *New England Journal of Medicine*, **307,** 293–297 (1982)

15 GRAY, R. K., ROSCH, J. and GROLLMAN, J. H. Arteriography in the diagnosis of islet cell tumors. *Radiology*, **97,** 39–44 (1970)

16 HAYASHI, M., FLOYD, J. C., Jr, PEK, S. and FAJANS, S. S. Insulin, proinsulin, glucagon and gastrin in pancreatic tumors and in plasma of patients with organic hyperinsulinism. *Journal of Clinical Endocrinology and Metabolism*, **44,** 681–694 (1977)

17 HOLST, S. S., HELLEND, S., INGEMANNSON, S., BANG PEDERSEN, N. and VON SCHENCK, H. Functional studies in patients with glucagonoma syndrome. *Diabetologia*, **17,** 151–156 (1979)

18 INGEMANSSON, S., LUNDERQUIST, A., LUNDQUIST, I., LOUDAHL, R. and TIBBIN, S. Portal and pancreatic vein catheterization with radioimmunologic determination of insulin. *Surgery, Gynecology and Obstetrics*, **141,** 705–711 (1975)

19 INGEMANSSON, S., LUNDERQUIST, A. and HOLST, J. Selective catheterization of the pancreatic vein for radioimmunoassay in glucagon-secreting carcinoma of the pancreas. *Radiology*, **119,** 555–556 (1976)

20 INGEMANSSON, S., HOLST, J., LARSSON, L. E. and LUNDERQUIST, A. Localization of glucagonomas by catheterization of the pancreatic veins and with glucagon assay. *Surgery, Gynecology and Obstetrics*, **145,** 509–516 (1977)

21 INGEMANSSON, S., HOLST, J., LARSSON, L. I., LUNDERQUIST, A. and NOBIN, A. Islet cell hyperplasia localized by pancreatic vein catheterization and insulin radioimmunoassay. *American Journal of Surgery*, **133,** 643–645 (1977)

22 INGEMANSSON, S., LARSSON, L. I., LUNDERQUIST, A. and STADIL, F. Pancreatic vein catheterization with gastrin assay in normal patients and in patients with Zöllinger-Ellison syndrome. *American Journal of Surgery*, **134,** 558–563 (1977)

23 KALLIO, H. and SUORANTA, H. Localization of occult insulin secreting tumors of the pancreas. *Annals of Surgery*, **189,** 49–52 (1979)

24 KOROBKIN, M. T., PALUBINSKAS, A. J. and GLICKMAN, M. G. Pitfalls in arteriography of islet cell tumors of the pancreas. *Radiology*, **100**, 319–328 (1971)
25 KOVAES, K., HORVATH, E., EZRIN, C., SEPP, H. and ELKAN, I. Immunoreactive somatostatin in pancreatic islet cell carcinoma accompanied by ectopic ACTH syndrome. *Lancet*, **1**, 1365–1366 (1977)
26 KREJS, G. J., ORCI, L., CONLON, M., RAVAZZOLA, M., DAVIS, G. R., RASKIN, P., COLLINS, S. M., McCARTHY, D. M., BAETENS, D., RUBENSTEIN, A., ALDOR, T. A. M. and UNGER, R. H. Somatostatinoma syndrome (biochemical, morphologic and clinical features). *New England Journal of Medicine*, **301**, 285–292 (1979)
27 LARSSON, L. I., GRIMELIUS, L., HAKANSON, R., REHFELD, J. F., STADIL, F., HOLST, J., ANGERVALL, L. and SUNDLER, F. Tumors producing several peptide hormones. *American Journal of Pathology*, **79**, 271–284 (1975)
28 LARSSON, L. E., SCHWARTZ, T., LUNDQUIST, G., CHANCE, R. E., SUNDLER, F., REHFELD, J. F., GRIMELIUS, L., FAHRENKRUG, J., SCHAFFALITZKY deMUCKADELL, D. and MOON, N. Pancreatic polypeptide in pancreatic endocrine tumors, possible implication in watery diarrhea syndrome. *American Journal of Pathology*, **85**, 675–682 (1976)
29 LARSSON, L. I., HIRSCH, M. A., HOLST, J., INGEMANSSON, S., KUHL, C., LENDKAER SENSEN, S., LUNDQUIST, G., REHFELD, J. F. and SCHAWARTZ, T. W. Pancreatic somatostatinoma: clinical features and physiological implications. *Lancet*, **1**, 666–668 (1977)
30 LARSSON, L. I. Gastrointestinal cells producing endocrine, neurocrine and paracrine messengers. *Clinics in Gastroenterology*, **9**, 485–615 (1980)
31 LUNDERQUIST, A. and TYLEN, U. Phlebography of the pancreatic veins. *Radiologie*, **15**, 198–202 (1975)
32 LUNDERQUIST, A., ERIKSSON, M., INGEMANSSON, S., LARSSON, L. I. and RIECHARDT, W. Selective pancreatic vein catheterization for hormone assay in endocrine tumors of the pancreas. *Cardiovascular Radiology*, **1**, 117–124 (1978)
33 MALAISSE-LAGAE, F., STEFAN, Y., COX, J., PERRELET, A. and ORCI, L. Identification of a lobe in the adult human pancreas rich in pancreatic polypeptide. *Diabetologia*, **17**, 361–366 (1979)
34 McINTOSH, C., ARNOLD, R., BOTHE, E., BECKER, H., KOBBERLING, J. and CREUTZFELD, W. Gastrointestinal somatostatin in man and dog. *Metabolism*, **27**, 1317–1320 (1978)
35 MILLAN, V. G., UROSA, C. L., MOLITCH, M. E., MILLER, H. and JACKSON, I. M. D. Localization of occult insulinoma by superselective pancreatic venous sampling for insulin assay through percutaneous transhepatic catheterization. *Diabetes*, **28**, 249–251 (1979)
36 MILLER, D. R. Functioning adenomas of pancreas with hyperinsulinism. *Archives of Surgery*, **90**, 509–520 (1965)
37 MITTY, H. A., EFREMIDIS, S., WESTKIN, M. G., DREILING, D. A. and RAYFIELD, E. J. Localization of insulinomas by radioimmunoassay of blood obtained by the transportal route. *Journal of Clinical Endocrinology and Metabolism*, **48**, 1035–1037 (1979)
38 deNUTTE, N., SOMERS, G., GEPTS, W., JACOBS, M. and PIPELEERS, D. Pancreatic hormone release in tumor associated hypersomatostinemia. *Diabetologia*, **15**, 227 (1978)
39 OBERG, K., LÖÖF, L., BOSTRÖM, H., GRIMELIUS, L., FAHRENKRUG, J. and LUNDQUIST, A. Hypersecretion of calcitonin in patients with the Vernes-Morrison syndrome. *Scandinavian Journal of Gastroenterology*, **16**, 135–144 (1981)

References 103

40 ORCI, L., MALAISSE-LAGAE, F., BAETEUS, D. and PENELET, A. Pancreatic polypeptide-rich regions in human pancreas. *Lancet*, **2**, 1200–1201 (1978)

41 PEK, S., FAJANS, S. S., FLOYD, J. C., Jr, KNOPF, R. F. and CONN, J. W. Failure of sulfonylureas to suppress plasma glucagon in man. *Diabetes*, **21**, 216–223 (1972)

42 REICHARDT, W. and CAMERON, R. Anatomy of the pancreatic veins. A post-mortem and clinical phlebographic investigation. *Acta Radiologica*, **21**, 33–41 (1980)

43 REICHARDT. W and INGEMANSSON, S. Selective vein catheterization for hormone assay in endocrine tumors of the pancreas. *Acta Radiologica*, **21**, 177–187 (1980)

44 ROBINS, J. M., BOOKSTEIN, J. J., OBERMAN, H. A. and FAJANS, S. S. Selective arteriography in localizing islet cell tumors of the pancreas. *Radiology*, **106**, 525–528 (1973)

45 SACKS, H., GRANT, B. J. and VINIK, A. I. Metabolism of synthetic human hepta-decapeptide gastrin by the isolated perfused rat livers. *South African Medical Journal*, **53**, 249–251 (1978)

46 SAID, S. I. and FALOONA, G. R. Elevated plasma and tissue levels of vasoactive intestinal polypeptide in the watery diarrhea syndrome due to pancreatic, bronchogenic and other tumors. *New England Journal of Medicine*, **293**, 155–160 (1975)

47 STEFANINI, P., CARBONI, M., PATRASSI, N. and BASOLI, A. Beta islet cell tumors of the pancreas: results of a study on 1067 cases. *Surgery*, **75**, 597–609 (1974)

48 STEFANINI, P., CARBONI, M., PETRASSI, N., De BERNARDINIS, N. P. and BLANDAMURA, V. The value of arteriography in the diagnosis and treatment of insulinomas. *American Journal of Surgery*, **131**, 352–356 (1976)

49 TURNER, R. C., LEE, E. C. G., MORRIS, P. J., HARRIS, E. A. and DICK, R. Localization of insulinomas. *Lancet*, **1**, 515–518 (1978)

50 UNGER, R. H. Somatostatinoma. *New England Journal of Medicine*, **296**, 998–1000 (1977)

51 VINIK, A. I., GRANT, B. J. and NOVIS, B. Gastrins in human antrum, duodenum, and peripheral circulation. *South African Medical Journal*, **49**, 225–257 (1975)

52 VINIK, A. I., HICKMAN, R. and GRANT, B. J. Endogenous and exogenous hepta-decapeptide gastrin transport across the pig liver. *South African Medical Journal*, **53**, 759–765 (1978)

53 VINIK, A. I., LEVITT, N. S., PIMSTONE, B. L. and WAGNER, L. Peripheral plasma somato-statin-like immunoreactive responses to insulin hypoglycemia and a mixed meal in healthy subjects and in noninsulin-dependent maturity-onset diabetics. *Journal of Clinical Endocrinology and Metabolism*, **52**(2), 330–337 (1980)

54 VINIK, A. I. and GLASER, B. Pancreatic endocrine tumors. In *Pancreatic Disease, Diagnosis and Therapy*, edited by T. L. Dent, pp. 427–461. New York, Grune and Stratton (1981)

55 ZÖLLINGER, R. M. and ELLISON, E. H. Primary peptic ulcerations of the jejunum associated with islet cell tumors of the pancreas. *Annals of Surgery*, **142**, 709–723 (1955)

7
Insulin tumours of the pancreas
L. P. Le Quesne and P. R. Daggett

The insulin secreting islet cell tumour of the pancreas (colloquially and hereinafter referred to as an insulinoma), the commonest cause of organic hyperinsulinism, is a rare lesion, but an important one, for its successful diagnosis and treatment can restore a patient completely to normal, whereas if overlooked it may cause permanent disability or even death as a result of repeated episodes of hypoglycaemia.

PATHOLOGY OF INSULINOMAS

The insulinoma occurs with an annual incidence of 0.5 to 1.25 per million of the population and is slightly commoner in women than in men[37]. Its peak incidence is in the fifth decade: it is rare in children and after the age of 60. It has been suggested that it arises from metaplastic change in pancreatic duct cells, rather than from the islets of Langerhans themselves[28]. By far the commonest finding is for there to be a discrete mass of β-cells. On rare occasions there are diffuse collections of β-cells throughout the pancreas, the condition of microadenomatosis (*see below*). Insulin tumours are rare in childhood, when the condition of hyperinsulinism is caused by a particular form of islet cell hyperplasia, known as nesidioblastosis[70].

The true insulinoma is usually single, although in up to 10% of all cases two or more have been said to occur[60]. Our own experience and that of others suggests, however, that this figure may be an overestimate: we have seen only one instance of multiple tumours in our series of 29 surgically treated patients. This individual suffered from type 1 multiple endocrine adenomatosis, a disorder in which pancreatic tumours are not infrequently multiple and which will be discussed subsequently. About 10% of all insulinomas behave as malignant neoplasms, metastasizing most often to the liver. Malignant insulinomas appear not to arise from benign adenomas, but develop *a priori* from nests of transformed duct epithelial cells[5]. As in the case of some other endocrine tumours, the diagnosis of malignancy on histological grounds may be difficult, and the true nature of the tumour may only be finally indicated by its biological behaviour. Although the prevalence of malignancy in insulinomas is quite high, it is less than with other types of islet cell tumours, and only about 12% of all islet cell carcinomas secrete insulin. The special problems of the management of malignant insulinomas will be described separately.

Insulinomas are usually 1.0 to 2.0 cm in diameter, but may be smaller or larger, with a range of 0.5 to 15.0 cm. They occur evenly distributed throughout the pancreas, although some 60% of those removed surgically are in the body and tail[16, 60]. The distribution of tumours in our own series is shown in *Figure 7.1*. In the past there has been considerable debate as to whether an insulinoma ever occurs outside the pancreas. It now appears certain that such tumours may develop, although they are exceedingly rare. They appear to arise in areas of pancreatic heterotopia and have been described in the stomach, duodenum, Meckel's diverticulum, ileum, gall-bladder and intestinal mesentery[22, 30, 47].

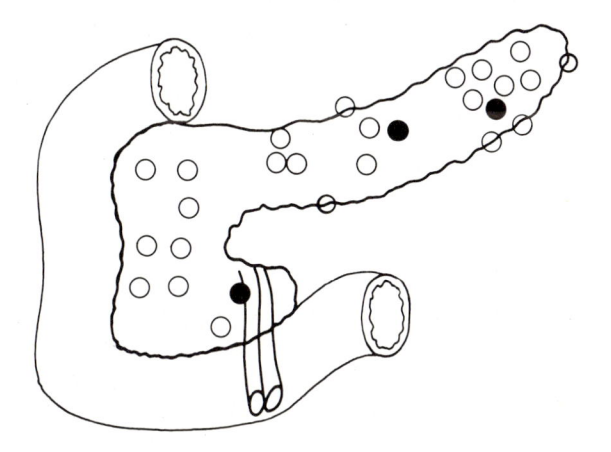

Figure 7.1 Diagram showing the distribution of tumours in 27 patients. The closed circles indicate tumours not felt at the first operation. (From Le Quesne *et al.*[34], courtesy of the Editor and Publishers, *British Journal of Surgery*)

Insulin secreting tumours are indistinguishable from other islet cell tumours on light microscopy, but their true nature can be revealed by electron microscopy, which shows the presence of the characteristic pro-insulin crystals within the cells. The histological appearances on light microscopy vary somewhat from tumour to tumour, and, furthermore, in a number of tumours there is evidence of cells secreting more than one hormone[48]. Pancreatic polypeptide (PP) may be found in a majority of insulinomas, though only in small quantities, but a suggestion that the plasma level of this substance might be useful as a marker in the diagnosis of insulin tumours has been discredited[43]. Insulinomas have also been known to secrete ACTH[31, 53] or to be associated with the carcinoid syndrome[1], particularly when the tumour is malignant. Even the 'pure' insulinoma shows different cytological patterns, and some contain amyloid[8].

Microadenomatosis

In this rare condition the pancreas is enlarged and diffusely involved[3]. The microadenomata may be little larger than a normal islet of Langerhans, but usually vary in size from 0.2 to 5.0 mm in diameter. The presentation, in clinical manifestations, does not differ from that of a solitary insulinoma, and there are no differences to be found on investigation. Effective treatment of this rare disorder requires extensive resection of the pancreas; although total pancreatectomy might be expected to be required, in practice a subtotal resection is often curative[20].

Multiple endocrine neoplasia (MEN)

Insulinomas in this condition (*see* Chapter 1) are usually benign, but often multiple, and there may even be diffuse microadenomatosis[67]. Insulin tumours as an expression of MEN type I tend to occur at an unusually early age, and when hyperinsulinism is diagnosed in children and adolescents a search must always be made for other endocrine disorders. Adenomas of all the glands capable of involvement in MEN type I are seldom synchronous and long-term follow-up is required to detect their development. In addition, first-order relatives should be screened for the various syndromes and kept under surveillance.

DIAGNOSIS

The symptoms of an insulinoma result from repeated, unpredictable attacks of hypoglycaemia of varying severity. Although well described and usually easy to recognize, the symptoms of hypoglycaemia may be confusing because of individual variation in response. The effects of a lowered blood glucose concentration (hypoglycaemia) result from (1) cerebral energy deprivation (neuroglycopenia), and (2) the effects of activation of the sympathetic nervous system. The clinical effects of the former include confusion, hunger, dizziness, bizarre behaviour, and paraesthesia, particularly around the mouth; in extreme examples there may be convulsions, proceeding to coma and death. The prominent features of the latter are tachycardia, pallor, sweating and pupillary dilatation.

Patients with an insulinoma may manifest any of these features[54], but in addition, presumably as an expression of the severity of the hypoglycaemia, may present with intermittent diplopia[18] or hemiparesis[2]. An important feature suggesting that the attacks of hypoglycaemia are due to an insulinoma is their timing, the attacks tending to occur before breakfast, late in the afternoon before the evening meal, or after vigorous exercise[4]. A further clue to the diagnosis is that the majority of subjects with an insulinoma gain weight, probably as a result of eating extra food in an effort to prevent hypoglycaemic attacks.

There are, however, many causes of a lowered blood glucose concentration (*Table 7.1*), some of which may cause diagnostic problems. In order to diagnose an insulinoma, it is necessary to show that inappropriate insulin production continues

Table 7.1 Causes of hypoglycaemia

	Underlying cause
Organic hyperinsulinism	Insulinoma
	Microadenomatosis
	Nesidioblastosis (in childhood)
Overdosage of hypoglycaemic agents	Insulin
(factituous hypoglycaemia)	Sulphonylureas (not biguanides)
Alimentary	After gastric operations
	Alcohol
Advanced liver disease	
Solid retroperitoneal tumours	
Endocrine disease	Hypoadrenalism
	Hypopituitarism
Congenital metabolic disorders	Leucine sensitivity
	Glycogen storage diseases

during hypoglycaemia. This means that a high serum insulin concentration must be demonstrable when the blood glucose level is low, preferably at a time when the patient is symptomatic. Methods of establishing the diagnosis of insulinoma and making a distinction from other causes of hypoglycaemia are reviewed in the ensuing sections of this chapter.

In the majority of cases the diagnosis of the presence of an insulinoma can now be made with confidence. This is the result of the development of reliable methods for the measurement of the concentration of insulin in the peripheral blood and, more recently, of that of the connecting C-peptide. Hitherto the diagnosis has rested on the use of a number of tests which, though now obsolete, are still sometimes used, and these tests are included to indicate their pitfalls and the reasons why they should no longer be used.

Outmoded tests

The glucose tolerance test

This investigation has no place in the diagnosis of an insulinoma[35]. It has, however, been widely advocated and used[71]. The glucose tolerance test (GTT) shows no diagnostic differences between normal subjects and those with an insulinoma, regardless of whether the glucose is given orally or intravenously, even when measurements of blood glucose are continued for 5 hours after the 50 g glucose load and combined with estimations of the serum insulin (the extended GTT). The only value of the glucose tolerance test in this context is in the diagnosis of essential reactive hypoglycaemia (*see below*), a disorder which is unlikely to be confused with an insulinoma.

The intravenous tolbutamide test

Tolbutamide releases insulin from normal and neoplastic β-cells, the response being exaggerated when there is an insulinoma. Blood samples are analyzed for glucose and insulin content at intervals for 3 hours after the intravenous injection of 1 g of sodium tolbutamide. In patients with an insulinoma the blood glucose level fails to return to its basal value or to 2.5 mmol/l (whichever is the lower) within 3 hours of the injection[17]. The serum insulin concentration in such cases is usually greater than 150 mU/l within 5 to 10 min of the injection, but similar levels may be achieved in patients with liver disease or simple obesity[12]. At least one fatality has followed severe hypoglycaemia induced by this test, and it should no longer be used.

The glucagon test

Glucagon releases insulin from β-cells and promotes glycogenolysis, thereby not producing severe hypoglycaemia. This test is therefore considerably safer than the tolbutamide test, but the responses of patients with an insulinoma are not sufficiently distinct for it to be diagnostically reliable[27]. In fasting normal subjects the serum insulin rises by 30–100 mU/l within a few minutes of the i.v. injection of 1 mg of glucagon. When there is an insulinoma, the insulin level exceeds 150 mU/l within 5 to 10 min of the injection, and rebound, mild hypoglycaemia is common, but false positive responses occur in obesity, acromegaly and when there is steroid excess[36].

Other tests

The oral administration of leucine produces a rise in serum insulin by 10 mU/l and a fall of glucose by 1.5 mmol/l in 40% of patients with an insulinoma[39].

The intravenous infusion of calcium gluconate produced a rise in serum insulin in 9 out of 10 insulinomas studied by Kaplan *et al.*[25], but this work has not been repeated. Neither of these tests has sufficient discriminant value to be reliable.

Current diagnostic methods

Glucose : insulin ratios

Current methods for diagnosis of insulinomas rely upon accurate measurement of glucose, insulin and C-peptide, and require an understanding of the normal relationship of these substances. Insulin is synthesized in the pancreatic islet β-cell as a precursor, pro-insulin. This is hydrolyzed to insulin itself and the connecting or C-peptide, both being released from the cell in equimolar amounts[52]. Insulin has a half-life in the circulation of 4 to 8 min, but that of C-peptide is much longer, probably in excess of 30 min[51]. Accordingly, the molar concentration of C-peptide is higher than that of insulin and its accurate measurement is therefore easier. Its concentration changes much less quickly than that of insulin and it can be used to provide a better guide to β-cell function. Insulin and C-peptide are released by several stimuli, by far the most important of which is glucose, acting through a glucoreceptor on the surface of the β-cell. Activity is suppressed by hypoglycaemia and falls to very low levels when the blood glucose concentration falls below 2.2 mmol/l. At this level of glucose concentration the concentration of endogenous insulin in the blood falls significantly within 10 min, and that of C-peptide within 1 hour, if hypoglycaemia is maintained[55]. In normal individuals who have fasted overnight the peripheral venous insulin concentration is always less than 15 mU/l and the corresponding glucose level usually between 2.5 and 4.0 mmol/l. When in the normal individual the blood glucose concentration is lowered to less than 2.0 mmol/l, the insulin level will be below 4 mU/l and may be undetectable by conventional assays. The level of C-peptide at this time will generally be below 0.2 pmol/l.

The cardinal diagnostic feature of organic hyperinsulinism is a disturbance of this normal relationship between the blood glucose concentration on the one hand and the insulin and/or C-peptide levels on the other. The only certain means of diagnosing an insulinoma is to show an inappropriately high serum level of insulin or C-peptide for a given blood glucose concentration, particularly when this is in the hypoglycaemic range. The reliable demonstration of this relationship requires careful attention to assay methods. Most routine laboratories provide a reliable glucose service, using glucose oxidase techniques and blood samples collected into sodium fluoride to inhibit glycolysis. Conventional insulin assays give maximum precision in the range 10 to 200 mU/l, and in order to detect the very low levels to be anticipated a special assay system must be used[65]. C-peptide assays are still evolving, but generally give reliable results down to the low level of 0.156 pmol/l[6]. The relationship between blood levels of glucose and insulin in normal subjects can be represented graphically, points above the line being designated 'inappropriate'. This is illustrated in *Figure 7.2*, which shows in addition our series of patients with a confirmed insulinoma.

If inappropriate hyperinsulinism can be shown during spontaneous symptomatic hypoglycaemia, the diagnosis of insulinoma is confirmed. For a valid interpretation of the results, samples for measurement of insulin (and preferably C-peptide as well) *must* be taken simultaneously with the specimen to be analyzed for glucose. The diagnosis is strengthened if the phenomenon can be demonstrated on two or more occasions.

If, as may often be the case, circumstances do not allow the taking of blood specimens to demonstrate inappropriate secretion of insulin during spontaneous hypoglycaemia, then the patient should be studied after a period of starvation. Of patients with an insulinoma, 90% will become hypoglycaemic after an overnight fast of 12 hours if the measurement is made on three consecutive nights[38]. In some patients it may be necessary to prolong the fast for 72 hours, culminating in a period of brisk exercise, a procedure which will unmask inappropriate insulin secretion in a further 8% of patients[41]. During these tests a number of patients may not

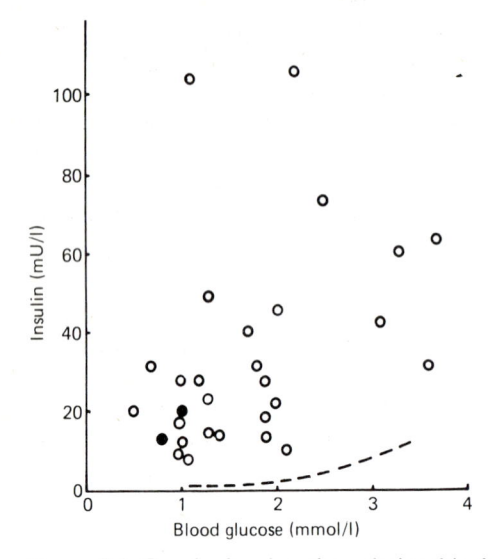

Figure 7.2 Graph showing the relationship between the serum insulin concentration and blood glucose concentration after an overnight fast in 29 patients with an insulinoma. Normal subjects will fall below the dotted line. In 2 patients (closed circles), the result after an overnight fast was equivocal, and the points shown represent the result of 36 hours starvation. (From Le Quesne *et al.*[34], courtesy of the Editor and Publishers, *British Journal of Surgery*)

manifest symptoms of hypoglycaemia. Such symptoms are not essential: the essential requisite is the demonstration of inappropriately high levels of insulin in the face of hypoglycaemia (i.e. a blood sugar level of less than 2.0 mmol/l).

It is important to bear in mind that fasting is potentially hazardous to a patient with an insulinoma. During fasting tests careful observation of the patient is essential, and the blood glucose level should be checked every 4 hours to forestall the development of severe hypoglycaemia.

Suppression tests

The first suppression tests measured the serum insulin concentration after the induction of hypoglycaemia with fish insulin, an agent which has biological activity but is not measured in the insulin radio-immunoassay[65]. An intravenous injection of fish insulin (0.15 U/kg body weight) is made and repeated after 30 min if the blood glucose level has not fallen to below 2.2 mmol/l. A blood sample to be analyzed for insulin and glucose is obtained before the first injection, and at 10-minute intervals until 20 minutes after adequate hypoglycaemia has been achieved. Glucose and insulin data must be interpreted together (*see Figure 7.2*) but, generally speaking, the diagnosis of insulinoma is supported if the insulin level remains about 4 mU/l when the blood glucose is below 2 mmol/l.

This technique has been rendered obsolete by the availability of the C-peptide assay. In the C-peptide test, an intramuscular injection of purified soluble insulin (such as Actrapid, Novo) is used (0.1 U/kg body weight). It is necessary to maintain a blood glucose level below 2.2 mmol/l for at least 30 min in order to allow previously secreted C-peptide to be cleared from the circulation. Frequent measurements of blood glucose (by Dextrostix) are essential, and samples for glucose and C-peptide measurement should be taken at the beginning of adequate hypoglycaemia, after 30 min, and if possible after 60 min. Glucose must not be given during this test unless judged essential, because it is a powerful stimulus to C-peptide release. Interpretation of this test depends upon the reference ranges of the local laboratory.

In normal subjects there is always suppression of C-peptide during hypoglycaemia, usually to below 0.2 pmol/l. In patients with an insulinoma this does not occur.

The suppression test should be used if hypoglycaemia has not been observed to occur spontaneously or has not been precipitated by fasting, or if there is any doubt about the diagnosis.

Differential diagnosis

As previously indicated (*see text* and *Table 7.1*), hypoglycaemia may be caused by conditions other than insulinoma, but their differentiation is usually straightforward.

Factitious hypoglycaemia

The deliberate induction of hypoglycaemia with insulin or a sulphonylurea is most commonly seen in members of the medical or related professions and their relatives. It is occasionally met with in the relatives of diabetic patients being treated with these agents. A high index of suspicion is required to make the diagnosis, but once considered, proof is usually a simple matter. Patients injecting themselves with insulin usually have circulating insulin levels far in excess of those found in cases of insulinoma. In addition, injected insulin contains very little C-peptide, whereas insulin produced endogenously will be associated with equimolar amounts of C-peptide. Thus the concentration of circulating C-peptide will be low when hypoglycaemia has been factitiously induced with insulin, but high when there is an insulinoma or when sulphonylureas have been consumed surreptitiously[61]. In the latter circumstance the only sure way of making the diagnosis is to detect the patient with the drug, or to show its presence in the blood by chromatography[63].

Alimentary hypoglycaemia

This term is used here to describe the well-known consequence of gastric drainage operations, which allow an unaccustomed glucose load to be presented to the jejunum. This not infrequently leads to rebound hypoglycaemia, but this possibility should be self-evident from the history and abdominal scar. Although not strictly alimentary, the condition of essential reactive hypoglycaemia may be considered under this heading. Reactive hypoglycaemia can be diagnosed during a prolonged glucose tolerance test, in which low blood glucose levels are found between 3 and 5 hours after the glucose load, usually preceded by unusually high insulin levels around 2 hours.

Alcohol

Ethanol can release insulin from the normal β-cell, and indeed this agent has been used as a provocative test in patients with an insulinoma. In normal subjects ethanol may cause quite profound hypoglycaemia, particularly when spirits are taken on an empty stomach[69]. Patients who experience this phenomenon are often thought to have an insulinoma, but differentiation is a simple matter on the basis of history.

Tumour hypoglycaemia

It is not known why some solid parenchymal tumours can, on rare occasions, cause hypoglycaemia. It is, however, apparent that circulating insulin levels are not high[68], and accordingly the distinction from an insulinoma is easy to make. Retroperitoneal sarcomata are the best-recognized cause of tumour hypoglycaemia and the association has been described as the Doege-Potter syndrome[32]. There is usually a large mass of tumour, and differentiation from insulinoma can be made clinically. Other tumours occasionally incriminated include primary liver cell carcinoma, adrenocortical carcinoma and teratomas in various sites.

To conclude, the cornerstone of the management of patients with a suspected insulinoma is the establishment, beyond doubt, of the diagnosis before embarking on any treatment or any attempt to localize the tumour. This can only be achieved by demonstrating unequivocally that the hypoglycaemia is accompanied by inappropriately high insulin secretion, as indicated by the level of insulin in the peripheral blood.

LOCALIZATION OF INSULINOMAS

Although about 90% of insulinomas can be isolated at laparotomy, a proportion which varies with the experience of the surgeon remain impalpable. On account of the problem posed by these 'occult' tumours, great attention has been focused upon methods for their preoperative identification.

Before attempting to localize an insulinoma within the pancreas, three questions should be considered. Has the diagnosis been made with complete confidence? Is it necessary to localize the tumour preoperatively in this patient? Finally, which, if any, of the available methods for localization can be relied upon to give the correct answer? The first question has been discussed and the second will be considered at the end of this section. The last question, that of the best method, must be examined in some detail.

Arteriography

This was first used by Olsson in 1963[44], and since then there have been reports both for and against its efficacy. When injections of contrast are made by hand or hydraulic pump into the coeliac axis, between 38% and 50% of tumours will be shown[33,50]. It is, however, clear that radiographic technique is all-important and that when injections of contrast are made into more distal radicles of the coeliac trunk as many as eight out of ten insulinomas may be shown[7,19]. Results as good as this are exceptional and involve the use of high resolution X-ray equipment and insertion of a catheter into the pancreatico-duodenal arteries. This requires time and great expertise and carries the risk of extravasation of dye and pancreatitis. Our own experience of arteriography is disappointing[34]. We have used it in 18 patients, and in only 10 of these was localization correct. In 4 the tumour was missed and in another 4 the site indicated by arteriography was at variance with the operative findings (*Table 7.2*). In the 9 instances of correct localization the tumour

Table 7.2 The results of four localization techniques*

	Angiogram n = 18	Transhepatic portal venous sampling n = 8	Ultrasound n = 11	CT scan n = 8
Localization correct	9	2	2	1
Localization false	4	5	2	3
True negative investigation	1	0	3	2
False negative investigation	4	1	4	2
Total number of technically correct investigations	10	2	5	3

* Data of Le Quesne and Daggett.

was felt easily at operation and the results of the investigation were superfluous. In our opinion, arteriography now has a very limited place in attempts to localize an insulinoma, unless the services of a skilled and enthusiastic radiologist are available.

Transhepatic portal venous sampling of blood

This procedure (*see* Chapter 6), when performed and interpreted correctly, gives the highest chance of accurate localization. The portal vein is entered by percutaneous puncture of the liver and the needle is advanced until blood can be withdrawn freely (technical details are described by Reichardt and Ingemansson[49]).

A fine polypropylene catheter is advanced down the needle, which can then be removed. The catheter can be guided into the splenic vein and the various other large veins draining the pancreas, its position being checked under screening with small injections of contrast. By this means samples of blood are withdrawn from known points close to the pancreas and analyzed for their content of insulin or other peptide hormones[23]. From these results and a knowledge of the catheter position a map can be built up showing the concentration of insulin in the portal venous system (*Figure 7.3*). The concentration rises sharply near to the vein draining the insulinoma, with progressively lower levels nearer to the liver.

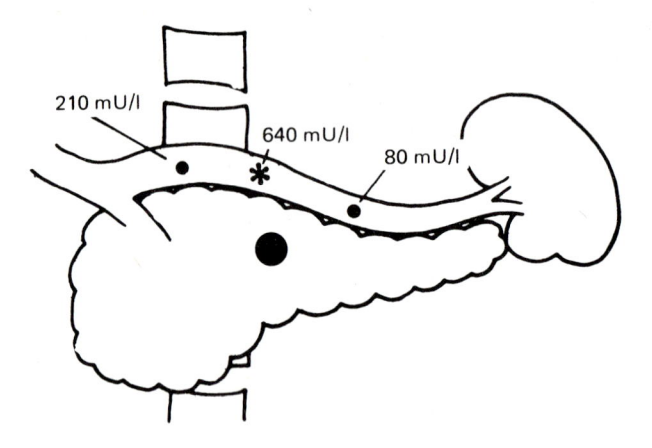

Figure 7.3 Diagrammatic representation of the findings of a transhepatic portal vein study, clearly indicating the site of the tumour (large closed circle). Note the magnitude of the peak. In the actual study more samples were taken than are represented in this diagram

When interpreting the results of this investigation, it is necessary to consider the radiological technique employed and the magnitude of the changes in insulin content within the portal system. The best results are obtained when the catheter samples are taken not only from the main portal and splenic veins but also from the inferior pancreatic and the several pancreatico-duodenal veins[42]. The concentrations of insulin in the veins draining the pancreas are normally much higher than in peripheral venous blood, as can be shown experimentally and deduced on theoretical grounds. Direct measurements in a number of species have shown a basal insulin secretion rate from the pancreas of 0.2 U/min per kg of body weight[14]. This is very similar to the production rate which can be calculated for man from indirect measurements.

The liver extracts 40% to 50% of the insulin from the blood on a single pass[14], but releases to the systemic circulation between 5.85 mU/min[62] and 9.5 mU/min[64]. The amount of insulin leaving the liver may thus be taken as the mean of these two figures, i.e. 7.68 mU/min. Allowing that half of the insulin delivered by the portal vein has been extracted, the production by the pancreas can be calculated as 15.35 mU/min (or, for a man of 70 kg, 0.22 mU/min per kg of body weight).

Pancreatic blood flow in man lies between 20 and 25 ml/min per 100 g of pancreatic tissue[15]. The adult human pancreas weighs 60 to 130 g, so that blood flows of 12.0 to 32.5 ml/min (mean 22.25 ml/min) might be expected. The insulin concentration in the veins draining the pancreas will thus be

$$\frac{\text{Total insulin production}}{\text{Total blood flow}} = \frac{15.35 \text{ mU/min}}{22.25 \text{ ml/min}} = 0.689 \text{ mU/ml} = 689 \text{ mU/l}$$

Pancreatic effluent blood enters the portal system by several large veins[49] and therein undergoes mixing by turbulent flow[9]. The portal vein carries 21 ± 4 ml (mean $\pm$ s.d.) of blood/min per kg of body weight[56], so that for an adult weighing 70 kg the flow would be 1470 ml/min. This will dilute the pancreatic effluent blood by a maximum factor of 66 by the time it reaches the liver. Accordingly, the concentration of insulin in the hepatic portal system can be as high as 689 mU/l close to a pancreatic vein, or as low as 10.4 mU/l at the hilum of the liver.

This presence of high insulin peaks in normal subjects, confirmed by Turner et al.[66], who recorded levels of over 500 mU/l, must be taken into account when interpreting results of this localization procedure for insulinomas. Failure to appreciate this may result in false claims to have localized the tumour, which we believe have been made by Pedrazzoli et al.[46] in 1980. We have been similarly misled ourselves in 5 of 8 patients in whom we have used the technique. We now believe that two conditions should be fulfilled. First, the procedure should be performed when the patient is fasted and does not have a glucose infusion running: this minimizes insulin production fron normal pancreatic tissue, but requires careful observation of the patient to forestall dangerous hypoglycaemia. Secondly, until there is clear evidence as to what constitutes a diagnostic peak, it is suggested that a value of 250 mU/l or more be considered significant, particularly if it is more than twice the level distal to it in the portal venous system. With these provisos transhepatic portal venous sampling has a high chance of localizing an insulin secreting tumour, but further experience is needed to define accurately the diagnostic criteria.

Intraoperative venous sampling

Cannulation of the splenic vein may be carried out under direct vision during laparotomy for removal of an insulinoma. Samples of blood may be analyzed in the operating theatre, using a special insulin assay which takes only 30 minutes[66]. A map can be built up as discussed previously, allowing identification of the insulinoma. Our experience, however, suggests that the surgeon can often find the tumour before the assay can even be set up. The technique has been rendered obsolete by the percutaneous transhepatic approach.

Other methods of localization

An attempt to make insulinomas more easily visible at operation was described by Keaveny, Tawes and Belzer[26] in 1971. They injected toluidine blue into the splenic and gastroduodenal arteries with the aim of producing *in vivo* staining of the tumour. This approach was not very successful and all the other methods of localization have used an imaging device. *Computerized tomography* (CT scanning) seldom produces first-class views of the pancreas. The difference in density between normal pancreas and an insulinoma is small[11], so that in view of the small size of most tumours only a minority can be expected to be detected by this technique. In our series of 8 patients scanned, a correct positive localization was made in only one (*see Table 7.2*). *Ultrasound* is equally disappointing and we have been able to show only two insulinomas correctly in a series of 11 patients examined. The resolution of ultrasound in the pancreas is of the order of 1 cm, and since many insulinomas are smaller than this it is not surprising that they were missed. Both ultrasound and CT scanning, however, may become more useful as the resolving power of the equipment improves. *Isotopic imaging* of the pancreas using selenomethionine is unreliable, even for diagnosis of large carcinomas, and is of no value in the detection of insulinomas. *Nuclear magnetic resonance* (NMR), the newest imaging technique, has not yet been applied to insulinomas. It can detect neoplasia within body cavities[45] and may eventually be useful for pancreatic tumours.

The place of localization

There is a high chance of an experienced surgeon being able to feel an insulinoma at operation, and in our own series this was the case in 26 of 27 tumours (*see Figure 7.1*). Stefanini *et al.*[59], however, have suggested that up to 10% of tumours may be impalpable and, based upon this type of experience, the recommendation has been made that preoperative localization should always be attempted[66]. The poor results from arteriography, CT scanning and ultrasound (*see Table 7.2*) indicate that these methods are seldom worth considering, unless one can obtain the help of a radiologist with particular interest and skill in the techniques required to demonstrate these small tumours by arteriography (*see above*). However, transhepatic portal venous sampling is a useful technique. In our opinion it is not indicated in all patients diagnosed as having an insulinoma, but should be performed (a) prior to the initial operation if the patient is intolerant to diazoxide (*see below*), or (b) before re-exploration in patients who have had a previous laparotomy which failed to reveal the tumour. The rationale for this approach is as follows: transhepatic sampling, a technique not free of complications, carries a 10–15% failure rate even in the best hands, while an experienced surgeon has a 90% chance of feeling the tumour. In the present state of experience with this technique, the use of this localization procedure prior to a laparotomy is therefore of doubtful value, except in the circumstances set out above, when the importance of removing the tumour at operation justifies an attempt to localize it by this means prior to laparotomy.

PRE- AND POSTOPERATIVE CARE

Once the diagnosis of insulinoma has been made, it is important to avoid further episodes of hypoglycaemia. This can be achieved by giving frequent high-carbohydrate snacks (including, if necessary, one at 3.00 a.m.) or with the drug diazoxide. This thiazide powerfully inhibits the release of insulin from the pancreatic islet β-cell and is effective in preventing episodes of hypoglycaemia when there is an insulinoma[4]. It may be used for long-term treatment when there is a contraindication to operation or when the tumour cannot be found at laparotomy, but some patients are intolerant to it. The main problem with diazoxide is that it can cause fluid retention, and this is usually manifest within 10 days of starting the drug. A trial of this substance should therefore be made in every patient with an insulinoma in order to detect those who will be intolerant[34]. If there are no problems, the surgeon knows that if he cannot locate the tumour, medical treatment will be possible. If there are side-effects, however, an attempt to localize the insulinoma prior to surgery should be made (see above). The initial dose of diazoxide is 50 mg three times a day, to be increased in increments of 50 mg until hypoglycaemic attacks are abolished. The maximum daily dose is 600 mg, but few patients require more than 300 mg daily.

During operation an infusion of 10% dextrose solution should be run to maintain the blood glucose concentration (measured every 15 min by Dextrostix) at, or above, 5 mmol/l. Immediately after removal of the insulinoma, the blood glucose level may rise and this has been claimed to be a useful pointer to the elimination of the abnormal source of insulin[13], but in our experience this rise may be slow to develop and is therefore not helpful whilst the patient is still on the operating table. In the postoperative period the blood glucose concentration should be measured every 2 hours during the first 24 hours, and less frequently thereafter, as indicated by the results. Mild diabetes is almost invariable, but only rarely needs treatment with insulin. It is caused by suppression of the normal pancreatic islets consequent upon the preceding hyperinsulinism, but usually resolves completely within 2 weeks[10].

As with any operation on the pancreas, there is a risk of serious complications. Stefanini et al.[60] reported 111 deaths in a series of 1076 patients, but our own mortality of 2 out of 29 individuals is probably more representative. Both deaths were from pancreatitis, the condition which was responsible for 37% of fatalities recorded by Stefanini. The other causes of death in that series included peritonitis (23%), respiratory failure (14%), hepatic failure (4%) and haemorrhage (4%). It is clear that mortality is substantially higher for re-exploration, and, indeed, one of our own fatalities followed a second laparotomy.

THE NEGATIVE LAPAROTOMY – WHAT TO DO

If the tumour cannot be found after mobilization and careful palpation of the pancreas[33] the surgeon must make the decision whether to abandon the effort and close the abdomen or to carry out a blind pancreatic resection. The role of the latter has been discussed by our group[40], and is now questionable. Simple resection of the body and tail will remove no more than 60% of occult insulinomas, and possibly many less.

Serial removal starting at the tail and working towards the body, combined with rapid but careful pathological examination, is no more successful. A rise in blood glucose level as the tumour is excised in this fashion is said to be helpful[29], but this approach has not been widely used.

If, at the first operation, the tumour cannot be found and it is known that hypoglycaemia can be prevented by diazoxide without deleterious side-effects, in our opinion the abdomen should be closed without resection of any pancreatic tissue and the patient treated with diazoxide. There is no evidence that the passage of time makes the insulinoma more easily palpable[59] so that there is no clear justification for a further laparotomy after any predetermined period, but a second attempt to locate and remove the tumour is clearly indicated if either the patient develops complications from the diazoxide or the symptoms can no longer be controlled by maximum dosage of the drug. Prior to this second operation transhepatic venous sampling should be performed (*see above*).

In our opinion blind distal pancreatectomy should only be performed (a) at the initial operation if the tumour cannot be located and it is known that the patient is intolerant to diazoxide, or (b) at the second operation if the tumour has not been located either by preoperative studies or at operation.

MALIGNANT INSULINOMAS

The usual histological criteria for malignancy cannot be applied to endocrine tumours in general or to those of the pancreas in particular, and the only sure sign is the presence of metastases. These are usually in the liver or local lymph nodes, deposits elsewhere being rather rare. Malignancy is not unusual in insulinomas, but probably not as common as the 10% incidence suggested[22,60] (Marks, personal communication). Malignant insulinomas produce frequent episodes of hypoglycaemia and the preceding history is likely to be shorter at the time of diagnosis than when the tumour is benign. Abdominal pain and weakness are common, but there are no specific features. Most malignant insulinomas are in the tail and body of the pancreas so that biliary obstruction seldom occurs[5]. Distinction between benign and malignant types cannot be made by biochemical testing, although the finding of chorionic gonadotrophin and its subunits in the blood is a useful pointer to the presence of a metastasizing tumour[24]. If at operation a malignant insulinoma is found, it should be removed if possible and consideration given to resection of hepatic metastases. This action alone may prolong survival from the untreated average of 1 year to 4 years[57]. Insulinomas are radio-resistant, but palliation can be achieved with the cytotoxic drug streptozotocin[21]. This has been given by intra-arterial infusion into branches of the coeliac axis, but this is unnecessary and good results can be obtained with intravenous administration. Streptozotocin causes irreversible damage to normal and neoplastic β-cells and can reduce tumour bulk in up to 50% of cases[5]. Its usefulness is, however, limited by renal and hepatic toxicity.

A major problem with malignant insulinomagly are continuing episodes of hypoglycaemia. These can be minimized by advising frequent, high-carbohydrate meals and by the use of diazoxide (*see p. 117*). When treating a malignant insulinoma, bendrofluazide (bendroflumethiazide) 10 mg daily should be given with the diazoxide in order to prevent problems of fluid retention. Other drugs, including phenytoin and corticosteroids, have been used to prevent insulin release from the tumour, but are generally unsuccessful. Similarly, conventional cytotoxic drugs such as cyclophosphamide, 5-fluorouracil and adriamycin have proved less successful than streptozotocin in reducing tumour bulk[26].

POSTOPERATIVE ASSESSMENT

Following the successful removal of an insulinoma, a temporary phase of mild glucose intolerance is common; the development of permanent diabetes is no more likely than in the general population. Hypoglycaemic attacks are abolished by removal of the abnormal insulin source and, if they recur postoperatively, indicate that a metastasis or second, benign tumour has been missed. Patients should be reassessed formally one month after surgery, at which time further measurements should be made of plasma glucose and insulin levels after overnight fasting: it should no longer be possible to demonstrate inappropriate hyperinsulinism at this time. After removal of a simple, benign insulinoma long-term follow-up is unnecessary, as 25-year review suggests that recurrence is very rare[58]. Patients, their families and medical advisers should, however, be warned to be on their guard for renewed symptoms.

Patients with a malignant insulinoma should of course be followed up indefinitely, and this is also advisable when there is a multiple endocrine neoplasia. In the latter case, regular review allows early detection not only of new insulinomas but also of the other endocrine syndromes which occur in this condition.

Acknowledgements

Many of the patients in the series which we describe were under the care of Dr J. D. N. Nabarro, whose knowledge and advice have been invaluable. We are indebted to Drs R. Turner and S. Bloom, and particularly to Professor V. Marks, for allowing us access to some of their data.

References

1 APPLEYARD, T. N. and LOSOWSKY, M. S. A pancreatic tumour with carcinoid syndrome and hypoglycaemia. *Postgraduate Medical Journal*, **46,** 159 (1970)

2 BEST, J. D., CHISHOLM, D. J. and ALFORD, F. B. Insulinoma: poor recognition of clinical features is the major problem in diagnosis. *Medical Journal of Australia*, **2,** 1–5 (1978)

3 BICKERSTAFF, E. R., DODGE, O. G., GOUREVITCH, A. and HEARN, G. W. Adenomatosis of the islets of Langerhans. *British Medical Journal*, **2**, 997 (1955)

4 BRITISH MEDICAL JOURNAL. Insulinomas (leading article). *British Medical Journal*, **1**, 927–928 (1981)

5 BRODER, L. E. and CARTER, S. K. Pancreatic islet cell carcinoma. I. Clinical features of 52 patients. *Annals of Internal Medicine*, **79**, 101 (1973)

6 CAYGILL, C. P. J., DAS, R. E. G. and BANGHAM, D. R. Use of a common standard for comparison of insulin C-peptide measurements by different laboratories. *Diabetologia*, **18**, 197 (1980)

7 CLOUSE, M. E., COSTELLO, P. and LEGG, M. A. Sub-selective angiography in localizing insulinomas of the pancreas. *American Journal of Roentgenology*, **128**, 741 (1977)

8 CREUTZFELDT, W., CREUTZFELDT, C., FRERICHS, H., TRACK, N. S. and ARNOLD, R. Histochemistry, ultrastructure and horomone content of human insulinomas. In *Hypoglycaemia* (Proceedings of European Symposium, Rome), edited by D. Andreani, P. J. Lefebvre and V. Marks, pp. 7–18. *Hormone and Metabolic Research Supplement Series*. Stuttgart, Georg Thieme Verlag (1976)

9 DREYER, B. Streamlining in the portal vein. *Quarterly Journal of Experimental Physiology*, **39**, 305 (1954)

10 DUNN, D. C. Diabetes after removal of insulin tumours of the pancreas: a long-term follow-up survey of 11 patients. *British Medical Journal*, **2**, 84 (1971)

11 DUNNICK, N. R., DOPPMAN, J. L., MILLS, S. R. and McCARTHY, D. M. Computed tomographic detection of non-beta pancreatic islet cell tumours. *Radiology*, **135**, 117–120 (1980)

12 FAJANS, S. S., SCHNEIDER, J. M., SCHTEINGART, D. E. and CONN, J. W. The diagnostic value of sodium tolbutamide in hypoglycaemia states. *Journal of Clinical Endocrinology and Metabolism*, **21**, 371–386 (1961)

13 FERRIS, D. O., MOLNAR, G. D., SCHNELLE, M., JONES, J. D. and MOFFITT, E. A. Recent advances in management of functioning islet cell tumour. *Archives of Surgery*, **1041**, 443–446 (1972)

14 FIELD, J. B. Insulin extraction by the liver. In *Handbook of Physiology*, **1**, (Section 7) American Physiological society (1972)

15 FOLKOW, B. and NEIL, E. *Circulation*, p. 468. Oxford University Press (1971)

16 FONKALSRUD, E. W., DILLEY, R. B. and LONGMIRE, W. P. Insulin secreting tumours of the pancreas. *Annals of Surgery*, **159**, 730–741 (1964)

17 FRERICHS, H. and CREUZFELDT, W. The intravenous tolbutamide test in the diagnosis of insulinoma. In *On the Intravenous Tolbutamide Test* (First Capri Conference), edited by W. Creutzfeldt and A. Czyzyk, pp. 163–173. Milan, Il Ponte (1967)

18 FRERICHS, H. and CREUTZFELDT, W. Insulin secreting tumours. *Clinics in Endocrinology and Metabolism*, **5**, 747–767 (1976)

19 GRAY, B. K., ROSCH, J. and GROLLMAN, J. H. Arteriography in the diagnosis of islet cell tumours. *Radiology*, **97**, 39–44 (1970)

20 HARRISON, T. S., CHILD, C. G., FRY, W. J., FLOYD, J. C. and FAJANS, S. S. Current surgical management of functioning islet cell tumours of the pancreas. *Annals of Surgery*, **178**, 485–495 (1973)

21 HERBAI, G. and LUNDIN, A. Treatment of malignant metastatic pancreatic insulinoma with streptozotocin. Review of 21 cases described in detail in the literature and report of complete remission in a new case. *Acta Medica Scandinavica*, **200**, 447–452 (1976)

22 HOWARD, J. M., MOSS, N. H. and RHOADES, J. E. Collective review. Hyperinsulinism and islet cell tumours of the pancreas with 398 recorded tumours. *Surgery, Gynecology and Obstetrics*, **90**, 417 (1950)

23 INGEMANSSON, S., LUNDERQUIST, A., LUNDQUIST, I., LOVDAHL, R. and TIBBLIN, S. Portal and pancreatic vein catheterization with radio-immunologic determination of insulin. *Surgery, Gynecology and Obstetrics*, **141**, 705–711 (1975)

24 KAHN, O. R., ROSEN, S. W., WEINTRAUB, B. D., FAJANS, S. S. and GORDEN, P. Ectopic production of chorionic gonadotrophin and its sub-units by islet cell tumours. *New England Journal of Medicine*, **297**, 565 (1977)

25 KAPLAN, E., RUBENSTEIN, A. H., EVANS, R., LEE, C. H. and KLEMENTSCHITSCH, P. Calcium infusion: a new provocative test for insulinomas. *Annals of Surgery*, **190**, 501 (1979)

26 KEAVENY, T. V., TAWES, R. and BELZER, F. O. A new method for intra-operative individualization of insulinomas. *British Journal of Surgery*, **58**, 233 (1971)

27 KUMAR, D., MEHTALIA, S. D. and MILLER, I. V. Diagnostic use of glucagon-induced insulin response. Studies in patients with insulinoma or other hypoglycaemic conditions. *Annals of Internal Medicine*, **80**, 697 (1974)

28 LAIDLAW, G. F. Nesidioblastoma, the islet cell tumour of the pancreas. *American Journal of Pathology*, **14**, 125 (1938)

29 LANDOR, J. H., LKACHKO, D. M. and LIE, T. H. Continuous monitoring of blood glucose during operation on islet cell adenomas. *Annals of Surgery*, **171**, 394 (1970)

30 LAROCHE, G. P., FERRIS, D. O., PRIESTLEY, J. T., SCHOLZ, D. A. and DOCKERTY, M. B. Hyperinsulinism: surgical results and management of occult functioning islet cell tumour: review of 154 cases. *Archives of Surgery*, **96**, 763 (1968)

31 LARSSON, L. I., GRIMELIUS, L., HAKANSON, R., REHFELD, J. F., STADL, F., HOLST, J., ANGERVALL, L. and SUNDER, J. Mixed endocrine pancreatic tumours producing several peptide hormones. *American Journal of Pathology*, **79**, 271 (1975)

32 LAURENT, J., DEBRY, G. and FLOQUET, J. *Hypoglycaemic Tumours*. Amsterdam, Excerpta Medica (1971)

33 LE QUESNE, L. P. Insulin tumours. In *Abdominal Operations*, edited by R. Maingot, p. 905. New York, Appleton-Century-Crofts (1980)

34 LE QUESNE, L. P., NABARRO, J. D. N., KURTZ, A. and ZWEIG, S. The management of insulin tumours of the pancreas. *British Journal of Surgery*, **66**, 373–378 (1979)

35 MARKS, V. Diagnosis of insulinoma. *Gut*, **12**, 385 (1971)

36 MARKS, V. and SAMOLS, E. Glucagon test for insulinoma: a chemical study of 25 cases. *Journal of Clinical Pathology*, **21**, 346 (1968)

37 MARKS, V. and SAMOLS, E. Insulinoma: natural history and diagnosis. *Clinics in Gastroenterology*, **3**, 559 (1974)

38 MARKS, V. and ROSE, F. C. *Hypoglycaemia*, ch. 7. Oxford, Blackwell (1981)

39 MARRACK, D., MARKS, V. and ROSE, F. C. A leucine-sensitive insulin-secreting tumour. *Lancet*, **2**, 1329 (1960)

40 MENGOLI, L. and LE QUESNE, L. P. Blind pancreatic resection for suspected insulinoma: a review of the problem. *British Journal of Surgery*, **54**, 748–756 (1967)

41 MERIMEE, T. J. and TYSON, J. E. Hypoglycaemia in man. Pathologic and physiologic variants. *Diabetes*, **24**, 161 (1977)

42 MILLAN, C. G., UROSA, C. L., MOLITCH, M. E., MILLER, H. and JACKSON, I. M. D. Localization of occult insulinoma by super-selective pancreatic venous sampling for insulin assay through percutaneous trans-hepatic catheterization. *Diabetes*, **28**, 249 (1979)

43 NELSON, R. L., SERVICE, F. J., ILSTROP, D. M. and GO, V. L. W. Are elevated pancreatic polypeptide levels in patients with insulinoma secondary to hypoglycaemia? *Lancet*, **2**, 659–661 (1980)

44 OLSSON, O. Angiographic diagnosis of an islet cell tumour of the pancreas. *Acta Chirurgica Scandinavica*, **126**, 346 (1963)

45 PARTAIN, C. L., JAMES, A. E. WATSON, J. T., PRICE, R. R., COULAM, C. M. and ROLLO, F. D. Nuclear magnetic resonance and computed tomography. *Radiology*, **136**, 767–770 (1980)

46 PEDRAZZOLI, S., FELTRIN, G., DODI, G., MIOTTO, D., PASTQUALI, C. and CEVESE, P. Usefulness of trans-hepatic portal vein catheterization in the treatment of insulinomas. *British Journal of Surgery*, **67**, 557–561 (1980)

47 PFEIFFER, D. B. and MILLER, D. B. Islet cell adenoma. 3 Cases, one extra-pancreatic, cured by operation. *Archives of Surgery*, **61**, 1096 (1950)

48 POLAK, J. M., ADRIAN, T. E., BRYANT, M. G., BLOOM, S. R., HEITZ, P. and PEARSE, A. G. E. Pancreatic polypeptide in insulinomas, gastrinomas, vipomas and glucagonomas. *Lancet*, **1**, 328–330 (1976)

49 REICHARDT, W. and INGEMANSSON, S. Selective vein catheterization for hormone assay in endocrine tumours of the pancreas. *Acta Radiologica Diagnostica*, **21**, 177–187 (1980)

50 ROBINS, J. M., BOOKSTEIN, J. J., OBERMAN, H. A. and FAJANS, S. S. Selective angiography in localizing islet cell tumours of the pancreas. *Radiology*, **106**, 525–528 (1973)

51 RUBENSTEIN, A. H., BLOCK, M. B., STARR, J., MELANT, F. and STEINER, D. F. Pro-insulin and C-peptide in the blood. *Diabetes*, **21** (Suppl. 2), 661–672 (1972)

52 RUBENSTEIN, A. H., MAKO, M. E., STARR, J. I., JOHN, D. S. and HORWITZ, D. L. Circulating pro-insulin in patients with islet cell tumours. In *Diabetes* (Proceedings of the Eighth Congress of the International Diabetes Federation), edited by W. J. Malaisse and J. Pirart, pp. 736–752. Amsterdam, Excerpta Medica (1973)

53 SADOFF, L., GORDON, J. and GOLDMAN, S. Amelioration of hypoglycaemia in a patient with malignant insulinoma during the development of the ectopic ACTH syndrome. *Diabetes*, **24**, 600 (1975)

54 SERVICE, F. J., DALE, A. J. G., ELVEBACK, L. R. and JIANG, N. S. Insulinoma: clinical and diagnostic features of 60 consecutive cases. *Mayo Clinic Proceedings*, **51**, 417–429 (1976)

55 SERVICE, F. J., HORWITZ, D. I., RUBENSTEIN, A. H., KUZUYA, H., MAKO, M. E., REYNOLDS, C. and MOLNAR, G. D. C-peptide suppression test for insulinoma. *Journal of Laboratory and Clinical Medicine*, **90**, 180 (1977)

56 SHERLOCK, S. *Diseases of the Liver and Biliary System*, ch. 9, p. 150. Oxford, Blackwell (1975)

57 SMRCKA, J., BRET, J., HAUER, J. and POLOMIS, V. Arteriography and successful removal of metastatic islet cell tumours in liver. *Diabetes*, **16,** 598 (1967)
58 SOGAARD, O. L. and AAGAARD, P. The results of surgical treatment of hyperinsulinism. *Danish Medical Bulletin*, **15,** 1 (1968)
59 STEFANINI, P., CARBONI, M., PATRASSI, N. and BASOLI, A. The surgical treatment of occult insulinomas: a review of the problem. *British Journal of Surgery*, **41,** 1 (1974)
60 STEFANINI, P., CARBONI, M., PATRASSI, N. and BASOLI, A. Beta cell tumours of the pancreas: results of a study of 1067 cases. *Surgery*, **75,** 597 (1974)
61 STELLON, A. and TOWNELL, N. H. C-peptide assay for factitious hyper-insulinism. *Lancet*, **2,** 148–149 (1979)
62 STERN, M. P., FARQUHAR, J. W., SIWERS, A. and REAVEN, G. M. Insulin delivery rate into plasma in normal and diabetic subjects. *Journal of Clinical Investigation*, **47,** 1947–1957 (1968)
63 SVED, S. McGILVERAY, I. J. and BEADOIN, N. Assay of sulphonylureas in human plasma by high performance liquid chromatography. *Journal of Pharmaceutical Sciences*, **65,** 1356–1359 (1976)
64 TURNER, R. C., GRAYBURN, J. A., NEWMAN, G. B. and NABARRO, J. D. N. Measurement of the insulin delivery rate in man. *Journal of Clinical Endocrinology and Metabolism*, **33,** 279–286 (1971)
65 TURNER, R. C. and HARRIS, E. Diagnosis of insulinomas by suppression tests. *Lancet*, **2,** 188–190 (1974)
66 TURNER, R. C., MORRIS, P. J., LEE, E. C. G., HARRIS, E. A. and DICK R. Localization of insulinomas. *Lancet*, **1,** 515–518 (1978)
67 VANCE, J. E., STOLL, R. W., KITABACHI, A. E., WILLIAMS, R. H. and WOOD, F. C. Nesidioblastosis in familial endocrine adenomatosis. *Journal of the American Medical Association*, **207,** 1679 (1969)
68 WALSH, C. H., WRIGHT, A. D. and COORE, H. G. Hypoglycaemia associated with an intrathoracic fibrosarcoma. *Clinical Endocrinology*, **4,** 393–398 (1975)
69 WRIGHT, J. and MARKS, V. Alcohol induced hypoglycaemia. *Advances in Experimental Medicine and Biology*, **126,** 479–483 (1980)
70 YAKOVAC, W. C., BAKER, L. and HUMMELER, K. Beta cell nesidioblastosis in idiopathic hypoglycemia of infancy. *Pediatrics*, **79,** 226 (1971)
71 YAGER, J. and YOUNG, R. T. Non-hypoglycaemia is an epidemic condition. *New England Journal of Medicine*, **291,** 907 (1974)

Editors' commentary on Chapter 7

This excellent review of insulin tumors of the pancreas emphasizes that the diagnosis of insulinoma or hypersecretion of insulin can be made with great accuracy today. We also consider the glucose/insulin ratio to be critical in establishing the diagnosis. Although we have assayed pro-insulin routinely, rather than C-peptide as described by the authors, each is equally valuable in addition to the measurement of insulin and glucose. We are pleased that the authors condemn the glucose tolerance test in screening patients for possible insulinomas and agree totally that it is usually of no value. We have also found suppression studies superfluous since glucose/insulin ratios and 72-hour fasts have become the tests accepted for definitive diagnosis.

Because localization is often not obtained by selective angiography we have become more enthusiastic and liberal in the use of percutaneous transhepatic venography with insulin sampling. With earlier diagnosis, more occult islet cell tumors are being discovered after conventional techniques for localization. It is our current feeling that, when angiography is negative, percutaneous transhepatic venography should be done prior to exploration. In addition, because of the increased incidence of multiplicity and microadenomatosis in patients with the MEN I syndrome, we believe that all such patients with organic hyperinsulinism should be studied regardless of the arteriographic findings. We agree that by careful exploration an experienced surgeon will discover most insulinomas at the time of operation when the disease is sporadic. This may not be true in MEN I patients, however, because of the high incidence of microadenomatosis. In some of these cases, hyperplasia, nesidioblastosis or multiple small adenomas can be diagnosed preoperatively by the transhepatic venous assay technique and a subtotal pancreatectomy appropriately planned.

8
Pancreatic transplantation
Paul McMaster

In 1922 the historic work by Banting and Best allowed a crude canine pancreatic extract to be used in the treatment of diabetes mellitus[3]. For the first time deaths in acute ketoacidotic coma could be prevented, and juvenile diabetics thrived instead of wasting away. The further refinement and development of purified insulin appeared to herald the end of diabetes as a major health problem. However, as many of these young diabetics entered middle age, it became clear that exogenous insulin administration alone would not control the ravages of diabetes[22].

THE PROBLEM OF DIABETES

Many of these diabetic patients developed progressive deterioration in small blood vessels, with thickening of the basement membrane and eventual vascular occlusion, in spite of careful dietary control and insulin injection. Some became blind, while others developed cardiac and cerebrovascular problems[22]. Peripheral vascular disease with gangrene requiring amputation became frequent, and impaired nerve function resulted in peripheral neuropathies, autonomic bladders and gastrointestinal problems. These difficulties, coupled with the increased risk of major infection, led to a much increased morbidity and age-related mortality[14], and often to death from renal failure.

Diabetes affects some 3% of the American population and is now the third commonest cause of death in the USA[3]. In Great Britain it is currently the commonest cause of new cases of blindness[22].

The failure of insulin injections alone to prevent these problems has led to studies to develop more successful and more sophisticated forms of diabetes management.

While a number of factors are clearly important in the development of progressive arterial destruction, the hypothesis has long been held that the microangiopathic devastation is in part related to disordered carbohydrate metabolism and that 'perfect control' would prevent or delay its development[23, 66, 75, 90]. While this probably represents an oversimplification, considerable effort is now being expended by clinicians to reduce the wide variations in carbohydrate control that occur on conventional insulin treatment. Newer insulin delivery systems with constant infusions by pumps are being introduced more widely clinically.

Is there really evidence that this hypothesis is true? Would perfect control prevent the progression of renal damage and vascular lesions? Increasing evidence suggests that this may be so. Firstly, extensive experimental studies have shown that the restoration of carbohydrate control by pancreas transplantation may delay or halt microangiopathic lesions in diabetic animals; in some models diabetic lesions actually disappear[32, 61, 100]. Secondly, diabetic patients transplanted with 'non-diabetic kidneys' soon develop renal glomerulosclerotic lesions[71], and patients made diabetic following major pancreatic surgery also develop retinal and renal microangiopathic complications[9, 17, 21]. Thirdly, clinical studies suggest that in some groups of insulin-requiring diabetics the onset and severity of microngiopathic lesions is directly related to the degree of control of their diabetes[41, 59, 66, 75].

Wide fluctuations of carbohydrate metabolism occur during conventional diabetic treatment[69], which is clearly unable to prevent major complications. If in the 1500 new cases of juvenile diabetes mellitus diagnosed each year in this country these major difficulties are to be avoided, then improved methods of management are urgently required.

The goal of pancreatic transplantation is total pancreatic endocrine replacement and re-establishment of islet function with the production of normal carbohydrate control and prevention of microangiopathic lesions.

PANCREATIC TISSUE IMPLANTATION

The original crude extracts of pancreatic tissue were obtained from the dog after exocrine obliteration by duct ligation, and several workers endeavoured to develop this approach for pancreatic fragment extraction and subsequent reimplantation. Tissues were reinjected into the groin or axilla of dogs[80], or the anterior chamber of the eye in mice[8]. In rats the testes were injected[20], and neonatal tissue was transplanted into the cheek pouch of the adult hamster made diabetic with alloxan[37]. Transient control of hyperglycaemia was achieved in a few of these models, but long-term successful implants were rare. More significant success was achieved when tissue extracted from duct-ligated rats was implanted into the anterior chamber of the eye, both as autografts and allografts[38].

Active programmes of research continue in rodent islet extraction and transplantation using various sources of islets (foetal, neonatal or adult islets) and altering the degree of purification (purified islet extracts or unpurified pancreatic tissue) in an attempt to improve the yield of islets and reduce their susceptibility to immunological destruction.

Pancreatic tissue preparation

Preparation of isolated adult islets of Langerhans

The progressive development in the techniques of islet extraction in rodents has allowed relatively reproducible techniques to be established.

Prior to islet extraction the acinar tissue is disrupted by retrograde injection of cold Hanks solution into the pancreatic duct via the common bile duct[49]. This forced disruption is followed by rapid chopping of the pancreatic tissue into small fragments and subsequent digestion with collagenase[70]. Following digestion and repeated washings, the islets can be separated from the residual tissue by centrifugation in Ficoll density gradient column, or they can be hand-picked using a dissecting microscope[27]. However, the yield of islet tissue is poor and as many as four donors are required to yield more than 1000 islets, not all of which will be functioning satisfactorily.

With minor modifications the same technique has been used in larger animals, although with less success. The dense, fibrous nature of the pancreatic tissue in the dog, monkey or human makes extraction more difficult and yields have tended to be even lower.

More recently the venous disruption technique in dogs has resulted in higher yields and this may prove a more reliable and successful method[16].

Alternative approaches

The poor yield of adult islet extraction and the major difficulties of harvesting purified islets have led to attempts at pancreatic tissue harvesting without individual identification of the islets. This technique has been used successfully in adult animals and using dispersed foetal and neonatal pancreatic tissue. The exocrine tissue can also be made to atrophy before attempts at separation from the islets by prior duct ligation, or by administration of pilocarpine or DL-ethionine, resulting in improved yields of viable islets[74]. In dogs prior treatment may not be necessary, as Mirkovitch and Campiche[67] were able to re-establish normoglycaemia after reimplantation of minced and collagenase-digested unpurified pancreatic tissue directly into the splenic pulp.

In *neonatal pancreatic tissue* there is a relatively lower exocrine activity and a high islet content. Minced and collagenase-digested neonatal tissue without separation could successfully be transplanted in mice, although the preparation technique and tissue dispersal time appear critical[57, 58].

Foetal pancreatic extraction techniques have also been studied and the ratio of endocrine tissue mass to exocrine enzyme activities appears favourable[7]. One foetal pancreas placed beneath the renal capsule and allowed to mature could ameliorate diabetes in the recipient[25, 81].

Results of experimental pancreas tissue transplantation

Adult islet transplantation

The last decade has seen numerous attempts to transplant isolated islets[2, 49, 70, 78]. Transplantation between genetically identical animals (isografting) was shown to be successful when islets were placed intraperitoneally in streptozotocin-induced diabetic animals, although a large number of donors were required. By increasing the number of transplanted islets the degree of carbohydrate control was also improved. However, the direct intraportal injection of embolized adult islets into the liver has proved to be most successful in rats[44]. In isografts, intraportal injection of over 1000 islets will re-establish normoglycaemia, with normal glucose tolerance curves and insulin levels[44, 56, 98]. Animals thrive, gain weight and do not develop microvascular complications[95]. Furthermore, some studies have shown that pre-existing diabetic complications do not progress, and may actually improve significantly[32, 60].

In rats the embolized islets lodge in the liver and produce limited hepatocyte dysfunction, but no serious long-term liver disruption occurs[33].

In larger animals extraction of islets has proved difficult and the viability yield has been poor[79]. The use of multiple donors is also less feasible. Mild diabetic states after pancreatectomy can, however, be improved in dogs by intraportal or intrasplenic embolization[24, 26, 46]. In monkeys improved carbohydrate control has also been achieved, but no truly normoglycaemic animals have been established[79].

While technical problems remain in large animals and man, of more fundamental importance is the apparent marked susceptibility of islets to immunological destruction when transplantation between strains is undertaken (allografts)[45, 73, 89].

In non-immunosuppressed allografts transplanted across weak or strong histocompatibility barriers, islet destruction by immunological activity is rapid. Across strong histocompatibility barriers, such as Fischer to ACI, normoglycaemia was re-established for only 2–3 days, a much shorter time than in other transplanted organs[73]. However, as rejection of islets has usually been defined as a return of hyperglycaemia, the number of functioning viable islets transplanted may be critical. Even so, it does seem that islets are destroyed more rapidly following transplantation than whole organs.

A number of attempts have been made to delay this rejection. Non-specific immunosuppressive agents seem less capable of delaying rejection of isolated islets; corticosteroids, cyclophosphamide and azathioprine produce only limited prolongation of grafts[4, 77, 99]. Antilymphocytic serum has been more successful in rodents[99], and the initial results of total lymphoid irradiation are encouraging[77]. It is perhaps disappointing that cyclosporin A seems no more effective than other agents[28] in preventing islet damage, particularly in view of its success in whole organ pancreas grafts[64].

Islets matured by prior culture under the renal capsule or *in vitro* may be less susceptible to damage because of their altered immune reaction[1]. Although results are somewhat conflicting, pre-culture may in some animal models also reduce islet destruction[42, 50].

Yet another approach has been to encapsulate islets in diffusion chambers intraperitoneally in an effort to isolate and protect them, and control of hyperglycaemia has been achieved experimentally[12, 91].

HUMAN ISLET TRANSPLANTATION

With the increasing development of animal models for islet preparation and separation it was natural that attempts should be made in man to overcome the problems of diabetes by islet transplantation. However, by and large the results have been disappointing[85, 86]. The basic collagenase digestion technique has been used and, although more difficult in man because of the fibrous nature and size of the gland, viable islets can be harvested. Yields have, however, been inconsistent, and, as multiple donors are impracticable, the standard Ficoll separation technique does not appear to yield consistently sufficient quantities of purified islets. Allografts seem particularly susceptible to immunological destruction and there have been few successes.

The best technique for islet extraction in man has yet to be established; currently most centres rely on unpurified pancreatic tissue obtained by collagenase techniques similar to those used in animal models *without* individual isolation and identification of islets.

Human pancreas autografting of unpurified pancreatic tissue

Chronic pancreatitis may require surgical treatment to control the complications of disease and relieve the intractable pain sometimes associated with chronic calcific pancreatitis. The removal of more than 90% of the pancreatic mass, leaving only the duodenal rim, will usually relieve the pain, although at a relatively high metabolic price. Exocrine insufficiency may require supplements, and many patients become frankly diabetic and require insulin. In these patients successful islet autografting would provide valuable metabolic support and avoid the particularly brittle and potentially unstable diabetes which may occur, and should not be hindered by immunological difficulties.

Unfortunately, islet preparations from the diseased pancreas have proved unreliable and the variable quantity of residual pancreatic tissue by the duodenum has made interpretation of the metabolic profiles achieved difficult[72, 82].

So far, 58 patients have undergone islet autotransplantation following total or near-total pancreatectomy, with the majority of cases undertaken in Genoa, Minnesota and Baltimore[82]. Valente *et al.*[97] have implanted autografts of unpurified pancreatic tissue into the portal vein following collagenase digestion in 16 patients. In 11 patients the graft was reimplanted immediately and in 5 cases implantation occurred after culture of pancreatic tissue for between 2 and 7 days. No exogenous insulin was required in 10 of these patients. The experience of other units has been less encouraging: only a third of the patients became insulin-independent and, again, there was the difficulty of assessing the role of the residual pancreas. However, insulin independence has been demonstrated following autografting in totally pancreatectomized patients, and in 2 patients insulin measurements of portal blood clearly showed no significant residual remnant activity[84].

However, in man the technique may not be as safe as in animals. An increase in portal pressure and deranged hepatocyte function have been reported, and on at least two occasions injections of unpurified pancreatic tissues have been followed by fatal disseminated intravascular coagulopathy[65, 68].

Foetal allografts

The success of foetal islet transplantation in animals has also encouraged early human studies in which foetal tissue has been harvested and transplanted. Groth et al.[34] in Stockholm have repeatedly infused islets into the portal system, although normoglycaemia could not be achieved.

Valente et al.[96] placed extracts of foetal pancreas in 11 patients intramuscularly and in 2 patients intraportally. Graft activity was assessed by insulin requirements and C-peptide contents. Somewhat varied responses were encountered, but more than 1 year after injection one patient still requires no exogenous insulin.

Unpurified pancreas allografts in man

Islet allografts used in man have been obtained by a number of tissue preparation techniques[87], but of 69 patients, who received 73 transplants, only 4 became insulin-independent[82].

In the first patient in Bordeaux, no immunosuppressive treatment was given, but the very short history of diabetes (less than 1 year) and the relatively high basic endogenous insulin levels make this case difficult to evaluate. Largiader, Kolb and Binswanger have, however, been able to withdraw insulin completely from a long-standing diabetic following intrasplenic injection of unpurified pancreas extract, although insulin was required in the first 3 months after transplantation[52]. Valente has treated 2 patients who became insulin-independent following allografting (personal communication). In the Minnesota study of 13 patients, none became insulin-independent, although in those with intraportal embolization insulin requirements were reduced[87].

This very low level of success in man is a clear reminder of the problems of transferring techniques developed for animal models to human clinical programmes. Failure may be due to the fundamental immunological difficulties, but the techniques of harvesting and preservation will need further development before the role of allografts in clinical transplantation can be truly assessed. In addition, the site of islet or unpurified tissue implantation will need to be carefully reviewed.

In man, elevated portal pressure has followed intraportal infusion and the fatal cases of disseminated intravascular coagulopathy clearly must give rise to caution[65, 84]. The intrasplenic or intramuscular routes would appear to present a safer approach, but how successful they are remains to be seen.

It would seem wise at this time to limit islet transplantation until successful techniques have been established in large animal *allograft* models.

ENDOCRINE SURGERY

Pancreas organ transplantation

Shortly following the work of Banting and Best[3] which so clearly demonstrated the role of the pancreas in the re-establishment of normoglycaemia the first attempts at experimental organ pancreas transplantation were undertaken. Using a tube anastamotic technique Gayet[29] was able to reduce the serum glucose of diabetic dogs for 12 hours after organ replacement. Subsequently vascular suture techniques were introduced and the combined approach of pancreatico-duodenal grafting slowly developed. In 1967 Largiader et al.[53] performed the first successful pancreatic duodenal graft in dogs.

Following the clinical introduction of non-specific immunosuppressive agents, the 1960s saw the early attempts at pancreas grafting in man. The first human pancreas transplant was performed in 1966 at the University of Minnesota by Kelly et al.[43]. This segmental pancreas allograft developed pancreatitis and a pancreatic fistula and ultimately failed; subsequent transplants in this initial series consisted of combined renal and pancreatico-duodenal allografts[54].

The 10 years following this first human pancreas transplant saw 57 pancreas grafts performed in 56 patients, predominantly in Minnesota, New York, Stockholm and London[82]. However, it soon became clear that the laboratory techniques which had been developed were not always satisfactory in man, with major problems developing due to exocrine pancreatic leakage and infection. Mortality in these immunosuppressed uraemic diabetics was high, and 52% of patients died shortly after transplantation. Only three grafts functioned for longer than one year[82]. The longest patient and graft survival was just over 4 years[31, 82].

These disappointing results led one early worker to comment that 'while islet transplantation was safe, it was ineffective. However, pancreas (organ) transplantation was metabolically efficient but dangerous'[51].

While the major problem confronting pancreas transplantation is immunological, too many of these early human attempts failed for purely technical reasons. New attempts had to be made in the laboratory to reduce the incidence of complications related to exocrine leakage and infection.

Recent laboratory studies of organ pancreas transplantation

The experimental vascular techniques are now well established, with the blood supply to the pancreas derived from the coeliac axis or splenic artery, and the venous return via the splenic and portal vein. Segmental grafting using this technique in the dog reduces the pancreatic haemodynamic flow, and vascular thrombosis is common[13]. Haemodynamic studies have suggested that a distal splenic artery to splenic vein fistula may improve blood flow and thus reduce thrombosis[10].

Studies were also undertaken to develop improved techniques for the control of exocrine secretion. These may be broadly divided into two categories:

(1) Ductal drainage techniques
(2) Ductal occlusion

PANCREATIC DUCTAL DRAINAGE TECHNIQUES

The initial attempts at exocrine drainage used the adjacent duodenum as a draining conduit to the exterior or into the bowel of the recipient animal, or the pancreas drained into a Roux-en-Y loop. Other intra-abdominal visceral drainage techniques were evaluated but most gave disappointing results in allografts, with duodenal necrosis, bleeding or infection[5, 40, 76, 93]. Recent studies using non-steroid immunosuppression have failed to reduce this relatively high incidence of duodenal breakdown[62].

Open duct drainage into the peritoneum has been established successfully in animals after pancreas transplantation. Pancreas enzymes draining directly into the peritoneal cavity are not activated by duodenal enzymes and in dogs did not produce serious complications[47]. The peritoneal cavity appears able to absorb the exocrine secretion, and pancreas allografts have been transplanted experimentally in animals with a low morbidity. In the intraperitoneal duct open technique, serum amylase levels are raised initially, but the pancreatic secretion diminishes gradually as the main duct closes, and amylase levels return to normal[48].

DUCT OCCLUSION

The technique of duct ligation in the transplanted graft has not proved successful[92], because of breakdown, leakage, or deterioration in islet function[39, 92]. However, its concept has led to studies in which complete ductal occlusion is accomplished by direct intraductal injection of an occluding agent. A number of synthetic polymers have been developed which will solidify after ductal injection and occlude even the minor ductuals, thus preventing leakage and leading to progressive exocrine atrophy and fibrosis. Dubernard *et al.* injected neoprene into the pancreatic duct *in situ* in the dog, which resulted in satisfactory endocrine function even in the presence of severe pancreatic acinar fibrosis[18, 19]. Kyriakides, Miller and Nuttal found this technique in transplanted diabetic animals to be associated with a low incidence of complications, although histological examination showed persistent inflammation and altered islet morphology[47]. Other occluding agents have been developed (prolamine[30], acrylic glues[55] and polyisoprene[64]), and duct injection has proved satisfactory in transplanted, immunosuppressed diabetic animals[64].

While laboratory research has continued in an effort to reduce technical problems, further attempts have been made to reduce the incidence of graft rejection. Non-immunosuppressed canine pancreas allografts are destroyed within a few days. The use of azathioprine, corticosteroids and antilymphocytic serum (ALS) in grafts not failing for technical reasons may extend graft survival for a short period[11, 15]. Total lymphoid irradiation, which has proved successful in other organ grafts, has now also been demonstrated to prolong pancreas graft survival.

However, the metabolic advantages of pancreas transplantation may be lost if corticosteroids are needed in high doses because of the disturbing action on carbohydrate control. Recent studies have shown significant prolongation of pancreas grafting with cyclosporin A, a non-steroid fungal metabolite[63, 64].

These laboratory developments, both in technique and in immunosuppressive management, are currently being evaluated clinically in several centres.

CURRENT PANCREAS TRANSPLANTATION IN MAN

During the last 3 years organ pancreas transplantation in man has been confined to segmental pancreas grafting.

While the ultimate goal of pancreas transplantation remains the successful total replacement of pancreatic endocrine function with a normal serum glucose and the prevention of microangiopathic complications, we remain some distance from this ultimate objective. Relatively few patients have been transplanted with a pancreas graft alone and the results have proved disappointing[35].

Patient selection

At present pancreas transplantation is usually confined to long-standing diabetics with major systemic complications including renal failure. Two approaches are being evaluated currently: (1) the combined renal and segmental pancreas graft; and (2) the delayed pancreas graft in successfully established renal transplant recipients.

The delayed pancreas graft, undertaken mainly at the University of Minnesota, has been performed between 6 months and 6 years after successful renal allografting. The pancreas graft has been used in young diabetic patients with renal allografts which show signs of microangiopathic deterioration. This delayed technique has the advantage of allowing a period of evaluation of the immunosuppressed diabetic patient with an organ graft, and, by simply grafting one organ at a time, may be associated with a lower surgical morbidity. It has also allowed, for the first time, donation from siblings or parents of live segments of pancreatic tissue[97].

Technique of combined pancreas and kidney transplantation

Donor

The pancreas is harvested from the donor at the time of removal of the kidney. Prior to laparotomy the donor is pretreated with 200 ml of 20% mannitol and fluid loading, aprotinin (Trasylol) 500 000 units intravenously, and heparin 10 000 IU.

After initial laparotomy both kidneys are fully mobilized and their vascular pedicle is dissected to their aortic and inferior vena caval origins. Each kidney is then removed in turn and preserved with hypertonic citrate at 4 °C. While maintaining donor circulation, attention is then directed to the pancreas. The gastrocolic omentum is divided, exposing the lesser sac and the anterior aspect of the pancreas. Mobilization of the spleen and tail of the pancreas allows identification of the distal splenic artery and splenic vein. Dissection at the lower border of the pancreas allows identification of the inferior mesenteric vein, which is ligated. Dissection above the pancreas identifies the splenic vein and coronary vein at its insertion to the portal vein. The coeliac axis is identified through the lesser omentum, and the hepatic artery, left gastric and splenic vessels are dissected free of lymphatic and neural tissues.

After transection of the neck of the pancreas the main pancreatic duct can be identified and intubated using a 14 Portex cannula, which is tied in place. The organ is then excised on its vascular pedicle and perfused initially with 250 ml of hypertonic citrate at 4 °C. Direct ductal instillation with natural latex polyisoprene is then undertaken until white speckles appear on the surface of the gland, indicating that the smallest ducts have filled. Between 4 and 6 ml of polyisoprene are required to occlude the ductal system completely.

Recipient operation

Prior to anaesthetic induction the recipient diabetic patient is given 500 000 units of Trasylol intravenously. Throughout the operation blood sugar control is maintained with a constant insulin infusion, and blood glucose is measured hourly. Following a standard renal transplantation, the iliac vessels on the opposite side are exposed and segmental pancreatic transplantation is undertaken. The coeliac axis or splenic artery is anastomosed directly end-to-side to the external iliac artery, and the splenic vein end-to-side to the external iliac vein. A window of peritoneum is opened, allowing part of the segmental graft to lie intraperitoneally with an omental wrap, and the wound is then closed with a single drain. In patients on continuous ambulatory peritoneal dialysis the omentum may have been removed and in this case the graft should be placed intraperitoneally so that any small leakage can be absorbed. Postoperatively, blood sugar is estimated hourly, and after 24 hours 4-hourly, and trasylol infusion is continued for 5 days. A continuous insulin infusion is continued until the blood glucose falls below 8 mmol/l.

Results

The present approach to segmental pancreas transplantation, based on newer technical and immunological developments, has resulted in a marked reduction in patient morbidity and mortality, although the techniques are yet far from perfect. Of 51 patients transplanted since 1977, only 10 have died of causes related to the transplantation, although, because of the advanced nature of the diabetic disease, only 34 patients are currently alive[97]. At present there are 3 patients whose pancreas grafts are functioning after more than 2 years and 16 with successful grafts for less than that period.

Successful techniques of open ductal drainage into the peritoneal cavity have proved difficult to establish in man. Of the 13 patients who received open duct grafts in Minnesota between 1978 and 1980, 4 developed ascites, peritonitis and systemic infection[97]. While in some patients peritoneal reaction was limited, the results of intraperitoneal implantation seem unpredictable. In contrast, ductal polymer injection has been associated with a lowering of morbidity and relatively few wound infections or leakages. However, the failure of some grafts more than 6 months after transplantation may in part be related to progressive dysfunction due to chronic pancreatic fibrosis[83,94]. In addition, one graft from an identical twin failed shortly after transplantation, following prolamine injection, with the gland showing intense interstitial fibrosis (Sutherland, personal communication). However, technical problems have been far fewer than in earlier series, and prevention of pancreatic rejection has now become the major clinical problem. The combined use of azathioprine, corticosteroids and ALS does not always prevent rejection, and so it is encouraging that cyclosporin A continues to show promise in preventing graft rejection. In our own recent studies of combined kidney and pancreas grafting, 4 of 8 pancreas grafts established without major technical problems functioned for more than 5 months, with patients requiring no exogenous insulin at all. One graft failed after 12 months, and 2 patients still have excellent pancreas and kidney function over 2 years after transplantation, without carbohydrate restriction or the need for exogenous insulin.

Metabolic effects of pancreas transplantation

The segmental pancreas graft is usually placed heterotopically on the iliac artery and vein, and thus insulin drains not into the portal vein and liver directly but into the systemic circulation. Experimental studies originally suggested that this heterotopic position, combined with a denervated gland, might result in altered carbohydrate physiology, with high systemic insulin levels and early relative hypoglycaemia[43]. Blood glucose and insulin studies after glucose tolerance tests were, however, conflicting[43,76]. Bewick et al. recently suggested that plasma glucose levels were in fact normal whether the pancreas graft was replaced orthotopically or heterotopically and that the liver was able to compensate for the route by which insulin arrived[6].

Human metabolic studies of the effects of pancreas transplants placed heterotopically have been limited, and their interpretation is difficult because of the different techniques used and the addition of corticosteroids. Following segmental transplantation, Gunnarsson et al.[36] observed near-normal serum glucose concentrations until rejection, and covariation of C-peptide and glucose, indicating an adequate feed-back mechanism. C-peptide estimation was used to differentiate between different causes of hyperglycaemia. They also observed a rise in postprandial blood glucose several days prior to graft rejection[36].

Sutherland, Rynasiewiz and Najarian[88] carried out metabolic studies after segmental grafting in patients whose serum C-peptide levels were less than 1 ng/ml (normal 2.5–10 mg/ml), with negligible urinary C-peptide excretion. Following successful grafting, serum C-peptide was normal and urinary C-peptide was normal or high, although this was clearly influenced by steroid administration. One of these patients had had a renal graft 6 years prior to pancreas grafting, and biopsy at the time of pancreas transplantation showed marked features of diabetic nephropathy. A biopsy of the same kidney 2 years after pancreas transplantation showed a clear decrease in the degree of mesangiomatrix thickening and intensity of staining of protein (Sutherland, personal communication).

Traeger et al.[94] noted delay and prolongation of the glucose tolerance curves after transplantation, which deteriorated further with time, although peripheral serum insulin and C-peptide levels were normal or high. Polyneuritis improved and nerve conduction velocity was accelerated after pancreas transplantation.

In patients with long-standing, insulin-requiring diabetes receiving combined grafts in the absence of steroid immunosuppression, McMaster et al.[23] noted near-normal 24-hour glucose serum profiles and a progressive fall in haemoglobin A,C. All exogenous insulin could be withdrawn although glucose tolerance tests showed a high glucose peak, with prolongation and elevation over 6 months after transplantation. A high fasting C-peptide was also noted, as well as an initial delay and subsequent elevation in C-peptide response to glucose challenge. Other metabolic profiles showed a similar pattern of glucose control, with a rise in postprandial lactate, a fall in glycerol concentration, and higher fasting β-hydroxybutyrate concentration.

THE FUTURE

Technical difficulties are slowly being overcome and improved methods of immunosuppression have led to a marked reduction in the morbidity and mortality of pancreas transplantation. With increased experience, earlier and better patient selection, and improved management, complications should be reduced further. As more patients are transplanted successfully the role of combined kidney and pancreas transplants or delayed pancreas grafting in diabetics in renal failure will become more clearly established. What is, however, already clear is that successful grafting obviates the need for exogenous insulin and frees the patient from the restrictions of dietary control. The influence of this liberation on morale and rehabilitation should not be overlooked in patients who have often had long periods of restricted activity and diet because of their renal failure and diabetes. Further studies will also show if the level of carbohydrate metabolism established in these patients will prevent or delay the progress of microangiopathic complications. If this does indeed happen then it will have played an important role in the management of diabetics in renal failure and given a valuable insight into the mechanism of microangiopathic complications.

However, before pancreas transplantation can be considered seriously in the management of insulin-dependent diabetics without renal failure, both the surgical techniques and immunosuppression must offer less risk than the outcome of the diabetic condition itself.

While pancreas organ transplantation is still at a relatively early stage of its development, progress during these last few years suggests that it may have a major role to play in the management of diabetes in the future.

Islet transplantation, however, which is a more attractive alternative aesthetically, still has to grapple with fundamental problems of islet cell procurement, storage and protection from aggressive rejection before its clinical application can be fully evaluated.

References

1 ANDERSON, A. and BOSCHARD, F. Culture of isolated pancreatic islets: its application for transplantation progress. *Transactions of the American Society for Artificial Internal Organs*, **23**, 342–345 (1977)

2 BALLINGER, W. F. and LACY, P. E. Transplantation of intact pancreatic islets in rats. *Surgery*, **72**, 175–186 (1972)

3 BANTING, F. G. and BEST, C. H. The internal secretion of the pancreas. *Journal of Laboratory and Clinical Medicine*, **7**, 251–266 (1922)

4 BELL, R. N., FERNANDEZ-CRUZ, L., BRIMM, J., LEE, S., SAYERS, H. and DELOFF, M. J. Prevention of glomerular basement membrane thickening in alloxan-diabetes. *Surgery*, **88**, 31–40 (1980)

5 BERGAN, J. J., HOEHN, J. G., PORTER, N. and DOG, L. Total pancreatic allografts in pancreatectomized dogs. *Archives of Surgery*, **90**, 521–526 (1965)

6 BEWICK, M., MUNDY, A. R., EATON, B. and WATSON, F. The endocrine function of heterotopic pancreatic allotransplantation in dogs. Normal and rejection. *Transplantation*, **31**, 15–18 (1981)

7 BROWN, J., CLARK, W. R., MOLNAR, G. and MULLEN, Y. S. Foetal pancreas transplantation for research of streptozotocin induced diabetes in rats. *Diabetes*, **25**, 56–64 (1976)

8 BROWNING, H. and RESNICK, P. Homologous and heterologous transplantation of pancreatic tissue in normal and diabetic mice. *Biology and Medicine*, **24**, 141 (1951)

9 BURTON, T. Y., KEARNS, T. P. and RYNEARSON, E. H. Diabetic retinopathy following total pancreatectomy. *Mayo Clinic Proceedings*, **32**, 735–739 (1957)

10 CALNE, R. Y., McMASTER, P., ROLLES, K. and DUFFY, T. J. Technical observation in segmental pancreas allografting; observations on pancreatic blood flow. *Transplantation Proceedings*, **13**(4) (Suppl. 2), 51–61 (1980)

11 CASTELLANOS, J., MANIFACIA, G., TOLEDO-PEREYRA, L. H., SHATNEY, C. H. and LILLEHEI, R. C. Consistent protection from pancreatisation in canine pancreas allografts treated with 5-fluorouracil. *American Journal of Surgery*, **19**, 305–311 (1975)

12 CHICK, W. L., PERRIS, J. J., LAURIS, V., LOW, D., CALLETT, P. M., PAWO, G., WHITTEMORE, A. D., LIKE, A. L., COTTON, C. K. and LYSAGHT, M. J. Artificial pancreas using living beta cells: effect on glucose homeostasis in diabetic rats. *Science*, **197**, 780–782 (1977)

13 COLLINS, J. Current state of transplantation of the pancreas. *Annals of the Royal College of Surgeons of England*, **60**, 21–27 (1978)

14 CROFFORD, O. B. Report of the National Commission on Diabetics to the Congress of the United States of America. NIH, 67–1018. Washington DC (1975)

15 DeGROVE, J., WESTBROEK, D. L., DIIJKHUIS, C. M., VRIESENDORY, H. M., McDIKKEN I. and ELLIEN-GERITSEN, W. Influence of HLA matching, ALS and 24 hour preservation on isolated pancreas allograft survivial. *Transplantation Proceedings*, **5**, 755–759 (1973)

16 DOWNING, R., SCHARP, D. W. and BALLINGER, W. F. An improved technique for the isolation and identification of mammalian islets of Langerhans. *Transplantation*, **29**, 79–83 (1980)

17 DOYLE, A. P., BALCERZAK, S. P. and JEFFREY, W. L. Fatal diabetic glomerulosclerosis after total pancreatectomy. *New England Journal of Medicine*, **270**, 623–624 (1964)

18 DUBERNARD, J. M., TRAEGER, J., NEYRA, P., TOURAINE, J. L., TRAUDIANT, A. and BLANC-BRUNAT, N. A new method of preparation of segmental pancreatic grafts for transplantation: trial in dogs and in man. *Surgery*, **84**, 633–639 (1979)

19 DUBERNARD, J. M., TRAEGER, J., NEYRA, P., TOURAINE, J. L., BLANC, N. and DEVONEC, M. Long term effect of neoprene injection in the canine pancreatic duct. *Transplantation Proceedings*, **2**, 1448–1499 (1979)

20 DUBOIS, A. M. and GONET, A. Effets de la graffe de pancreas foetal sur la glycémie et la régéneration des ilots de Langerhans de rats alloxanisés ou pancreatectomiés. *Acta Anatomica (Basel)*, **41**, 336 (1960)

21 DUNCAN, L. J. P., MacFARLANE, A. and ROBSON, J. S. Diabetic retinopathy and nephropathy in pancreatic diabetes. *Lancet*, **274**, 822–826 (1958)

22 EDITORIAL. Diabetic complications. *British Medical Journal*, **1**, 941 (1978)

23 ENGERMAN, R., BLOODWORTH, J. M. B. and NELSON, S. Relationship of microvascular disease in diabetes to metabolic control. *Diabetes*, **26**, 760–769 (1977)

24 FELDMAN, S. D., DODI, G., HARD, K., SCHARP, D. W., BALLINGER, W. F. and LACY, P. E. Intrasplenic islet isografts. *Surgery*, **82**, 386–394 (1977)

25 FELDMAN, S. D., SCHARP, D. W., LACY, P. E. and BALLINGER, N. F. Foetal pancreas isografts cultured and uncultured to reverse streptozotocin induced diabetes mellitus. *Journal of Surgical Research*, **29**, 309–318 (1980)

26 FINCH, D. R. A., WISE, P. H. and MORRIS, P. J. Successful intrasplenic transplantation of syngenic and allogenic isolated pancreatic islets. *Diabetologia*, **13**, 195–199 (1977)

27 FINKE, E. H., LACY, P. E. and OHO, J. Use of reflected green light for specific identification of islets of Langerhans after collagenase digestion. *Diabetes*, **28**, 612–613 (1979)

28 GARVEY, J. F. W., McSHANE, D., POOLE, M. D., MILLARD, P. R. and MORRIS, P. J. The effects of Cyclosporin A on experimental pancreas allografts in the rat. *Transplantation Proceedings*, **12**, 266–269 (1980)

29 GAYET, R. and GUILLAMIE, M. La régulation de la secretion interne pancreatique par un processus humanol, demonstré par des transplantations de pancreas. *Comptes Rendus des Séances de la Societé Biologie et de ses Filiales*, 1613–1614 (1927)

30 GEBHARDT, C. and STOLTE, M. Pankreasgang-Okklusion durch Injektion einer schnellhärtenden Aminosäurelösung. *Langenbecks Archiv für Chirurgie*, **346**, 149–166 (1978)

31 GLIEDMAN, M. L., GOLD, M., WHITTAKER, J., RIFKIN, H., SOBERMAN, R., FREED, S., TELLIS, V. and VEITH, F. J. Clinical segmental pancreatic transplantation with ureter-pancreatic duct anastomosis for exocrine drainage. *Surgery*, **74**, 171–180 (1973)

32 GRAY, B. N. and WATKINS, E. Prevention of vascular complications of diabetes by pancreatic islet transplantation. *Archives of Surgery*, **111**, 254–257 (1976)

33 GRIFFITH, R. C., SCHARP, D. W., HARTMAN, B. K., BALLINGER, W. F. and LACY, P. E. A morphologic study of intra-hepatic portal vein islet isografts. *Diabetes*, **26**, 201–214 (1977)

34 GROTH, C. G., ANDERSON, A. BJORKEN, C., GUNNARSSON, R., HELLERSTROM, C., LUNDGREN, G., PETERSON, B., SWENNE, I. and OSTMAN, J. Attempts at transplantation of foetal pancreas to diabetic recipients. *Transplantation Proceedings*, **13**(4) (Suppl. 2), 208–212 (1980)

35 GROTH, C. G., LUNDGREN, G., ARNER, P., COLLSTE, H., HARDSTEDT, C., LEWANDER, R. and OSTMAN, J. Rejection of isolated pancreatic allografts in patients with diabetes. *Surgery, Gynecology and Obstetrics*, **143**, 933–940 (1976)

36 GUNNARSSON, R., ARNER, P., LUNDGREN, G., OSTMAN, J. and GROTH, C. G. Assessment of pancreatic graft function. *Transplantation Proceedings*, **12**(4) (Suppl. 2), 107–111 (1980)
37 HOUSE, E. L. and JACOBS, M. S. Effect of pancreatic homograft on the blood of normal and diabetic hamsters. *Anatomical Records*, **144**, 259 (1962)
38 HULTQUIST, G. T. and THORELL, J. Isolation of pancreatic islet tissue by transplantation. *Nordisk Medicin*, **69**, 47 (1963)
39 IDEZUKI, Y., GOETZ, F. C. and LILLEHIE, R. C. Late effect of pancreatic duct ligation on beta cell function. *American Journal of Surgery*, **117**, 33–39 (1969)
40 INOV, T., ORA, K. and MORI, S. Manifestation of rejection of pancreatic dudodenal allografts. *Transplantation*, **6**, 503–513 (1968)
41 JOB, D., ESCHWEGE, E., CUYOT-AGENTON, C., AUBRY, J. D. and TCHOBROVESKY, G. Effect of multiple daily insulin injections on the course of diabetic retinopathy. *Diabetes*, **25**, 463–469 (1976)
42 KEDINGER, M., HAFFEW, K., GRENIER, J. and ELROY, R. *In vitro* culture reduces immunogenicity of pancreatic endocrine islets. *Nature*, **270**, 736–738 (1977)
43 KELLY, W. D., LILLEHEI, R. L., MERKEL, F. K., IDEZUKI, Y. and GOETZ, F. C. Allotransplantation of the pancreas and duodenum along with the kidney in diabetic nephropathy. *Surgery*, **61**, 827–837 (1967)
44 KEMP, C. B., KNIGHT, M. J., SCHARP, D. W., BALLINGER, W. F. and LACY, P. E. Effect of transplantation site on the results of pancreatic isografts in diabetic rats. *Diabetologia*, **9**, 486–491 (1973)
45 KOLB, E., URFER, K. and LARGIADER, F. Early rejection of allotransplanted pancreatic islets in the dog. *Transplantation Proceedings*, **11**, 543–548 (1979)
46 KRETSCHMER, G. I., SUTHERLAND, D. E. R., MATAS, A. J., CAIN, J. L. and NAJARIAN, J. S. The dispersed pancreas: transplantation without islet purification in totally pancreatectomised dogs. *Diabetologia*, **13**, 495–502 (1977)
47 KYRIAKIDES, G., MILLER, J. and NUTTAL, F. Q. Intra-peritoneal segmental pancreatic allografts with unligated ducts in pigs. *Transplantation Proceedings*, **11**, 527–529 (1979)
48 KYRIAKIDES, G. K., SUTHERLAND, D. E. R., OLSON, L., MILLER, J. and NAJARIAN, J. S. Segmental pancreatic transplantation in dogs. *Transplantation Proceedings*, **11**, 530–532 (1979)
49 LACY, P. E., WALKER, M. M. and FINK, C. E. J. Perfusion of isolated rat islets *in vitro*. *Diabetes*, **21**, 987–998 (1972)
50 LACY, P. E., DAVIE, J. M. and FINKE, E. H. Induction of rejection of successful allografts of rat islets by donor peritoneal exudate cells. *Transplantation*, **28**, 415–420 (1979)
51 LARGIADER, F. Pancreas transplantation (editorial). *European Surgical Research*, **9**, 399 (1977)
52 LARGIADER, F., KOLB, E. and BINSWANGER, O. A long-term functioning human pancreatic islet allotransplant. *Transplantation*, **29**, 76–77 (1980)
53 LARGIADER, F., LYONS, G. W., HIDALGO, F., DIETZMAN, R. H. and LILLEHI, R. C. Orthotopic allotransplantation of the pancreas. *American Journal of Surgery*, **113**, 70–76 (1967)

54 LILLEHEI, R. C., SIMMONS, R. L., NAJARIAN, J. S., WEIL, R., UCHIDA, H., RUIZ, J. O., KJELLSTRAND, C. M. and GOETZ, F. C. Pancreatecto-duodenal allotransplantation. Experimental and clinical experience. *Annals of Surgery*, **172**, 405–436 (1970)

55 LITTLE, J. M., LAVER, C. and HOGG, J. Pancreatic duct obstruction with an aerglate glue. A new method of producing pancreatic exocrine atrophy. *Surgery*, **8**, 243–249 (1977)

56 MARQUET, R. I. and HEYSTEK, G. A. The effect of immunosuppression treatment in the survival of allogenic islets of Langerhans in rats. *Transplantation*, **20**, 428–431 (1975)

57 MATAS, A. J., SUTHERLAND, D. E. R., STEFFES, M. W. and NAJARIAN, J. S. Minimal collagenase digestion: amelioration of diabetes in the rat with transplantation of one neonatal pancreas. *Transplantation*, **22**, 71–73 (1976)

58 MATAS, A. J., SUTHERLAND, D. E. R., PAYNE, W. D., ECKHARDT, J. and NAJARIAN J. S. A mouse model of islet transplantation using neonatal donors. *Transplantation*, **24**, 389–393 (1977)

59 MATAS, A. J., SUTHERLAND, D. E. R., STEFFES, M. W. and NAJARIAN, J. S. Islet transplantation. *Surgery, Gynecology and Obstetrics*, **145**, 757–772 (1977)

60 MAVER, S. M., SUTHERLAND, D. E. R. and STEFFES, M. W. Pancreatic islet transplantation: effects on the glomerular lesions of experimental diabetes in the rat. *Diabetes*, **23**, 748–753 (1974)

61 MAVER, S. M., STEFFES, M. W., MICHAEL, A. L. and BROWN, D. M. Studies of diabetic nephropathy in animals and man. *Diabetes*, **25**, 850–857 (1976)

62 McMASTER, P. Unpublished data (1981)

63 McMASTER, P., CALNE, R. Y., GIBBY, O. M. and EVANS, D. B. Pancreatic transplantation in man. *Transplantation Proceedings*, **13**(4) (Suppl. 2), 58–61 (1981)

64 McMASTER, P., PROCYSHIN, A., CALNE, R. Y., VALDES, R., ROLLES, K. and SMITH, D. Prolongation of canine pancreas allograft survival with Cyclosporin A. *British Medical Journal*, **280**, 444–445 (1980)

65 MEHIGAN, D. G., BALL, W. R., ZUDEMA, G. D., EGGLESTON, J. G. and CAMERON, J. L. Disseminated intravascular coagulopathy after islet allotransplantation. *Annals of Surgery*, **191**, 287–293 (1980)

66 MIKI, E., FUKUDA, M., KAZA, T. and KOSAKA, K. Relation of course of retinopathy to control of diabetes. *Diabetes*, **18**, 773–780 (1969)

67 MIRKOVITCH, V. and CAMPICHE, M. Intrasplenic autotransplantation of canine pancreatic tissue: maintenance of normoglycaemia after total pancreatectomy. *European Surgical Research*, **9**(3), 173–190 (1977)

68 MITTAL, Y. K., TOLEDO PEREYRA, L. H., PARMA, M., RAMASWAMY, K., PURI, V. K., CORTEZ, J. A. and GORDON, D. Acute portal hypertension and disseminated intravascular coagulation following pancreatic islet autotransplantation after subtotal pancreatectomy. *Transplantation*, **31**(4), 32 (1981)

69 MOLNAK, G. D., TAYLOR, W. F. and HO, M. M. Day to day variation of continuous monitored glycaemia. *Diabetologia*, **8**, 342–348 (1972)

70 MOSKALEWSKI, S. Isolation and culture of the islets of Langerhans of the guinea pig. *General and Comparative Endocrinology*, **5**, 342–353 (1965)

71 NAJARIAN, J. S., SUTHERLAND, D. E. R., SIMMONS, R. L., HOWARD, R. J., KJELLSTRAND, C. M., RAMSAY, R. C., GOETZ, F. C., FRYD, D. S. and SOMMER, B. G. Ten year experience with

renal transplantation in juvenile onset diabetes. *Annals of Surgery*, **190**(4), 487–500 (1979)

72 NAJARIAN, J. S., SUTHERLAND, D. E. R. and STEFFES, M. W. Isolation of human islets of Langerhans for transplantation. *Transplantation Proceedings*, **7**, 611–613 (1975)

73 NASH, J. R., PETERS, M. and BELL, P. R. F. Comparative survival of pancreatic islets, heart, kidney and skin allografts in rats with and without enhancement. *Transplantation*, **24**, 70–73 (1977)

74 PAYNE, W. L., SUTHERLAND, D. E. R., MATAS, A. J., GORECKI, P. and NAJARIAN, J. S. DL-Ethionine treatment of adult pancreatic donors. *Annals of Surgery*, **189**, 248–256 (1979)

75 PIRART, J. Diabetes mellitus and its degenerative complications. *Diabetes*, **2**, 168–188; 252–263 (1978)

76 RUIZ, J. O., UCHIDA, J., SCHULTZ, L. S. and LILLEHEI, R. C. Function studies after auto- and allotransplantation and denervation of pancreatico-duodenal segments in dogs. *American Journal of Surgery*, **123**, 236–242 (1972)

77 RYNASIEWICZ, J. J., SUTHERLAND, D. E. R., KAWAHARAK, K. and NAJARIAN, J. S. Total lymphoid visualisation. Prolongation of pancreas and islet allografts in rats. *Surgical Forum*, **31**, 359–360 (1980)

78 SCHARP, D. W., KEMP, C. B., KNIGHT, M. J., BALLINGER, W. F. and LACY, P. E. The use of Ficoll in the preparation of viable islets of Langerhans from the rat pancreas. *Transplantation*, **16**, 686–689 (1973)

79 SCHARP, D. W., MURPHY, J. J., NEWTOWN, W. T., BALLINGER, W. F. and LACY, P. E. Transplantation of islets of Langerhans in diabetic Rhesus monkeys. *Surgery*, **77**, 100–105 (1975)

80 SELLE, W. A. Studies on pancreatic grafts made with a new technique. *American Journal of Physiology*, **113**, 118 (1935)

81 SPENCE, R. K., PERLOFF, L. J. and BARKER, C. F. Foetal pancreas in treatment of experimental diabetes in rats. *Transplantation Proceedings*, **2**, 533–536 (1979)

82 SUTHERLAND, D. E. R. International human pancreas and islet transplant registry tabulation. *Transplantation Proceedings*, **12** (Suppl.), 229–236 (1980)

83 SUTHERLAND, D. E. R. Pancreas Transplant Register update. *Transplantation Proceedings*, **12**(4) (Suppl. 2), 229–235 (1981)

84 SUTHERLAND, D. E. R., GOETZ, F. C. and NAJARIAN, J. S. Review of world's experience with pancreas and islet transplantation. *Transplantation Proceedings*, **13**(1), 241–297 (1981)

85 SUTHERLAND, D. E. R., MATAS, A. J. and NAJARIAN, J. S. Pancreatic islet cell transplantation. *Surgical Clinics of North America*, **58**, 365–382 (1978)

86 SUTHERLAND, D. E. R., MATAS, A. J., KRETSCHMER, G. I. and NAJARIAN, J. S. Clinical applications and future of islet transplantation. In *Transplantation and Clinical Immunology*, edited by J. L. Touraine *et al.* **10**, 227–231 (1979)

87 SUTHERLAND, D. E. R., MATAS, A. J., GOETZ, F. C. and NAJARIAN, J. S. Transplantation of dispersed pancreatic islet tissues in humans. *Diabetes*, **29** (Suppl. 1), 31–44 (1980)

88 SUTHERLAND, D. E. R., RYNASIEWICZ, J. I. and NAJARIAN, J. S. Current status of pancreas and islet transplantation. *Handbook of Diabetes Mellitus*, edited by M. Brownlea (1979)

89 SUTHERLAND, D. E. R., RYNASIEWICZ, J. J., KAWAHARA, K., GORECKI, P. and NAJARIAN, J. S. Rejection of islets versus immediately vascularised pancreatic allografts: a quantitative comparison. *Journal of Surgical Research*, **29**, 240–247 (1980)

90 TCHOBROVESKY, G. Relation of diabetic control to development of microvascular complications. *Diabetologia*, **15**, 143–152 (1978)

91 THEODOROU, N. A. and HOWELL, S. L. An assessment of diffusion chambers for use in pancreatic islet transplantation. *Transplantation*, **27**, 350–353 (1979)

92 TOLEDO-PEREYRA, L. H. and CASTELLANOS, J. Role of pancreatic duct ligation for segmental pancreas autotransplantation. *Transplantation*, **28**, 469–475 (1979)

93 TOLEDO-PEREYRA, L .H., CASTELLANOS, J., LAMPE, E. W., LILLEHEI, R. C. and NAJARIAN, J. S. Comparative evaluation of pancreas transplantation technique. *American Surgeon*, **182**, 567–571 (1975)

94 TRAEGER, J., DUBERNARD, J. M., RUITTON, A. M., MALIK, M. C. and TOURAINE, J. L. Clinical experience with 15 neoprene-injected pancreatic allografts in man. *Transplantation Proceedings*, **13**(1), 298–304 (1981)

95 TRIMBLE, E. F., KARAKASH, C., MALAISSE-LAGAE, F. and VISGATINE, I. Effects of intraportal islet transplantation on the transplanted tissues and recipient pancreas. I. Functional studies. *Diabetologia*, **19**, 341–347 (1980)

96 VALENTE, U., FERRO, M., BAROCCI, S., CAMPISI, C., PARODI, F. and CATALDI, L. Report of clinical cases of human foetal pancreas transplantation. *Transplantation Proceedings*, **13**(4) (Suppl. 2), 213–217 (1980)

97 VALENTE, U., FERRO, M., CAMPISI, C., CATALDI, L., FONTANA, I., De ROSA, E., CAMA, A. and JOSATTI, E. Report of clinical cases of islet autotransplantation. *Transplantation Proceedings*, **13**(4) (Suppl. 2), 202–204 (1980)

98 VIALETTES, B., LASSMANN, V., VAGRE, P. and SIMON, M. C. Islet transplantation in diabetic rats. *Acta Diabetologica*, **16**, 1–8 (1979)

99 VIALETTES, B., SUTHERLAND, D. E. R., PAYNE, W. A., MATAS, A. J. and NAJARIAN, J. S. Synergistic effect of donor specific soluble membrane antigen injection and ALG administration on the survival of islet allografts in rats. *Transplantation*, **25**, 336–338 (1978)

100 WEIL, R., NOZAWA, M., KOSS, M., WEBER, C., REEMTSMA, K. and McINTOSH, R. M. Pancreatic transplantation in diabetic rats: renal function, morphology, ultrastructure and immunohistology. *Surgery*, **78**, 142–148 (1975)

Editors' commentary on Chapter 8

Renal failure is a significant cause of death in young diabetics, and amounts to about 20% of all deaths in diabetics under the age of 40 years.

Diabetic patients with renal failure are not good candidates for maintenance dialysis: proneness of the diabetic to infection, the difficulties associated with vascular access and progressive microvascular disorders all contribute to the poor outcome of maintenance dialysis, and only some 30% of diabetic patients on haemodialysis will survive for 3 or more years. The graft survival of cadaveric renal transplantation in these patients is also very poor, with a graft survival rate as low as 45%. Those patients who do manage to retain a successful transplant run into serious problems with diabetic control due to the administration of steroids, and they are not often well rehabilitated. There has, therefore, been reluctance to accept diabetic patients in renal failure on to transplant programmes.

There is no doubt that the ideal method of management would be the transplantation of pancreatic islets, but the technical problems of harvesting sufficient islets from the donor pancreas and the difficulties of preservation and re-implantation are so significant that this method of treatment is still in a very experimental stage. Attention has been turned again to vascularized pancreatic transplants carried out at the same time as the renal grafts.

Since 1977 there are records of 128 pancreatic transplants in pancreatic patients. Twenty-four of these grafts continue to function beyond 1 year and one is actually still functioning at 3½ years after transplantation. The problems of ablating the exocrine secretion of the pancreas appear to be more easily controlled and the biochemical profiles of patients who have had successful grafts are certainly very dramatic in their normality. Very little can be said at the present time about the effect of pancreatic grafts on the microvascular complications of diabetes in the transplanted kidney and it will take some time to find answers to this question. However, early reports on the improvement in small vessel pathology following successful combined pancreatic and kidney grafts are encouraging.

The technical problems of vascularized pancreatic grafts have not yet been overcome and this explains why only about one in six continue to function. Blood flow through the graft must be adequate, and several groups have demonstrated the need for either additional splenic arterial anastomosis or arteriovenous fistulae adjacent to the graft.

Patient selection will always be the main problem but the fact that more diabetic patients are starting on continuous ambulatory peritoneal dialysis suggests that the population of diabetic patients in renal failure on maintenance dialysis will rise so that there could well be an increase in demand for pancreatic transplantation in the future. The present pilot studies are therefore to be encouraged.

9
Surgical considerations in the MEN I syndrome

Norman W. Thompson

INTRODUCTION

Multiple endocrine adenomatosis (MEA) type I, or Wermer's syndrome, is a familial disorder characterized by involvement of the pituitary, pancreas and parathyroid glands with hyperplasia or neoplasms. The syndrome is genetically transmitted as an autosomal dominant defect with high penetrance but variable expressivity. Furthermore, clinical evidence of involvement may be synchronous or metachronous. Because the involved endocrine organs may develop hyperplastic changes, adenomas or carcinomas, the syndrome is now referred to as multiple endocrine neoplasia (MEN) type I. The clinical presentation of this disorder is related to the variable secretion of one or more polypeptide hormones or amines. Several endocrinopathies may be clinically apparent simultaneously, for example Cushing's syndrome and the Zollinger-Ellison syndrome. In addition to the principal endocrine organs affected by the genetic defect, other abnormalities have been described in the MEN I syndrome. The adrenal glands are involved with hyperplasia secondary either to pituitary or, in some cases, ectopic ACTH secretion. There is also an increased incidence of both functioning and non-functioning adrenocortical adenomas. Also seen with a higher frequency than could be expected by chance alone are carcinoid tumors involving the gastrointestinal tract, the bronchus and the thymus[3, 29, 41]. Multiple lipomas are another feature of the disease seen in some families.

The following case illustrates many of the acute surgical problems associated with the MEN I syndrome. This patient's syndrome had remained unrecognized until fatal complications had developed. This was particularly unfortunate, as each of her major endocrine problems was amenable to surgical therapy. Her necropsy findings support the concept of the MEN I syndrome as an 'all or none' phenomenon involving the pituitary, endocrine pancreas and parathyroid glands.

Case 1. EH, a white female aged 51, was admitted to hospital elsewhere in August 1970 because of acute pain associated with ureteral calculi. In addition she had had persistent nausea and some vomiting, and had noted diarrhea for several months prior to admission.

Her first renal stones caused symptoms 4 years before, and subsequently she had had a dozen episodes of ureteral colic and spontaneous passage of small stones. Recurrent urinary tract infections had been treated with antibiotics.

During 3 weeks in hospital her serum calcium levels ranged from 16 to 18 mg/dl (4 to 4.5 mmol/l). Despite intermittent episodes of disorientation, nausea, vomiting and persistent abdominal pain, vigorous efforts to lower the serum calcium level were not pursued. Apparently urgent parathyroidectomy was not considered. After 3 weeks she began to have melena and then hematemesis. During a 24-hour period, 12 units of whole blood were administered. She was then given intravenous phosphates to lower her serum calcium and immediately went into shock from which she could not easily be resuscitated. When transferred to the University Hospital she was in irreversible shock. On arrival her systolic blood pressure was 80 mmHg. Despite all efforts, she remained hypotensive until her death several hours later. Based on the history and physical findings, a clinical diagnosis of MEN I syndrome was made. She had obvious Cushing's syndrome, hyperparathyroidism, and suspected peptic ulcer disease associated with a possible gastrinoma. Her death was considered to be a direct result of severe hypercalcemia associated with the administration of intravenous phosphate solutions. At necropsy, a small pituitary adenoma was found and both adrenal glands showed marked cortical hyperplasia. The parathyroid glands were all enlarged, particularly the right superior, which weighed 90 g and extended from the angle of the mandible to the clavicle (*Figures 9.1 and 9.2*). A duodenal ulcer 2 cm in size penetrated into the head of the pancreas, which was normal except for a localized 1.5 cm gastrinoma (*Figures 9.3 and 9.4*). There were no metastases. Both renal veins were thrombosed, a recognized complication of hypercalcemic crisis. Microscopic examination confirmed the gross findings and in addition showed severe metastatic calcification involving lungs, heart, kidneys and pancreas.

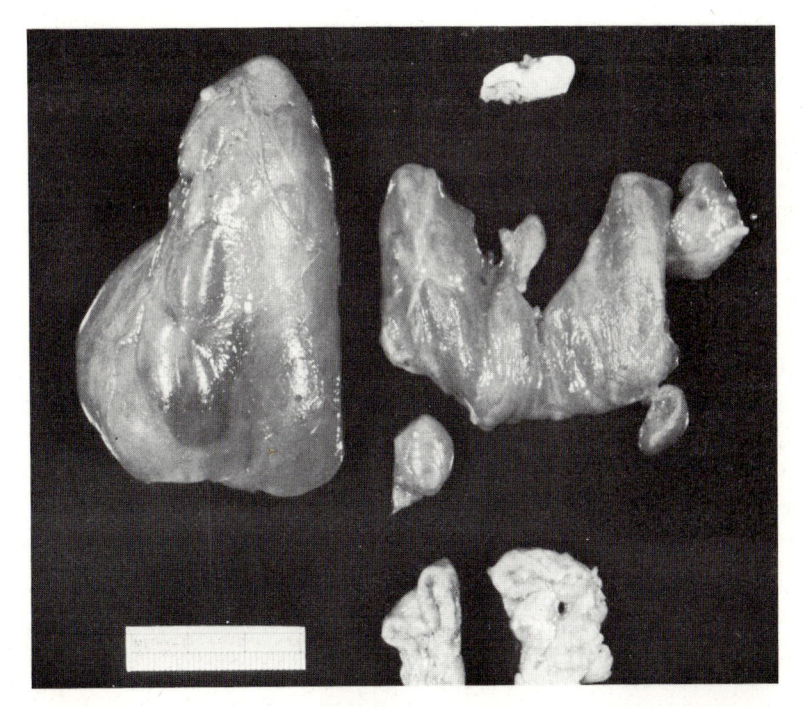

Figure 9.1 Case 1: Autopsy findings, endocrine glands. Microadenoma of pituitary, asymmetrical parathyroid hyperplasia. Huge (90 g) right superior parathyroid. Note normal thyroid gland. Adrenal glands: bilateral cortical hyperplasia, Cushing's disease

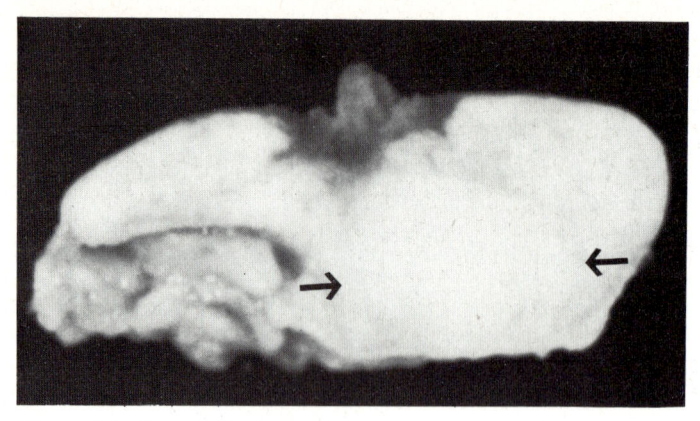

146 *Surgical considerations in the MEN syndrome*

Figure 9.2 Case 1: Pituitary glands. The arrows indicate a 0.5 cm microadenoma

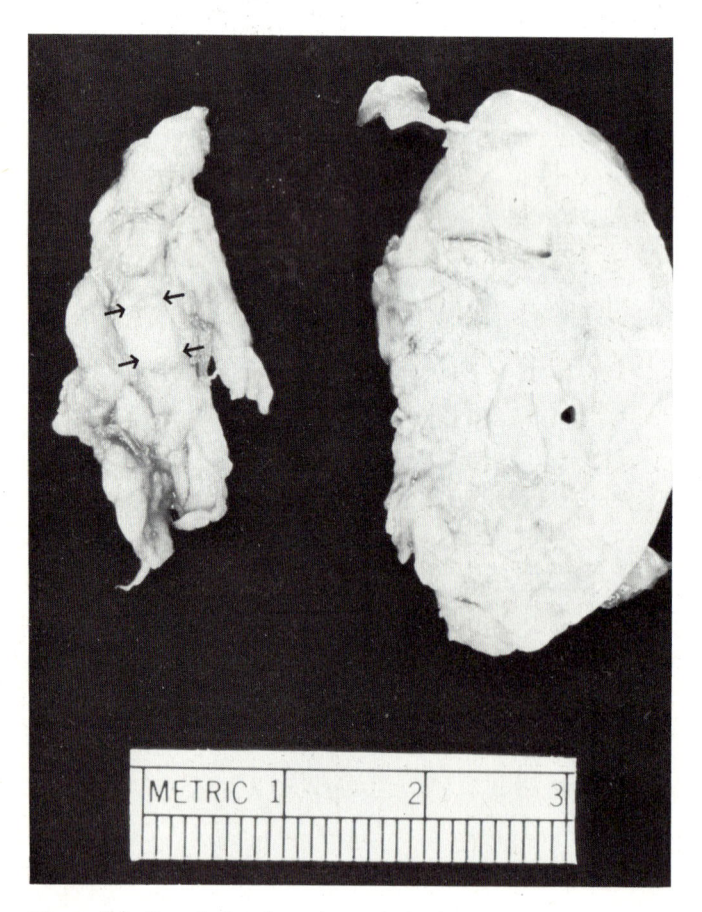

Figure 9.3 Case 1: Sections through the head of the pancreas. The arrows indicate a 0.6 cm islet cell tumor (gastrinoma). The remainder of the pancreas was normal

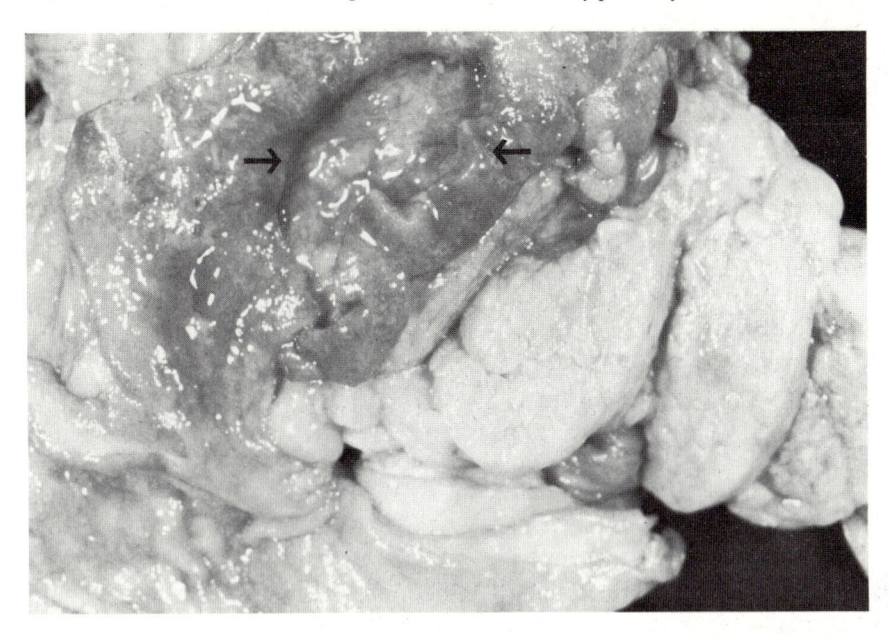

Figure 9.4 Case 1: Gross specimen of duodenum and head of pancreas. The arrows indicate a 2.5 cm ulcer in the first portion of the duodenum penetrating into the head of the pancreas

The synchronous appearance of all three common endocrinopathies associated with the MEN I syndrome represents a dramatic presentation of this disease. The successful management of such cases requires clinical experience, a sense of urgency, the appropriate selection of diagnostic studies and skillful surgical intervention. The following sections will consider details of surgical management of each of the endocrine organs involved in this syndrome.

SURGICAL CONSIDERATIONS OF PARATHYROID INVOLVEMENT IN THE MEN I SYNDROME

In 1954 Wermer, in a classic paper, delineated the components of the MEN I syndrome[40]. Although he classified the enlarged parathyroids frequently seen in this syndrome as adenomas, subsequent documentation has shown that the histological changes are those of chief cell hyperplasia involving all of the parathyroids[1, 20, 21, 28, 32]. The parathyroid glands have been found to be involved in at least 90% of cases, and all hypercalcemic patients with a suspected MEN I syndrome should be assumed to have parathyroid involvement. Hyperparathyroidism is the most frequent clinical manifestation of the MEN I syndrome and, in most cases, the first finding.

The majority of patients are hypercalcemic when the MEN I syndrome is diagnosed initially. During the past decade nearly all MEN I patients identified by screening asymptomatic family members at risk have had hypercalcemia as the first biochemical finding. Because of the frequent involvement of the parathyroid glands, routine periodic screening of family members should obviously always include estimations of serum calcium and/or parathyroid hormone levels. It is our policy also to evaluate all new patients with the Zollinger-Ellison syndrome, insulinomas, and other islet cell tumours for possible hyperparathyroidism, even if there is a negative family history for endocrinopathies.

MEN I patients with hyperparathyroidism have symptoms similar to those of patients with non-familial parathyroid disease caused by adenomas. Many patients identified by screening families with this syndrome show relatively mild symptoms or are asymptomatic at the time of diagnosis. Symptoms of lethargy, weakness, nervousness, constipation, anorexia, polyuria, polydipsia, and nocturia are common. The frequency of mild symptoms early in the disease has led some to conclude that hyperparathyroidism is unlikely to be of consequence to patients with the MEN I syndrome. This has not been our experience, however. Some patients may first present with severe hypercalcemia associated with significant bone or renal complications. Until recently, patients with gastrinomas as a component of the MEN I syndrome frequently had a history of recurring renal stones or even nephrectomy prior to the diagnosis of the syndrome. We have had several patients whose first manifestations of the MEN I syndrome were due to brown tumors of bone. In contrast to most patients with non-familial primary hyperparathyroidism, MEN I patients usually have evidence of hyperparathyroidism before the third or fourth decades. We identified recently four members of one family who were hypercalcemic before the age of 15 years. Biochemical changes and parathyroid hormone levels in MEN I patients are similar to those found in the usual patient with primary hyperparathyroidism. Families with hyperparathyroidism and paradoxical hypocalciuria have recently been reported[15, 24, 25, 36]. This is an entirely separate syndrome, which is transmitted as an autosomal dominant trait and must be differentiated from the MEN I syndrome. Hypercalcemia is frequently found in these patients during childhood. This newly described familial disease, called 'familial hypocalciuric hypercalcemia', is currently being identified in asymptomatic children by careful screening of families known to be affected. This syndrome can frequently be diagnosed during the first decade of life. The hypercalcemia does not respond to subtotal parathyroidectomy. Fortunately the hypercalcemia is rarely severe, and the symptoms and complications of hyperparathyroidism are rare. It should not be confused with the MEN I syndrome, as surgical intervention is meddlesome, futile and rarely necessary.

MEN I syndrome patients with biochemical evidence of hypercalcemia and elevated parathyroid hormone levels should undergo neck exploration. Left untreated, parathyroid disease in these patients frequently causes bone and renal disease. At operation all four parathyroid glands should be identified and a careful search made for additional glands. It should be assumed that hyperplasia is present and that all glands are involved, even though some may be normal in size. It is not unusual, particularly in younger partients, to find two or more glands of normal size. The pathological findings may be confusing.

Castelman, Schantz and Roth[7] were the first to describe the pathological findings in primary chief cell hyperplasia which may occur independent of the MEN I syndrome. They particularly noted the distribution of chief or oxyphil cells in cords, sheaths in a follicular arrangement replacing the stroma fat cells. This histological picture is difficult, if not impossible, to distinguish from that of a solitary adenoma. In the MEN I syndrome, the hyperplasia may not involve all glands equally, and characteristically there is asymmetry of the parathyroid glands. This appearance may cause the surgeon to mistake the lesion for an adenoma when microscopically all of the parathyroid glands are abnormal. In such cases the intraoperative diagnosis of hyperplasia by biopsy of a normal sized gland is of more than academic interest. Failure to recognize hyperplasia in patients with MEN I will result in inadequate resection of parathyroid tissue and inevitable recurrence of hypercalcemia. The interpretation of frozen section biopsy specimens from parathyroid glands of normal appearance is notoriously difficult, and even experienced endocrine pathologists may err in labeling normal glands as hyperplastic and hyperplastic glands as normal. Such errors in interpretation have led surgeons to perform subtotal parathyroidectomies for adenomas, and excision of a single enlarged gland when chief cell hyperplasia was present. When the pathologist is unable to make a definite intraoperative diagnosis, the surgeon may have to base his operative decision on the patient's family history and/or knowledge of other endocrine disorders. Because conventional staining of histological sections may be insufficient for consistent interpretation, new diagnostic methods have been developed[30, 43]. The use of parenchymal fat stains to assess the functional state of glands has been advocated. This test is based on the assumption that a diminution in the amount of parenchymal fat indicates hyperfunction of a parathyroid gland. This change may be seen in either adenomas or hyperplastic glands. Thus the finding of an enlarged parathyroid gland plus one or more normal sized glands with decreased parenchymal fat indicates asymmetric parathyroid hyperplasia rather than adenoma. Other methods that are being developed include flow cytometry to differentiate hyperplastic from normal parathyroid glands. Although none of these tests have been universally accepted, there is hope that the surgeon will benefit from these efforts. Eventually intraoperative interpretation of biopsies of parathyroid glands should become more reliable than has been the case. These tests, when applied routinely during parathyroid operations, may correctly diagnose diffuse hyperplasia, particularly in patients without a known family history of endocrinopathies. After all parathyroids have been identified on naked eye examination and verified by frozen section biopsy, a subtotal parathyroidectomy should be performed. Usually, excision of three and a half or more glands is required. The vascular integrity of each parathyroid gland should be assessed prior to its excision. One readily accessible parathyroid gland is selected for partial excision. A well vascularized remnant, equivalent in size to a normal parathyroid gland weighing 30–50 mg, is left. The remnant is marked carefully with one or two metal clips attached to its capsule, well away from its vascular pedicle. These may be used for identification should a future operation for recurrence become necessary. We have usually selected an inferior parathyroid gland and gently attached it to the thyroid capsule, away from the recurrent laryngeal nerve. When it is clear that the remnant is viable, the remaining glands are completely excised. Currently some surgeons perform total parathyroidectomy, autografting a portion of one gland into a forearm muscle[38, 39]. This alternative has gained popularity because of the reported high incidence of recurrence of hypercalcemia in patients with the MEN I syndrome[28]. The technique, popularized by Wells[38, 39], has the advantage of providing easy access to the parathyroid graft (using only a local anesthetic) should graft hypertrophy eventually cause recurrence. We have not adopted this technique for MEN I patients because we have encountered only one recurrence in a patient in which an adequate subtotal parathyroidectomy was believed to have been performed. Parathyroid reoperations in MEN I patients have been necessary for other reasons, however. The most common causes of failure have been the following: (1) The parathyroid disease was erroneously assumed to be due to an adenoma because of the finding of a single enlarged gland and frozen section misinterpretation of biopsies from other normal sized glands. In each of our own cases where this occurred the permanent sections were correctly interpreted, and these patients were carefully evaluated for other evidence of the MEN I syndrome even when the family history had initially been considered negative. (2) Intraoperative recognition of multigland disease was noted, but the surgeon excised fewer than three glands, apparently fearing possible hypocalcemia. (3) At least three glands were excised, but there was failure to identify a supernumerary fifth gland. At reoperation, the fifth gland, or less frequently a missing fourth gland, was found in the upper portion of the thymus, easily accessible from the neck incision.

In our experience, and that of others, MEN I patients have an increased incidence of supernumerary (fifth or even sixth) parathyroid glands compared to the general population (15% versus 6%). Failure to identify a supernumerary fifth gland would not prevent persistence or recurrence of hypercalcemia in a patient having a total parathyroidectomy and forearm autograft.

Because of the high incidence of supernumerary glands in patients with the MEN I syndrome, we routinely perform cervical thymectomies, even when four or five parathyroids have already been identified. If hypercalcemia persists or recurs following subtotal parathyroidectomy in these patients, selective venous catheterization with venous sampling for parathyroid hormones should be considered for localization once other causes of hypercalcemia have been ruled out.

When asymmetrical parathyroid hyperplasia is encountered in a patient with no known family history or other features of an endocrinopathy, the possibility of MEN I should be suspected. In this group of patients we initiate an endocrine evaluation which includes pituitary function studies and gut hormone analysis. In the routine patient with primary hyperparathyroidism and no family history or other specific endocrine findings, we do not obtain these studies before parathyroidectomy. Because only the rare patient with primary hyperparathyroidism has other endocrinopathies, this policy has eliminated many costly and time-consuming preoperative studies. By focusing attention on a selected group of patients with asymmetrical parathyroid hyperplasia, however, the diagnosis of pancreatic islet cell disease and pituitary hyperfunction has been made at an early stage. If no evidence of involvement is initially found, annual repetition of these studies may be rewarding. The metachronous expression of the MEN I syndrome is particularly apparent in younger patients who are followed for a period of years. It should be assumed that other manifestations of the MEN I syndrome will eventually develop[21].

SURGICAL CONSIDERATIONS OF PANCREATIC ISLET CELL DISEASE IN THE MEN I SYDROME

The currently available evidence suggests that the pancreas will be involved in all patients with the MEN I syndrome. In a careful search of the English language literature during the 25-year period from 1953 to 1978, Majewski and Wilson[21] found 37 patients for whom complete multisystem pathological data were reported. The endocrine involvement included the parathyroids, pancreas and pituitary in all cases. These authors concluded that the MEN I syndrome was an 'all or none' phenomenon. Although the evidence from autopsy studies is clear, the involvement in clinical cases is less apparent. Synchronous involvement of each of these endocrine glands during clinical evaluation has been relatively infrequent, particularly in younger patients. In our experience virtually all patients with proven MEN I syndrome demonstrated hyperparathyroidism when this was specifically searched for with serum calcium and parathyroid hormone levels. In younger individuals this aspect of the disease may be asymptomatic. The second most common manifestation of the syndrome is that of pancreatic islet cell disease, usually identified one to two decades later than hypercalcemia. The exceptions are patients presenting with islet cell syndromes being evaluated for the first time. These patients usually have hyperparathyroidism and a gut hormone syndrome synchronously. Pituitary adenomas, with or without symptoms, may also be present. Only one of our patients has had a pituitary adenoma as the first finding in a subsequently proven MEN I syndrome. This patient, a girl of 16 years, underwent a hypophysectomy for a large tumor causing optic nerve compression and headaches. At the age of 22 years she became hypercalcemic and had a subtotal parathyroidectomy for four-gland hyperplasia. She first had symptoms of peptic ulcer disease at the age of 27 years and was proved to have a Zollinger-Ellison syndrome due to islet cell hyperplasia the following year. Patients such as this support the concept that all of the endocrine glands associated with the syndrome will eventually become involved, provided the patient survives long enough. The importance of periodic endocrine screening of MEN I patients and their relations cannot be overemphasized. Follow-up study of suspected MEN I patients and screening of MEN I family members now allows earlier detection of pancreatic islet involvement than was possible a decade ago.

The most common functional manifestation of the MEN I pancreatic islet cell involvement is the Zollinger-Ellison syndrome[12, 20, 42]. These patients present with either peptic ulcer symptoms, diarrhea, or both. Next in frequency are patients with hypoglycemia from insulin excess due either to β-cell hyperplasia or insulinomas. More recently MEN I patients have been identified with glucagonomas, VIPomas, somatostatinomas and pancreatic polypeptide secreting tumors (PPomas). Some of these patients are entirely asymptomatic and the diagnosis has been established on the basis of hormone assays and subsequent localization studies. Pancreatic polypeptide (PP) has been found to be a common secretory product of islet cell hyperplasia, microadenomas or gross pancreatic tumors in the MEN I syndrome and is currently recommended as a marker in screening studies for the disease[10, 11]. Although PPomas remain an infrequent isolated tumor of islet cells, hypersecretion of PP in either the basal or food-stimulated state occurs in the majority of MEA I patients with islet cell disease. Recent studies have shown that many MEN I patients with islet cell disease secrete excesses of more than one hormone. In some cases a single tumor may be responsible, whereas in others multiple tumors producing different secretory products may be present. In most cases the clinical syndrome will represent the predominant hormone secreted, if that is one causing symptoms. If, however, the hormone is PP, the patient is asymptomatic. The metachronous development of functional syndromes has also been reported[10, 42]. We have seen 2 patients with MEN I syndromes who after the surgical treatment of gastrinomas developed hypoglycemia due to insulinomas. Adding to the diagnostic dilemma in the MEN I syndrome is the fact that some patients may develop islet cell tumors not secreting any currently identifiable peptides[10]. These patients may not be diagnosed until metastatic liver disease becomes apparent. There appears to be no pattern of islet cell involvement even within the same family, emphasizing that screening the asymptomatic family members of known Zollinger-Ellison MEN I patients by serum gastrin levels is insufficient to detect pancreatic disease. For example, we have studied one family in which three involved members had a gastrinoma, a PPoma and a malignant non-functional islet cell tumor with hepatic metastases. Clinical evidence of islet cell disease usually appears in the fourth or fifth decade of life in MEN I patients. Recently we have, through hormonal screening, been able to detect the presence of islet cell disease in the third decade, usually in completely asymptomatic patients. The most commonly elevated hormones in these patients have been PP or gastrin, or both. As emphasized earlier, these patients usually have coexisting hypercalcemia. In patients with hypergastrinemia, surgical treatment of the hyperparathyroidism may cause the baseline serum gastrin to return to normal. Postoperative proof of islet cell disease requires a positive response to the provocative secretin stimulation test. Because asymptomatic MEN I pancreatic islet cell disease has been detectable, by the use of hormone immunoassays, for only a few years, conclusions as to how best to manage such cases are still evolving. Current theories regarding the management of the functional islet cell syndromes associated with the MEN I syndrome will be discussed, using examples encountered in recent practice.

The Zollinger-Ellison component of the MEN I syndrome

In Chapter 10 Dr Zollinger has presented a comprehensive and authoritative review of the diagnosis and management of gastrinomas in the post-cimetidine era. The current controversies of medical and surgical alternatives are also reviewed thoroughly. This discussion will address the specific problems associated with the Zollinger-Ellison syndrome as a component of the MEN I syndrome.

It is currently estimated that the Zollinger-Ellison syndrome is associated with the MEN I syndrome in approximately 30% of all cases. The incidence has varied from 10% to nearly 50% of patients undergoing surgery for gastrinomas. In a recent report, Friesen[9] noted that 7 of 23 patients operated upon for gastrinomas had the MEN I syndrome. In the largest surgical series reported from one hospital[2], 19 of 66 patients (29%) had the MEN I syndrome. In 11 of these patients the diagnosis of gastrinoma was made after the diagnosis of primary hyperparathyroidism had been established. Our experience has been similar in that gastrinomas are being found more frequently and at an earlier stage when known MEN I patients with hyperparathyroidism or new patients found to have parathyroid hyperplasia rather than adenomas are investigated for hypergastrinemia. The diagnosis of the Zollinger-Ellison syndrome can be established with precision by using gastrin immunoassays and the provocative secretin stimulation test in patients who have gastric hyperacidity[8, 9, 18, 22, 23, 34, 35, 42, 44]. The availability of radioimmunoassays for gastrin, combined with an increased clinical awareness of the possibility of these syndromes, has led to earlier recognition of the disease. It is clear that a number of the patients currently being diagnosed would not have been recognized a decade ago. Some of these patients may be asymptomatic or have only minimal symptoms of peptic ulcer disease or diarrhea. Patients with the classic findings of the syndrome have become infrequent and we have seen only one patient with a jejunal ulcer during the past 5 years. Cimetidine, so frequently used in the treatment of patients with any symptoms suggesting peptic ulcer disease, may be partly responsible for the change in the clinical pattern of the syndrome[4, 26, 27, 34, 44].

When the Zollinger-Ellison syndrome is diagnosed in a patient with hypercalcemia and biochemical evidence of primary hyperparathyroidism, it is our policy to treat the hyperparathyroidism as the first priority. If peptic ulcer disease is present, intensive medical treatment with cimetidine is initiated. In some cases there may be marked improvement after the hypercalcemia has been corrected. Occasionally parathyroidectomy alone may indefinitely relieve hypergastrinemia and its associated sequelae. As an example of this phenomenon, the following case is presented.

Case 2. FK, a white female aged 62, was first admitted to the University Hospital in 1974. During the preceding 4 years she had noted some loss of memory and generalized weakness. These were her chief complaints. The cause of her weakness was thought to be diarrhea: she had had six to eight watery stools per day intermittently, and then persistently for the past 3 years. In addition she had aortic insufficiency and aortic stenosis, with a heart block that had recently been treated by the placement of a permanent pacemaker. During the 3 months prior to her admission her serum calcium levels had been found to be in the range of 12–14 mg/dl (3.0–3.5 mmol/l). A 12-hour gastric analysis revealed a secretion of 180 mEq/l of hydrochloric acid. Serum gastrin analysis showed a concentration of 1100 pg/dl (ng/l). Shortly after admission a subtotal parathyroidectomy was performed, leaving the equivalent of one normal parathyroid gland. She was found to have asymmetrical parathyroid hyperplasia involving all four glands. Her diarrhea ceased immediately after operation. From 1974 to 1978 her serum calcium levels ranged from 8.2 mg/dl to 9.6 mg/dl (2.1–2.4 mmol/l). During that time 11 serum gastrin analyses were performed and all were under 200 pg/dl (ng/l). In 1976 she underwent successful aortic valve replacement. Although there was no MEN I family history at the time of diagnosis in 1974, one sister was subsequently found to be hypercalcemic and has had subtotal parathyroidectomy. One other sister and two brothers are apparently free of any endocrinopathy. This patient has remained asymptomatic, with no evidence of hypergastrinemia or gastric hyperacidity during an 8-year period, despite the biochemical evidence of gastrinoma prior to her parathyroidectomy. Because of her cardiac status and age, as well as the complete lack of symptoms, she has not been considered a candidate for pancreatic exploration. We still consider it most likely that she has a small gastrinoma or islet cell hyperplasia that has been 'dormant' since the correction of her hypercalcemia.

154 *Surgical considerations in the MEN syndrome*

This patient showed an exceptional response to parathyroidectomy. Although short-term palliation is likely to occur in most cases, definitive treatment of the gastrinoma should be considered. This is particularly true in younger patients, where the malignant potential of the pancreatic component of the MEN I syndrome must be seriously considered. The following patient emphasizes the complex surgical aspects of the MEN I syndrome that may present synchronously.

Case 3. VS, a white female aged 48, was admitted to the University Hospital in February 1977 because of hypercalcemia and diarrhea. Serum calcium levels ranged from 12.7 to 13.8 mg/dl (3.18 to 3.45 mmol/l). The diarrhea had started approximately 1 year before and was initially intermittent but had become progressively more severe, with 10 to 12 watery bowel movements a day. She had no symptoms of peptic ulcer disease. Although she had not gained weight, she had noted a change in fat distribution, particularly in the supraclavicular regions and in the mid-abdomen. Facial hirsutism had been present for about 6 months. A 12-hour gastric aspiration obtained 1500 cc (ml) of gastric fluid containing 140 mEq of hydrochloric acid. Selective visceral angiograms showed an 11 cm vascular tumor in the distal pancreas (*Figure 9.5*). No metastases were demonstrated, although it was apparent that the splenic vein was occluded. An additional finding was an 8 cm vascular tumor involving the left adrenal gland. An upper gastrointestinal series demonstrated no ulcer, but hypertrophic gastric folds as well as the small bowel findings typical of the Zollinger-Ellison syndrome with gastric hypersecretion.

Pertinent laboratory studies showed hypercalcemia, hypophosphatemia and elevated parathyroid hormone concentrations. Serum cortisol was elevated, as were the levels of urinary 17-hydroxy- and 17-ketosteroids. The serum ACTH level was normal.

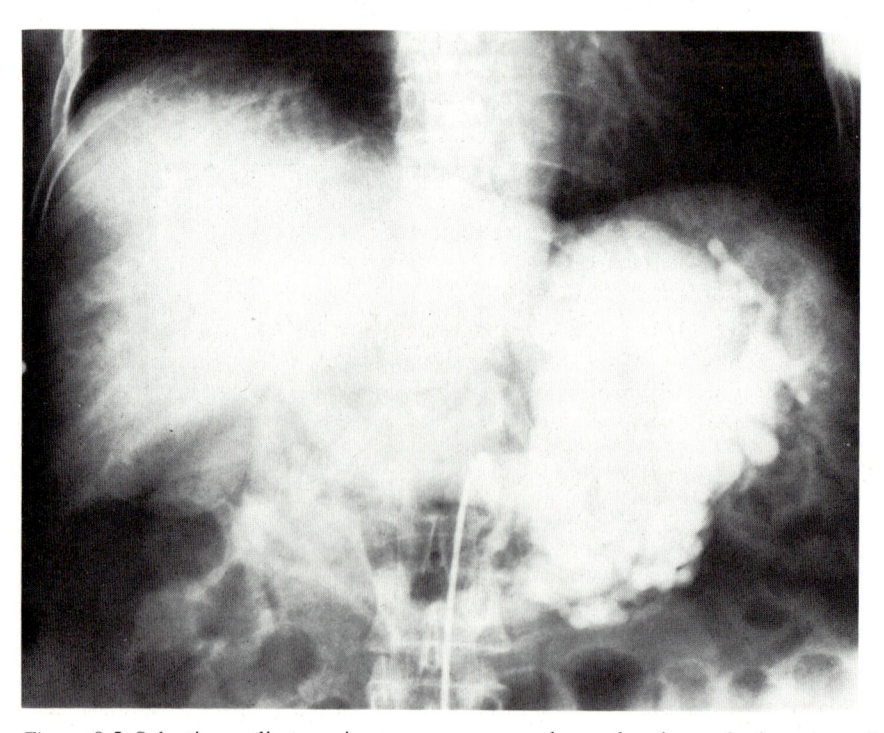

Figure 9.5 Selective celiac angiogram – venous phase showing splenic vein collaterals (varices) and a large pancreatic tumor of the distal body and tail (11 cm gastrinoma)

A diagnosis of the MEN I syndrome with hyperparathyroidism, gastrinoma, and Cushing's syndrome was made. The latter syndrome was felt to be due to a functioning adrenal cortical tumor rather than either pituitary-dependent Cushing's disease or the ectopic ACTH syndrome. There was no family history of the syndrome in either siblings or parents.

On 17 March 1977 a subtotal parathyroidectomy was performed after asymmetrical parathyroid hyperplasia had been demonstrated. Approximately 5 g of hyperplastic parathyroid tissue was excised. The patient's recovery was uneventful and she became normocalcemic. On 22 March 1977 a distal pancreatectomy and splenectomy, total gastrectomy with end-to-side Roux-en-Y esophagojejunostomy, and left adrenalectomy were performed (*Figures 9.6 and 9.7*). The remaining head, neck and proximal body of the pancreas appeared normal. There was no evidence of metastatic gastrinoma in either lymph nodes or the liver.

During the past 5 years the patient has remained normocalcemic and essentially asymptomatic. She has no further clinical or biochemical evidence of Cushing's disease. Corticosteroid replacement therapy was discontinued 6 months after the operation. Furthermore, serum gastrin levels have been less than 100 pg/dl (ng/l). Secretin-stimulated gastrin levels, measured on two occasions, have remained normal.

This patient presented with the synchronous appearance of hyperparathyroidism, autonomous adrenocortical hyperfunction due to an adenoma, and a very large gastrinoma, initially thought to be malignant, causing severe diarrhea. Despite the tumor's large size, causing occlusion of the splenic vein, it was macroscopically and microscopically benign. There has been no evidence to suggest metastatic disease in a 5-year period of follow-up. In this patient with MEN I there has been no other evidence of pancreatic islet cell disease. In retrospect, the total gastrectomy, which was then a standard procedure in this clinical setting, was probably unnecessary. Because of the recent introduction of selective pancreatic venous sampling to localize the source of hypergastrinemia, and the additional armamentarium of histamine-2 receptor blockers, a similar patient today would be treated by pancreatic resection and adrenalectomy. Fortunately this patient, like many others with the Zollinger-Ellison syndrome, has tolerated her total gastrectomy very well, without any significant sequelae.

The two major problems in managing the Zollinger-Ellison syndrome are gastric acid hypersecretion and the malignant potential of the gastrinoma. Unfortunately, the ideal therapy, namely surgical excision of a localized tumor with permanent return of the serum gastrin level to normal, has not been possible in most cases in the past because the gastrinoma had or was suspected to have spread beyond surgical cure at the time of diagnosis[2, 33, 42, 44]. Before the advent of cimetidine, failure to remove the total stomach, even when a gastrinoma was grossly excised, frequently led to early postoperative disasters because of the continued hypersecretion of gastric acid[44]. This was particularly true in the MEN I patients because of the multicentric occurrence of the tumors, the diffuse disease of the pancreatic islets, or the presence of lymph node or liver metastases[5, 37, 42]. The effectiveness of cimetidine in controlling acid secretion, increased clinical awareness, the availability of serum gastrin immunnoassays, and more precise tumor localization techniques have evoked a re-evaluation of the standard surgical management by total gastrectomy[4, 6, 9, 17, 23, 26, 27, 33, 34, 35, 44]. Our current efforts are to identify the potentially curable surgical patients, avoiding total gastrectomy when this appears

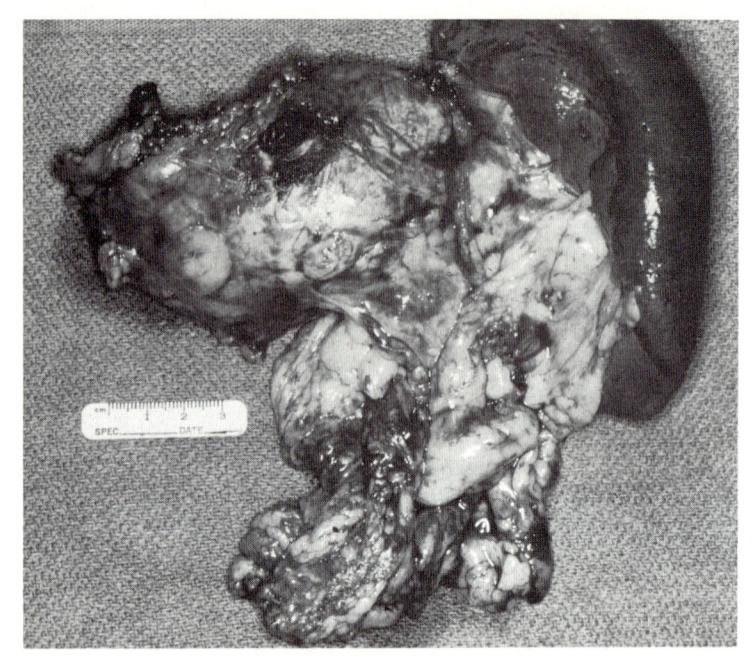

Figure 9.6 Operative specimen from a 60% distal resection of the body and tail of the pancreas with the spleen. The encapsulated tumor (gastrinoma) was 11 cm in diameter

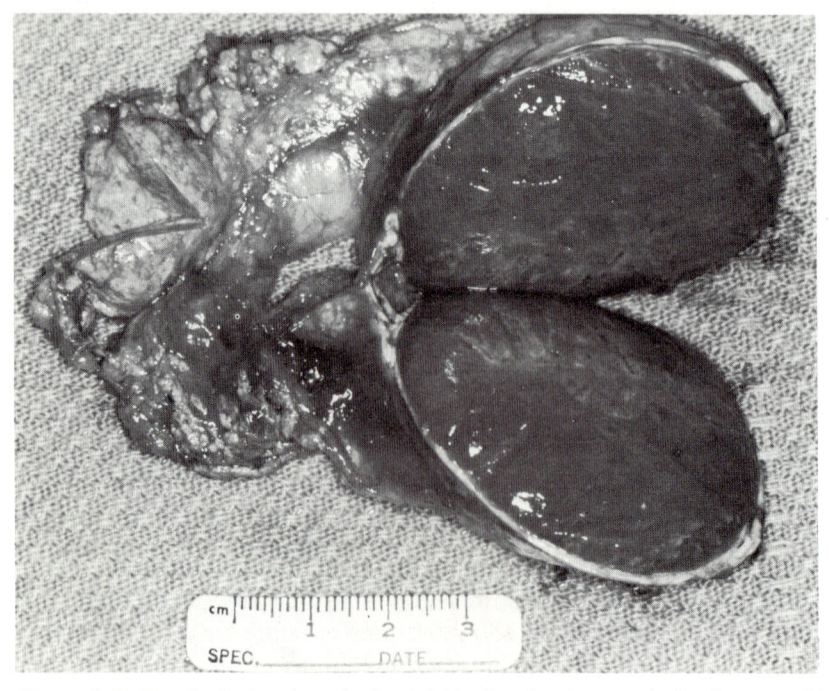

Figure 9.7 Case 3: Left adrenal gland including benign cortical adenoma. Note nodular cortical hyperplasia in remaining gland

feasible. Unless metastatic disease is detected by conventional diagnostic studies, including visceral angiography, percutaneous transhepatic portal venous hormone sampling for gastrin and pancreatic polypeptide as well as other gut hormones is carried out and interpreted before a surgical procedure is planned. If the source of gastrin hypersecretion is localized and grossly confirmed at operation, the tumor or the involved portion of the pancreas is excised. In the presence of diffuse disease, confirmed at operation in a good-risk patient, we continue to believe that total gastrectomy and excision of gross tumor, when practical, offers the patient the best long-term palliation. In older or poorer risk patients, well controlled on cimetidine, our policy is to continue conservative management when surgical cure of the gastrinoma appears unlikely. Surgical alternatives in MEN I patients are listed below.

(1) Gastrinoma excision or partial pancreatectomy
(2) Total gastrectomy, tumor excision
(3) Total gastrectomy and biopsy*
(4) Exploration, biopsy, highly selective vagotomy and cimetidine*
(5) Exploration, biopsy antrectomy, vagotomy and cimetidine*
(6) Parathyroidectomy and cimetidine
(7) Exploration, biopsy and cimetidine*
(8) Cimetidine**

The presence of hypergastrinemia in the MEN I patient poses special problems in surgical management because of the higher incidence of diffuse disease (microadenomatosis, islet cell hyperplasia or multiple tumors) than in patients with the sporadic appearance of the Zollinger-Ellison syndrome, in which a single gastrinoma is the most common etiology. Furthermore, whether gastrinomas are more likely to be malignant with metastases in the MEN I syndrome is another question that has not been sufficiently investigated. The presence of hypergastrinemia in one of our patients after distal pancreatectomy and total gastrectomy during a 5-year period was considered evidence of lymphatic and/or liver metastases. A subsequent venous hormone sampling study, however, demonstrated that the source of gastrin was the remaining pancreatic head. At exploration during a hysterectomy, no evidence of liver or peripancreatic disease was found. The remaining pancreatic head felt thicker than normal but there were no discrete palpable tumors. Her serum gastrin continues to remain in the 1000 pg/dl (ng/l) range. She is believed to have functioning microadenomatosis or hyperplasia of the remaining islet cells. However, in Friesen's recent report of 23 patients with the Zollinger-Ellison syndrome, 4 of the 8 deaths in patients with non-resectable gastrinomas occurred in MEN I patients[9]. Two of the patients with liver metastases survived for 9 and 11 years after total gastrectomy, with regression of the tumor to a non-detectable status for 6 and 11 years. Bonfils et al.[2] recently reported 92 patients who were diagnosed at the Hôpital Bichat in Paris during a 16-year period. In 13 of these

---

* Metastases present.
** No effect on gastrin level or tumor growth.

patients there was definite evidence of islet cell hyperplasia as the cause of the syndrome. There were 19 patients with the MEN I syndrome, but unfortunately no detailed information as to how many of these patients had hyperplasia and/or metastatic disease at the time of surgery was given. Since starting to use portal venous sampling, we have studied 6 patients with proven Zollinger-Ellison syndromes who were MEN I family members. In 2 MEN I patients, each with two tumors localized by transhepatic venous hormone sampling, excision failed to permanently correct the hypergastrinemia or an abnormal response to secretin. In the 4 other patients there was diffuse hypergastrinemia elicited from the pancreas. Several of these patients have had total gastrectomies and distal pancreatectomies which confirmed the diffuse islet cell involvement predicted by venous sampling. Whether or not these preliminary results in MEN I hypergastrinemic patients will apply to all familial cases remains to be determined. If so, surgical removal of the primary source of gastrin, short of total pancreatectomy, will not be possible. We do not believe that total pancreatectomy is justified because of the morbidity and mortality of the operation, and the possibility that undetected gastrinoma metastases may necessitate total gastrectomy at a later date. Another question that remains to be answered is whether the pancreatic component of the MEN I syndrome in patients in whom it occurs sporadically is any different from that in patients with a very clear family history. We are currently reviewing 3 patients in this category who are apparently cured of their pancreatic disease several years after distal pancreatectomy. Certainly careful documentation and long-term follow-up will be necessary to answer some of these provoking questions. At present it would appear that most patients with the MEN I syndrome remain at risk throughout their life for developing new islet cell tumors even when apparently cured for extended periods of time. This consideration, however, should not discourage the attempt to cure an islet cell tumor encountered in this syndrome. The malignant potential of these tumors poses a long-term threat. In Friesen's report there were 3 patients who had excisions of gastrinomas as separate definitive procedures[9]. In one of his patients excision of a pancreatic gastrinoma was the initial procedure. Associated islet cell hyperplasia subsequently required a distal pancreatectomy and total gastrectomy, which resulted in a 16-year tumor-free period with normal serum gastrin. Two of his other patients with the MEN I syndrome had excisions of gastrinomas as separate procedures after total gastrectomy with concomitant excision of pancreatic gastrinomas. These patients were considered to have developed new primary tumors during their follow-up period. It is concluded that with aggressive diagnostic, localization and surgical techniques most patients with the Zollinger-Ellison syndrome in association with the MEN I syndrome will receive significant long-term palliation, if not cure.

Insulinoma and other islet cell tumors

The second most common pancreatic endocrinopathy associated with the MEN I syndrome is caused by hyperinsulinism. In most cases this is due to one or more discrete insulinomas, with or without associated islet cell hyperplasia or nesidioblastosis[19, 31, 37, 42]. Although we have seen organic hypoglycemia caused by nesidioblastosis in several adult patients, none have had the MEN I syndrome[13]. Because more than one insulinoma is rare in patients with sporadic insulinomas, the finding of two or more insulinomas should alert the surgeon to the possibility that the patient has an MEN I syndrome, if this has not already been identified.

There are two significant differences in the surgical consideration of insulinomas and gastrinomas in the MEN I syndrome. Complete excision of insulinoma(s) from the pancreas is usually feasible and leads to permanent cure of the inappropriate secretion of insulin. Although malignant insulinomas may occur in the MEN I syndrome, the great majority are benign at the time of diagnosis. In both conditions associated hypersecretion of other peptide hormones by the endocrine pancreas may also occur. This hypersecretion may occur from hyperplastic islets, microadenomas or concomitant neoplasms[10, 11, 12, 17]. The diagnosis of insulinoma has been facilitated by the availability of insulin immnoassay and can be made with certainty in virtually all cases[10, 13, 14, 16]. Because the source of insulin hypersecretion may not be discrete (single insulinoma) in MEN I patients, preoperative localization studies are mandatory in all cases. Selective visceral angiography will usually not demonstrate insulinomas less than 1.5 cm in size and may fail to demonstrate a significant number of larger ones. We believe, however, that this study should be done in every patient, as other important useful information can be obtained, e.g. regarding the presence of metastases and the individual patient's arterial anatomy. Transhepatic selective portal venous sampling for insulin as well as other hormones should be strongly considered in these cases where diffuse islet cell disease is not uncommon[17]. Although local excision of an insulinoma may be possible in MEN I patients, it is more likely that partial pancreatectomy will be required because of multiplicity, islet cell hyperplasia or other adenomas secreting another polypeptide.

It should be emphasized that MEN I patients are at risk for the development of insulinoma throughout their lifetime and that such tumors may develop years after treatment of another islet cell tumor. The diagnosis may be overlooked or delayed in a patient who has been treated by total gastrectomy for the Zollinger-Ellison syndrome. Symptoms of hypoglycemia may be attributed to dumping or changes in dietary habits. We have had 2 patients who developed insulinomas following previous resections for gastrinoma, and another with concomitant insulinoma, gastrinoma, PPoma and glucagonoma.

Many patients with the MEN I syndrome have hypersecretion of pancreatic polypeptide as a marker of pancreatic involvement[11]. In our experience the most common finding in such patients is diffuse microadenomatosis, hyperplasia or nesidioblastosis, with or without another functioning neoplasm. Hypersecretion of pancreatic polypeptide alone is not associated with a recognized clinical syndrome. It should, however, be considered a source of concern when found in an asymptomatic MEN I patient. Exactly what should be done in these patients is not clear if pancreatic CT scan and arteriography are considered normal. If either of these studies demonstrates a pancreatic mass, exploration and surgical excision are indicated after selective portal venous hormone sampling. Unfortunately PPomas may be quite large and associated with metastatic spread to the liver at the time of diagnosis. Periodic screening for pancreatic polypeptide should be performed in all known MEN I patients. We have had the misfortune of following one MEN I patient during a 5-year period when his pancreatic polypeptide hormone level was markedly elevated. Because he was entirely asymptomatic and selective arteriogragraphy was considered normal, surgical exploration was not recommended. When he developed acute abdominal pain and duodenal obstruction, a celiotomy was performed and a localized adenocarcinoma found in the head of the pancreas. In addition he had diffuse microadenomatosis, several adenomas about 1 cm in size, and nesidioblastosis involving the entire pancreas. Whether the adenocarcinoma arose from the islet cell involvement as an example of reverse nesidioblastosis is not clear. With the exception of the adenocarcinoma, the entire pancreas was virtually replaced with islet cells or islet cell tumors. Despite a total pancreatectomy, the patient died from multiple metastases within 6 months. Whether earlier operation might have prevented this outcome is not known. The findings suggested that nothing short of total pancreatectomy would have excised his involved islet cell disease, which was not macroscopically apparent. Cases such as this emphasize the dilemma which the surgical management of islet cell disease in the MEN I syndrome often poses.

SURGICAL CONSIDERATIONS OF THE PITUITARY INVOLVEMENT IN THE MEN I SYNDROME

Pituitary manifestations of the MEN I syndrome are less frequent than those of the other endocrine organs involved. If the concept of the 'all or none' phenomenon is correct, however, then all patients with the syndrome have or will develop micro- or macroadenomas. Microadenomas are defined as benign pituitary tumors 1 cm in diameter or less, and may be chromophobe, basophil or acidophil in cellular consistency. Many pituitary tumors are non-secretory and almost all are slow growing, benign lesions. Depending on the cell type and polypeptide produced, several different clinical syndromes may develop. The most common sporadic pituitary adenoma, and the one most commonly seen in MEN I patients, is the prolactin cell adenoma. In women the most common clinical syndrome is one of menstrual irregularity associated with infertility and galactorrhea, which may be present in 30–80% of cases. In men a prolactin cell adenoma may be associated with loss of libido, headaches, impotence and visual disturbances, if large enough. Galactorrhea occurs in 30% or less of male patients. Benign pituitary adenomas may become large enough to produce associated mass effects. Most commonly these are loss of visual acuity, visual field defects, cranial nerve palsies, and headaches. The headaches are usually retro-orbital or bitemporal. The visual field defects characteristically start with bitemporal hemianopia and loss of the superior temporal quadrants. Computerized tomographic scanning with third generation scanners (GE 8800) is capable of detecting adenomas as small as 2–3 mm. Because hyperprolactemia is not life-threatening, the best management of the small adenoma is debatable. Treatment with bromocriptine is frequently successful and is currently widely used. Transsphenoidal adenoma excision, however, is considered the treatment of choice for small adenomas, as it is a curative procedure in most cases. In patients with larger lesions associated with mass effects hypophysectomy may be required.

Cushing's disease, or pituitary-dependent adrenocortical hyperplasia, may occur in MEN I patients also. These patients sometimes present with a characteristic Cushing's syndrome. The therapeutic options available include transsphenoidal microadenoma excision, hypophysectomy, mitotane medical therapy with or without pituitary irradiation, and bilateral adrenalectomy. In most cases, unless the pituitary adenoma is large, transsphenoidal hypophysectomy is currently considered the procedure of choice. When growth hormone is the secretory product of the tumor, acromegaly may develop. Once again, the choice of treatment depends on the individual patient and must be based on his overall condition, age, and size of tumor. The options include medical therapy with bromocriptine, pituitary irradiation, and transsphenoidal surgical excision. Hypophysectomy is reserved for patients with large tumors extending beyond the sella turcica or associated with compression symptoms.

References

1 BALLARD, H. S., FRAME, B. and HARTSOCK, R. J. Familial multiple endocrine adenoma–peptic ulcer complex. *Medicine*, **43**, 481 (1964)
2 BONFILS, S., LANDOR, J. H., MIGNON, M. and HERVOIR, P. Results of surgical management in 92 consecutive patients with Zollinger-Ellison syndrome. *Annals of Surgery*, **194**, 692–697 (1981)
3 BORDI, C. Nonantral gastric carcinoids and hypergastrinemia. *Archives of Surgery*, **116**, 1238 (1981)
4 BRENNAN, M. F., JENSEN, R. T., WESLEY, R. A., DOPPMAN, J. L. and McCARTHY, D. M. The role of surgery in patients with Zollinger-Ellison syndrome (ZES) managed medically. *Annals of Surgery*, **196**, 239–245 (1982)
5 BROWN, R. E. and STILL, W. J. S. Nesidioblastosis and the Zollinger-Ellison syndrome. *American Journal of Digestive Disease*, **13**, 656–663 (1968)
6 BURCHASTH, F., STAGE, J. G., STADIL, F. et al. Localization of gastrinomas by transhepatic portal catheterization and gastrin assay. *Gastroenterology*, **77**, 444–450 (1979)
7 CASTELMAN, B., SCHANTZ, A. and ROTH, S. Parathyroid hyperplasia in primary hyperparathyroidism. *Cancer*, **38**(4), 1668–1675 (1976)
8 CLAIN, J. E. Diagnosis and management of gastrinoma (Zollinger-Ellison syndrome). *Mayo Clinic Proceedings*, **57**, 265–266 (1982)
9 FRIESEN, S. R. Treatment of the Zollinger-Ellison syndrome: a 25-year assessment. *American Journal of Surgery*, **143**, 331–338 (1982)
10 FRIESEN, S. R. Tumors of the endocrine pancreas. *New England Journal of Medicine*, **306**, 580–590 (1982)
11 FRIESEN, S. R., KIMMEL, J. R. and TOMITA, T. Pancreatic polypeptide as a screening marker for pancreatic polypeptide apudomas in multiple endocrinopathies. *American Journal of Surgery*, **139**, 61–72 (1979)

12 GELSTON, A. L., DELISLE, M. B. and PATEL, Y. C. Multiple endocrine adenomatosis Type I: occurrence in octagenarian with high levels of circulating pancreatic polypeptide. *Journal of the American Medical Association*, **247**, 665–666 (1982)
13 HARNESS, J. K., GEELHOED, G. W., THOMPSON, N. W. *et al.* Nesidioblastosis in adults. *Archives of Surgery*, **116**, 575–580 (1981)
14 HARRISON, T. S. Insulin secreting lesions of the pancreas. In *The Pancreas*, edited by W. S. Keynes and R. G. Keith, pp. 221–240. New York, Appelton-Century-Crofts (1981)
15 HEATH, H., III and PURNELL, D. C. Urinary cyclic 3'–5' adenosine monophosphate responses to exogenous and endogenous parathyroid hormone in familial benign hypercalcemia and primary hyperparathyroidism. *Journal of Laboratory and Clinical Medicine*, **96**(6), 974–984 (1980)
16 HERMAN, R. E. and COOPERMAN, A. M. Endocrine disease of the pancreas. In *Surgery of the Pancreas*, edited by A. M. Cooperman and S. O. Hoerr, pp. 205–225. St. Louis, Missouri, C. V. Mosby (1978)
17 INGEMANSSON, S. G. Pancreatic and intestinal vein catheterization with hormone assay. *Bulletin of the Department of Surgery* (*University of Lund, Sweden*), **13**, 1–13 (1977)
18 KEITH, R. G. Gastrinomas and other non-insulin producing inslet cell lesions. In *The Pancreas*, edited by W. S. Keynes and R. G. Keith, pp. 241–259. New York, Appelton-Century-Crofts (1981)
19 LAIDLAW, G. F. Nesidioblastoma, the islet tumor of the pancreas. *American Journal of Pathology*, **14**, 125–139 (1938)
20 LAMERS, G. B. H. W. and FROELING, P. G. A. M. Clinical significance of hyperparathyroidism in familial multiple endocrine adenomatosis type I (MEA I). *American Journal of Medicine*, **66**, 422–424 (1979)
21 MAJEWSKI, J. T. and WILSON, S. D. The MEA I syndrome: an all or none phenomenon? *Surgery*, **86**, 475–484 (1979)
22 MALAGELADA, J. R., DAVIS, V. S., O'FALLON, W. M. and GO, V. L. W. Laboratory diagnosis of gastrinoma. I. A prospective evaluation of gastric analysis and fasting serum gastrin levels. *Mayo Clinic Proceedings*, **57**, 211–218 (1982)
23 MALAGELADA, J. R., GLANZMAN, S. L. and GO, V. L. W. Laboratory diagnosis of gastrinoma. II. A prospective study of gastrin challenge. *Mayo Clinic Proceedings*, **57**, 219–226 (1982)
24 MARX, S. J., POWELL, D., SHIMKIN, P. M., WELLS, S. A. KETCHAM, A. S., McGUIGAN, J. E., BILEZIKIAN, J. P. and AURBACH, G. D. Familial hyperparathyroidism – mild hypercalcemia in at least nine members of a kindred. *Annals of Internal Medicine*, **78**, 371 (1973)
25 MARX, S. J., SPIEGEL, A. M., BROWN, F. M. and AURBACH, G. D. Family studies in patients with primary parathyroid hyperplasia. *American Journal of Medicine*, **62**, 698–706 (1977)
26 McCARTHY, D. M. Report on the United States experience with cimetidine in Zollinger-Ellison syndrome and other secretory states. *Gastroenterology*, **74**, 453–458 (1978)
27 McCARTHY, D. M. The place of surgery in Zollinger-Ellison syndrome. *New England Journal of Medicine*, **302**, 1344–1347 (1980)

28 PRINZ, R. A., GAMVZOS, O. I., SELLU, D. and LYN, J. A. Subtotal parathyroidectomy for primary chief cell hyperplasia of the multiple endocrine neoplasia type I syndrome. *Annals of Surgery*, **193,** 26–29 (1981)

29 ROSALI, J. HIGA, E. and DAVIE, J. Mediastinal endocrine neoplasm in patients with multiple endocrine adenomatosis (previously unrecognized association). *Cancer*, **29,** 1075–1083 (1972)

30 ROTH, S. I. and GALLAGHER, M. J. The rapid identification of 'normal' parathyroid glands by the presence of intracellular fat. *American Journal of Pathology*, **84,** 521–528 (1976)

31 SHERMETA, D. W., MENDELSOHN, G. and HALLER, J. A. Hyperinsulinemic hypoglycemia of the neonate associated with persistent fetal histology and function of the pancreas. *Annals of Surgery*, **191,** 182–186 (1980)

32 SNYDER, N., SCURRY, M. T. and DEISS, W. R. Jr. Five families with multiple endocrine adenomatosis. *Annals of Internal Medicine*, **80,** 231 (1974)

33 STADIL, F., STAGE, G., REHFELD, J. F, ESEN, and FISCHERMAN, K. Treatment of Zollinger-Ellison syndrome with streptozotocin. *New England of Medicine*, **294,** 1440–1446 (1976)

34 STAGE, J. G., STADIL, F. and FISCHERMAN, K. New aspects in the treatment of the Zollinger-Ellison syndrome. In *Cimetidine*, edited by W. Creutzfeldt, pp. 137–148. Amsterdam, Excerpta Medica (1978)

35 STAGE, J. G. and STADIL, F. The clinical diagnosis of the Zollinger-Ellison syndrome. *Scandinavian Journal of Gastroenterology*, **14** (Suppl. 53), 79–91 (1979)

36 THORGURSSON, U., COSTA, J. and MARX, S. J. The parathyroid glands in familial hypocalciuric hypercalcemia. *Human Pathology*, **12**(3), 229–237 (1979)

37 VANCE, J. E., STOLL, R. W., KITABCHI, A. E., BUCHANAN, K. D., HOLLANDER, D. and WILLIAMS, R. H. Familial nesidioblastosis as the predominant manifestation of multiple endocrine adenomatosis. *American Journal of Medicine*, **52,** 211–227 (1972)

38 WELLS, S. A., Jr, ELLIS, G. J., GUNNELLS, J. C., SCHNEIDER, A. G. and SHERWOOD, L. M. Parathryoid autotransplantation in primary parathyroid hyperplasia. *New England Journal of Medicine*, **295,** 57–62 (1976)

39 WELLS, S. A., FARNDON, J. R., DALE, J. *et al*. Long term evaluation of patients with primary parathyroid hyperplasia managed by total parathyroidectomy and heterotopic autotransplantation. *Annals of Surgery*, **192**(4), 451–458 (1980)

40 WERMER, P. Genetic aspects of adenomatosis of endocrine glands. *American Journal of Medicine*, **16,** 221–225; 363 (1954)

41 WILLIAMS, E. D. and CELESTIN, L. D. The association of bronchial carcinoid and pluriglandular adenomatosis. *Thorax*, **17,** 120–127 (1962)

42 WILSON, S. D. Wermer's syndrome: multiple endocrine adenopathy type I. In *Surgical Endocrinology: Clinical Syndromes*, edited by S. R. Friesen, pp. 265–283. New York, J. P. Lippincott (1978)

43 WOLTERING, E. A., EMMOT, R. C., JAVALDPOUR, N., MARX, S. and BRENNAN, M. F. (ABOCH) Cell surface antigens in parathyroid adenoma and hyperplasia. *Surgery*, **90**(1), 1–10 (1981)

44 ZOLLINGER, R. M., ELLISON, E. C., FABRI, P. F. Primary peptic ulceration of the jejunum associated with islet cell tumors: twenty-five years' experience. *Annals of Surgery*, **192,** 422–430 (1980)

10
Current views on the surgery of gastrinoma in the post-cimetidine era
Robert M. Zollinger and Helene P. Ayres

Total gastrectomy was advised as a life-saving procedure when the concept of the ulcerogenic islet cell tumor was introduced in 1955[38]. Removal of all acid-secreting surface was the only certain method of controlling the exaggerated gastric hypersecretion associated with gastrin-induced hyperplasia of the parietal cell mass. Control of the acid factor was not possible with antacids available at that time or by irradiation to the fundus of the stomach. The survival of patients having less than a total gastrectomy was minimal, and many patients underwent repeated operations in a futile attempt to control hypersecretion and recurrent ulcer.

This therapeutically static situation persisted for almost two decades until the H_2-receptor antagonists were introduced in the early seventies. Metiamide, introduced in 1972, was followed by cimetidine in 1976 in England and in 1977 in the United States[1]. Metiamide, though effective, was associated with granulocytopenia, which made it unacceptable for general clinical use. Cimetidine, on the other hand, provided immediate dramatic and effective clinical relief of symptoms, which ensured its widespread acceptance. The appearance of an agent that lowered gastric acidity challenged the traditional therapy of total gastrectomy for gastrin-producing islet cell tumors.

Cimetidine is well tolerated and has infrequent and minor side effects. It is usually taken orally in a dose of 300 mg with meals and at bedtime, but it can be taken intravenously or in rectal suppositories. The maximum concentration occurs in 1 to 1½ hours, and it is effective for approximately 4 hours. Most of the drug is excreted in the urine within 24 hours, but some is excreted in the bile. Given in the usual doses, cimetidine inhibits not only fasting secretion but also secretion induced by sham feeding, pentagastrin, fundic distension, insulin, caffeine, and eating[14]. The drug is also effective in depressing the cephalic vagal phases of gastric secretion. The volume of gastric juice is reduced, as are hydrogen-ion concentration and pepsin. While it has no effect on basal gastrin levels, it may increase the postprandial concentration of gastrin. It does not appear to have an effect on lower esophageal sphincter pressure, gastric emptying, or pancreatic secretion.

While cimetidine has been dramatic in providing almost immediate relief to the patient with gastric hypersecretion, there have been scattered reports of various side effects. These have been minimal and have included headaches, diarrhea, skin rashes, and elevations in serum creatinine, as well as antiandrogenic effects[37], i.e. gynecomastia[30] and reduction in sperm count[33]. Clinically, the occasional elderly patient receiving cimetidine may exhibit mental confusion, as may very young patients and those on large doses. Large doses of cimetidine should be avoided in the elderly patient with renal or liver impairment. A creatinine level above 3.0 mg/100 ml (265 μmol/l) or a creatinine clearance below 30 ml/min is an indication for increasing the interval of the 300 mg dose of cimetidine to 12 hours[17].

More recently, attention has been called to the effect of the cimetidine on liver metabolism. Feely, Wilkinson and Wood[12] reported that cimetidine acutely reduced liver blood flow by 25% during fasting in normal subjects. There was a reduction of one third when 300 mg of cimetidine was given four times a day. They emphasized the therapeutic implications for patients with liver disease, as well as for those being given drugs that are highly extracted by the liver. It has been emphasized that cimetidine is a potent inhibitor of the P450 mixed function oxidase microsomal enzyme system of the liver[25]. This impairs the elimination of many drugs, including warfarin-type anticoagulants, diazepam, phenytoin, and chlordiazepoxide. A cumulative effect may result, since the cimetidine reduces the oxidative metabolism of many drugs, including propranolol[12]. These authors caution against the simultaneous use of cimetidine and propranolol because of the dangers of the cumulative effect of the latter on cardiovascular function.

Roberts et al.[28] have reported that cimetidine impairs the elimination of theophylline and antipyrine in healthy subjects. The clinician must remain alert to the potential dangers of giving cimetidine in combination with certain other drugs, especially anticoagulants, antidepressants, and certain vasodilators. However, others have questioned the reported effects on liver blood flow by cimetidine[15,16]. Benzodiazepines, lorazepam, and oxazepam are unaffected because they use glucuronidation pathways[7]. Cimetidine should not be given to pregnant or post-partum women since it crosses the placental barrier and is excreted in milk[14].

The effectiveness of the H_2-receptor antagonist precludes the need for an urgent decision concerning surgical exploration, which formerly prevailed. It is logical and usually clinically safe to give cimetidine while various diagnostic tests are being carried out and the diagnosis of gastrinoma is confirmed or refuted. Additional time is safely provided for parathyroid evaluation as well as assessment of possible involvement of the adrenals and the pituitary gland. Cimetidine, along with medical supervision of the diet, should result in a healing trend in any ulcerations, control of diarrhea, and improved nutrition. This approach is also useful in patients with recurrent ulceration, including a gastrojejunal colic fistula following one or more previous gastric operations.

But many factors must be considered when recommending cimetidine therapy as the only long-term treatment of the patient with gastrinoma. Will the patient comply for 5 to 10 years or longer? Unlike the ulcer patient, the gastrinoma patient must take medication at regular times without fail, and perhaps in ever-increasing dosage as tumor growth and hypergastrinemia increase. The monitoring of cimetidine dosage has depended mostly on assessment of symptom-response, although Straus, Greenstein and Yalow[32] have suggested that the effectiveness of cimetidine treatment for gastrinoma can be monitored objectively by plasma secretin levels. They reported a patient with gastrinoma who remained clinically symptom-free for 6 months on a dose of 900 mg of cimetidine daily while the plasma secretin levels remained undetectable.

The tendency for both patient and physician to be pleased with the result of cimetidine therapy influences both to continue medical therapy indefinitely, despite the fact that the gastrinoma almost always has a malignant potential[35]. Should cimetidine be routinely given until the patient fails to obtain relief or until the tumor has progressed to the extent of producing localized symptoms? The question is often raised, why risk surgical intervention that may include total gastrectomy as well as hemipancreatectomy unless survival following operation is definitely superior to that after prolonged H_2-receptor antagonist therapy? Evidence is lacking that either cimetidine therapy or total gastrectomy alters the growth pattern of the gastrinoma, although Friesen[13] has suggested that tumor regression may rarely follow total gastrectomy.

There are, however, several circumstances in which prolonged cimetidine therapy should be considered. When the diagnosis is questionable and the secretin stimulation ('push') test is not available for further evaluation, surgical treatment should be postponed. Family obligations, the current economic position of the patient, a serious primary disease involving the vascular system, patients – especially women – who have long been underweight, the patient's refusal to undergo surgery, and the presence of associated hyperparathyroidism all temporarily contraindicate urgent surgical intervention. In time, some of these factors may cease to have significance. The value of cimetidine in preoperative preparation cannot be overemphasized.

Despite all the factors to be considered, it is impossible to determine the extent of the gastrinoma or to learn whether local excision of a solitary tumor or substantial debulking of the tumor and metastases is possible without surgical exploration. Only by surgical means can a few patients be cured and the lives of many more be extended.

PREOPERATIVE DIAGNOSIS

The firmness of the diagnosis and the likely location of the tumor are always of primary concern to the surgeon. In addition to the clinical history, it is essential to verify the presence of free hydrochloric acid in the stomach. Repeated elevations of the serum gastrin levels in the presence of hyperchlorhydria support the diagnosis. The provocative secretin stimulation test has become of increasing importance in confirming the diagnosis of gastrinoma while ruling out other causes of hypergastrinemia. It is of particular value when the serum gastrin is elevated only minimally; the test is not of similar assistance when the gastrin levels are elevated to 1000 pg/ml or above because the diagnosis is more obvious[19]. The test results may be influenced by the type and amount of secretin given.

The secretin challenge test is done by giving 2 Clinical units GIH secretin per kg body weight to the patient in a fasting state over a period of 30 s. It is important that a skin test be performed first by administering 1/10 cc (0.1 ml) of secretin intradermally to form a wheal with a nearby similar injection of saline. When an obvious reaction occurs at the site of the injection, secretin is not given. A venous heparin well is inserted when the fasting gastrin is drawn, and additional samples are taken at 1, 3, 5, 7, 10, 15, and 30 min. The gastrin level rises within several minutes in a positive test, which makes early venous sampling after the injection so important (*Figure 10.1*).

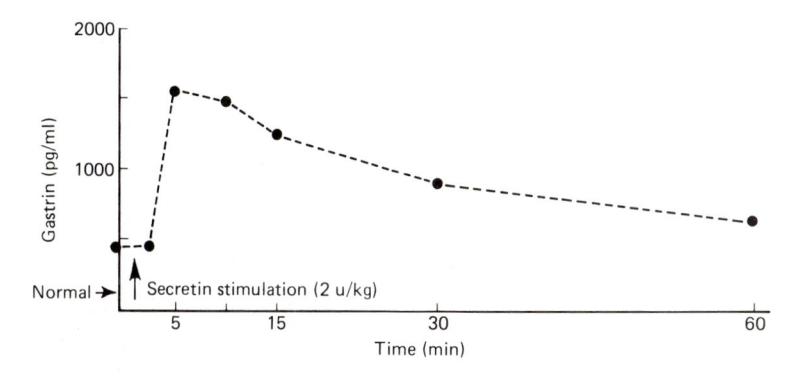

Figure 10.1 The curve of a positive secretin stimulation ('push') test indicates the presence of a gastrinoma

When the maximum gastrin levels during the secretin stimulation test exceed the fasting level by 200 pg or more, the diagnosis of gastrinoma is justified. The hypergastrinemia associated with a retained gastric antrum or antral G-cell hyperplasia, or following a protein meal, kidney failure, and other conditions, does not elevate in response to secretin stimulation. While calcium gluconate or magnesium sulfate can also be used as a provocative test, the time required is several hours longer, and the diagnostic gastrin levels are not as precise as when secretin is given, especially when the gastrin levels are only modestly elevated. Secretin stimulation is desirable in order to minimize negative abdominal exploration. A strongly positive test does provide moral support for the surgeon to diligently explore both sides of the pancreas and to proceed to control the acid factor by appropriate surgical measures.

When operating for a malignancy, the surgeon is anxious to secure as much localization as possible of the tumor or tumors, as well as the metastases. Because the gastrinoma tends to be small and multiple, with hormone-producing metastases as well, angiography or venous sampling for comparative gastrin levels has not been as helpful in demonstrating this tumor as in locating other endocrine tumors, such as insulinoma. However, experience is increasing in the use of selective percutaneous transhepatic venous sampling for gastrin levels[31]. A plastic catheter is directed by the roentgenologist into the portal vein[22] and splenic vein in order to obtain venous samples from the tail, body and head of the pancreas. On occasion, such serial gastrin determinations can be effective in localizing solitary hormone-producing tumors.

Subtotal body scanning has not been as diagnostically productive as was hoped because of the small size of the tumor. Computerized tomographic scanning of the liver and spleen can detect liver metastases, but less frequently pancreatic tumors. Ultrasound scanning may prove to be more valuable: a promising preliminary report indicates that intraoperative use of ultrasound, B-mode, high-resolution scanning and a hand-held gas-sterilized transducer can reveal even such a small mass as a sonolucent area[29].

A complete endocrine survey is important, especially if more than one member of the family has a similar history and symptoms. Special emphasis is directed toward the status of the parathyroid glands. Abnormal parathyroid glands are present in one fifth to one fourth of all patients with gastrinoma. The multiple endocrine neoplasia syndrome (MEN type I), also known as Wermer's syndrome, consists of neoplasia or hyperplasia of pancreatic islet cells, the parathyroids and the pituitary (*see* Chapter 9). The MEN II, or Sipple syndrome, consists of involvement by pheochromocytoma, thyroid carcinoma, parathyroid adenoma or hyperplasia, and occasionally mucosal neurofibromatosis. However, there is enough overlapping to warrant considering adrenal involvement in MEN I and pancreatic islet cell tumors in MEN II. Cameron and Spiro[3] reported a patient having a gastrinoma associated with the MEN II syndrome. They suggested that 'type I and II are classifications which are neither absolute nor exclusive and that multiple endocrine adenomata should be regarded as a spectrum of endocrine disorders'. The apud concepts of Pearse[23,24] regarding the neuroectodermal origin of these tumors explain the various combinations of endocrine tumors. The incidence of hyperparathyroidism is the highest, and can approach 20 to 25% of patients. Other endocrine tumors are far less frequent. The current trend is to advise parathyroid exploration while the gastric hypersecretion is controlled by cimetidine. The gastrin levels usually fall noticeably when the serum calcium is returned to normal, but slowly rise as the tumor growth progresses.

The newer diagnostic tests have contributed to the establishment of the diagnosis of islet cell tumor perhaps five or more years earlier than was possible formerly. The added survival resulting from earlier diagnosis must be taken into consideration in any evaluation of current therapy.

SURGICAL TREATMENT

There is a consensus that the hypercalcemia associated with hyperparathyroidism should be corrected by parathyroidectomy before the gastrinoma is attacked surgically. Correction of the hyperparathyroidism results in lowering of the serum calcium levels, with more effective control of the gastric hypersecretion with cimetidine as the islet cell tumor grows and continues to gradually increase the hypergastrinemia. Cimetidine removes the danger from the excessive gastric hypersecretion while repeated calcium determinations and parathyroid hormone levels can be evaluated. The parathyroid adenoma may be located by nuclear scan[5], as well as by ultrasonography[29] and arterial venous sampling[9]. Because hyperparathyroidism tends to recur during long-term follow-up observation, it is desirable to visualize all parathyroid glands at the time of operation. Consideration should be given to the removal of three and one-half parathyroids. Certainly any enlarged parathyroid gland should be excised. Autotransplantation may accompany extensive parathyroid resections.

Adequate cimetidine therapy[8, 18] can be continued for some months before a decision is made for or against abdominal exploration. The hypercalcemia associated with hyperparathyroidism does not contraindicate the secretin stimulation tests, but the provocative calcium gluconate test should be avoided.

It has been observed that the incidence of renal calculi suggesting hyperparathyroidism is greater than the incidence of hypercalcemia. This variant tends to be associated with those gastrinoma patients who have had a long clinical history of diarrhea. This observation is consistent with the increased frequency of renal calculi in chronic diarrhea and steatorrhea from other causes[39].

Cimetidine and vagotomy have afforded the surgeon more latitude in recent years, without a routine commitment to total gastrectomy[4]. A decision to perform an operation is based on several factors. First, it is always hoped, regardless of how unrealistic it may be, that a solitary tumor will be found, especially in the submucosa of the duodenum or in the left half of the pancreas (*Figure 10.2*). While there is no doubt that a few patients are permanently cured when only a solitary tumor exists, the incidence of success is about 1 in 20, or 5% (*see* Chapter 9).

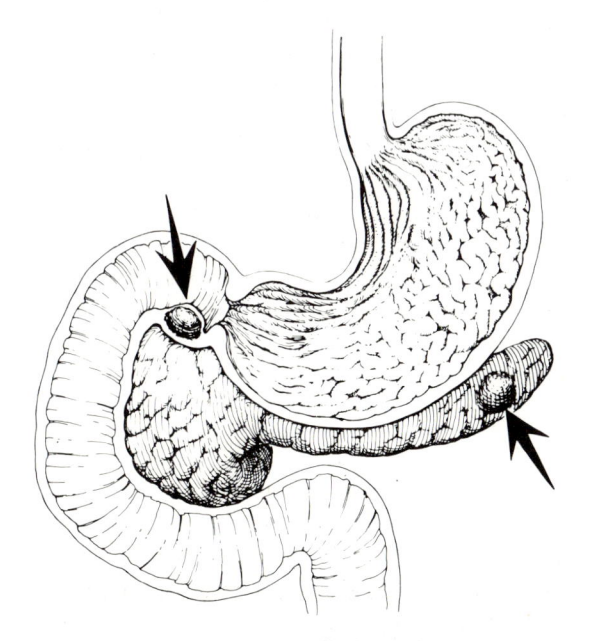

Figure 10.2 Solitary tumors (indicated by arrows) are quite uncommon. Carcinoid tumors in the first portion of the duodenum are more likely to be solitary than those within the pancreas. There is a 5% chance of a solitary tumor occurring in the first portion of the duodenum or within the pancreas which, when excised, corrects the hypergastrinemia

Second, the surgical exploration determines the extent of local invasion as well as the distribution of metastases. Biopsies are taken for histological confirmation of the diagnosis.

Third, if no tumor is found by careful palpation and inspection, a truncal vagotomy and pyloroplasty or a highly selective vagotomy[26] is performed in order to decrease the volume of gastric secretion and enhance cimetidine therapy. A vagotomy should be performed whenever the stomach is not totally resected.

Fourth, total gastrectomy with Roux-en-Y reconstruction is indicated when extensive tumor is found, with or without metastases, when residual tumor remains, when cimetidine therapy has failed, and in the very young. The patient should be a reasonably good surgical risk, and the surgeon should be experienced in the major technical procedures on the stomach and pancreas.

The pros and cons of long-term therapy with H_2-receptor antagonists versus surgical exploration should be carefully explained to the patient. Certainly, patients who have gained complete relief of discomfort find it difficult to accept a reason for the complete removal of the stomach. And many physicians tend to agree. However, it remains logical to advise surgical exploration in every patient, unless their physical condition contraindicates any type of major surgical procedure.

The patient must be informed that he is most likely to have a malignant lesion[2] that will stimulate an excess production of hydrochloric acid as long as he lives. He can be reassured that the gastrinoma and its metastases tend to grow slowly. But the suggestion that a solitary islet cell tumor will be completely removed is hardly warranted, since the chances are probably not more than 4 or 5 in 100. It is more logical to face the fact that the entire stomach may be removed, along with the spleen, adjacent lymph nodes, and the left half of the pancreas. However, he should be made aware that just as cimetidine and freedom from distress have no effect on the growth of the tumor, neither does total gastrectomy, although Friesen[13] and others[4] have documented a few patients whose tumors have apparently receded after total gastrectomy.

The decision for or against surgical exploration and possible gastrectomy is particularly challenging in children. While in youngsters, as in adults, cimetidine relieves symptoms and permits recovery from the acute consequences of gastric hyperactivity, and averts the dangers of gastrointestinal hemorrhage or perforation, the prospect of strict long-term adherence to a demanding regimen of medication justifies consideration of surgical treatment. Of 15 children under 16 years of age collected in a tumor registry in the United States during the pre-cimetidine era[36], 8 had less than total gastrectomy and 6 died, 5 from complications of recurrent ulceration. All 7 children having total gastrectomy remained alive, though metastatic or multiple tumors, or both, were present in all 7 at the time of total gastrectomy. Presumably gastrin-producing tumor may remain in these patients, but one child in whom gastrin increased for 6 years began to exhibit lowered levels after 8 years, and 2 other patients had progressively lower levels each year following total gastrectomy.

The current preoperative preparation of the patients with gastrinoma is usually not as complicated as in former years, when fulminating complications often followed previous surgical procedures. A period of therapy with the H_2-receptor antagonists tends to heal ulcerations, with subsidence of extensive inflammatory involvement about the duodenum or jejunum beyond the ligament of Treitz. Furthermore, H_2-receptor antagonist therapy prevents the tremendous losses of fluids and electrolytes resulting from severe gastric hypersecretion as well as diarrhea. The weight of the patient is carefully monitored as a check on the extent of the possible fluid losses. The blood volume is restored; the fluid and electrolyte balance is assured; and vitamins B and C are given. Antibiotics may be given. A low mortality can be attained if attention is paid to all details of preoperative preparation.

OPERATIVE TECHNIQUE

The lower chest and abdomen are shaved and the patient is placed in a moderate reverse Trendelenburg position following intratracheal intubation and induction of anesthesia. A small-lumen tube (F No. 16) is inserted intranasally into the stomach.

A midline incision is made, which extends up over the xyphoid and beyond the umbilicus on the left side. An elongated xyphoid is often excised, and bleeding on either side controlled by transfixing sutures. The stomach appears more vascular than normal, and feels to palpation like a sponge. The duodenum is enlarged and duodenal deformity may or may not be evident. Ulcerations in the second or third portions of the duodenum are not unusual. The jejunum beyond the ligament of Treitz should be inspected, since ulceration in this area is not at all uncommon. The liver is examined for metastases. Occasionally a very large metastatic lymph node filled with tumor is located just above the first portion of the duodenum.

Special attention is given to the first portion of the duodenum for signs of recent or past ulceration, and it is carefully palpated in search of a small gastrinoma beneath the mucosa. The duodenum is mobilized by the Kocher maneuver, which permits more accurate digital palpation of the head of the pancreas. The greater omentum is reflected upward in order to define the relatively avascular cleavage plane just above the colon. This plane is divided, with a minimal number of blood vessels to be divided and ligated. The lesser sac is entered, and the transverse colon as well as both flexures are freed from the greater omentum to enhance visualization of the head, body, and especially the tail of the pancreas, which may extend into the hilus of the spleen. With the stomach retracted upward, a careful visual as well as digital examination of the pancreas is carried out. The relatively avascular peritoneal attachment along the inferior border of the pancreas can be incised and the posterior aspect of the body of the pancreas easily mobilized by blunt finger dissection.

Occasionally a gastrinoma is overlooked in the very end of the tail of the pancreas, which may be closely adherent to the hilus of the spleen. Blind resection of the left half of the pancreas is no longer advocated. Solitary tumors easily exposed can sometimes be enucleated, but the bed of the tumor must be thoroughly inspected for bleeding, as well as leakage of pancreatic juice from a sizable duct. An effort should be made to control the bleeding carefully, as well as to avoid a postoperative pancreatic fistula.

When the body and tail of the pancreas contain numerous tumors, it is worth while to resect the involved portion of the gland. Total pancreatectomy is not indicated because of the high incidence of functioning metastases that would continue to cause complications from marked gastric hypersecretion, as well as the endocrine problems that ensue. There is clinical evidence that the excision of tumor tissue does tend to prolong the average survival of patients[39]. Easily exposed tumors in the head of the pancreas may be locally enucleated and the tumor bed edges carefully approximated. Some have advocated a Whipple procedure when portal segmental hormone studies have suggested localization of tumor within the head of the pancreas[31]. All detectable lymph nodes should be excised, including the occasional large one filled with metastasis which has been found occasionally just above the duodenum. Prolonged survival of more than 5 years may follow resection of a localized metastasis found on the surface of the liver.

Since the introduction of the H_2-receptor antagonists, the surgeon can direct the initial major technical effort toward removing as much tumor and metastasis as can be done with reasonable safety for the patient. There remain two choices regarding the procedures to be performed on the stomach. A vagotomy should always be done when any stomach remains, and there is nothing to be gained by adding a subtotal resection. The second choice is total gastrectomy.

A vagotomy tends to decrease the acid output by approximately one half. Richardson et al.[27] emphasized the effect of vagotomy in a small series of patients with gastrinoma who showed a definite decrease in gastric hypersecretion following vagotomy. In 1956, Ellison reported a patient with an ulcerogenic islet cell tumor who underwent vagotomy by Zollinger in 1947; the 12-hour overnight gastric secretion was reduced by one half, and the milliequivalents of hydrochloric acid were lowered from 129 to 58 mg[10]. These observations suggest that some type of vagotomy should be done when less than a total gastrectomy is performed. Because localized tumors do occur in the region of the pylorus, it seems logical to perform a vagotomy and pyloroplasty. This facilitates visual as well as digital examination of the mucosa of the first portion of the duodenum adjacent to the pylorus. Tumors buried in the submucosa may become apparent only on microscopic study.

When total gastrectomy is performed, the first 3 cm of the duodenum should be included in the specimen. The lumen of the duodenal portion of the specimen may be filled with a moist gauze sponge so that the pathologist will include the entire circumference of the duodenum in his study. The lumen of the duodenum is digitally palpated in search of a possible tumor nodule and closed in two layers with interrupted silk or synthetic sutures or a stapler. All gastrosplenic vessels are ligated close to the gastric side, and the peritoneum over the lower end of the esophagus is divided. A better exposure is obtained if the avascular triangular ligament of the left lobe of the liver is divided, and the left lobe folded upward against the remaining liver. With the xyphoid removed, the left lobe mobilized, and the patient placed in a reverse Trendelenburg position, a reasonable exposure of the esophagogastric junction can be achieved. The vagus nerves are divided and both ends ligated. If the patient has had a previous vagotomy, great care is taken to avoid fraying the muscular wall of the esophagus. With traction on the stomach, the esophagus is anchored in three or four places to the margins of the hiatus. This prevents retraction of the esophagus when it is divided near the gastric junction. This hiatus posterior to the esophagus should be closed with three or four interrupted sutures.

Since the esophagus lacks a peritoneal surface, it is advantageous to place a series of mattress sutures through the lower esophageal wall adjacent to the line of division. These sutures provide a cuff which improves the anastomosis with the jejunal mucosa. Furthermore, fraying of the non-peritonealized esophageal wall is avoided and bleeding controlled.

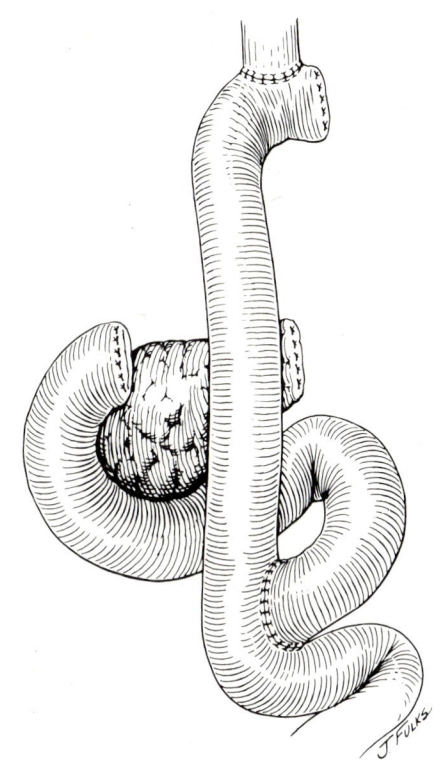

Figure 10.3 The Roux-en-Y type of anastomosis is preferred. Hemipancreatectomy with resection of mestastases is performed commonly

Although many types of reconstruction have been advocated, it is no longer considered advantageous to construct a pouch as a substitute stomach. The Roux-en-Y type of anastomosis is the preferred type of reconstruction (*Figure 10.3*). The jejunum is divided beyond the ligament of Treitz. The mobilized arm, 15 to 20 cm in length and with good arterial pulsations, is passed through an opening made in the mesocolon just to the left of the middle colic vessels. The end of the jejunum is closed with two layers of silk, and an end-to-side anastomosis is performed. The jejunum should be anchored to the diaphragm posterior to the esophagus and again anteriorly after a two-layer closure of the anastomosis. Some prefer the use of a stapler for the anastomosis. The proximal jejunum is anastomosed to the arm going to the esophagus, and all openings in the mesenteries are closed. The Levin tube may be directed around toward the closed duodenal stump. Drainage is used only if a partial pancreatic resection is performed or a tumor is enucleated from the pancreas.

POSTOPERATIVE CARE

The immediate postoperative care is related to the extent of the surgical procedure. Intravenous cimetidine therapy should be given on a regular schedule until oral intake is permitted to all patients having less than a total gastrectomy. Blood amylase determinations are performed postoperatively and repeated daily in patients having procedures on the pancreas until values are normal. Fluid and electrolytes are replaced as in any major postoperative patient. The nasal suction tube remains in place until bowel action has returned. Antibiotics may be given. Collections in the left subphrenic space must not be overlooked. Serum gastrin levels should be measured and repeated every 6 months, and later annually. The initial postoperative gastrin levels tend to fall, but by far the majority continue to rise ever so slowly in the ensuing months. It is unwise to accept early low gastrin levels after any surgical procedure as solid evidence that all tumor has been removed. At least 5 years of observation is required to be certain that the gastrinoma has not persisted or recurred.

Patients having a total gastrectomy should have repeated instruction regarding their diets before leaving the hospital. Six small feedings a day can eventually be replaced by a regular three-meals-a-day diet. The nutritional consequences of total gastrectomy for gastrinoma are surprisingly good compared to those after total gastrectomy for carcinoma of the stomach. Perhaps the chronic hypergastrinemia stimulates the appetite and has a trophic effect on the mucosa of the small intestine. It has proved useful to readmit patients undergoing total gastrectomy for several days of dietary observation every 3 months during the first year after operation. They must be firmly indoctrinated to the necessity of monthly injections of vitamin B_{12} for the rest of their lives. Approximately two thirds of these patients will sustain their ideal weight.

Patients who have postoperative gastrointestinal complaints should have barium studies to evaluate the adequate patency of the esophageal anastomosis. Some may require dilation of the anastomosis. A few patients develop cholecystitis and cholelithiasis. It is surprising how extensive the gastrin-producing tumors involving the pancreas may be without producing pain, in contrast to observations made in carcinoma of the pancreas.

Patients having less than a total gastrectomy with or without vagotomy will inevitably require a resumption of cimetidine therapy for the rest of their lives. For a variety of reasons, some patients in this group will no doubt require reoperation and total gastrectomy because of recurrent uncontrollable symptoms or failure to continue the recommended schedule of medication.

Blood studies, including gastrin and calcium as well as prolactin levels, especially in patients with the MEN I syndrome, should be performed every 6 months for several years, then on a yearly basis. Hypercalcemia may recur owing to recurrent hyperparathyroidism. An increase in the occurrence of kidney stones has been observed in patients whose chief preoperative complaint had been diarrhea for years without evidence of hypercalcemia[39]. Tumor activity can be evaluated from the results of the provocative secretin test when the gastrin levels are less than 1000 pg/ml. The 5 to 7 min gastrin elevation tends to increase each year when tumor is present. Fabri et al.[11] have advocated measuring the percentage of the G-17 component in the total gastrin. A value of more than 20% for this fraction appears to indicate significantly increased tumor activity. When the fasting gastrin level exceeds 1000 pg, the possibility of performing scans and a liver-pancreas arteriogram should be considered.

THE ROLE OF CHEMOTHERAPY

A progressively mounting gastrin level should raise the question of chemotherapy with streptozotocin. There is no evidence that irradiation to the tumor is beneficial. Indeed, some patients survive for well over 5 years despite extensive pancreatic involvement as well as metastases to regional lymph nodes and, in some instances, verified multiple metastases to the liver.

The gastrinoma and its functioning metastases have failed to yield the secret of their malignant potential to either the clinician or the pathologist. Metastases are common and have been estimated to be present in perhaps three-fourths of all cases. So far, microscopic studies have not been helpful in evaluating which tumor is fast growing and which tumor will grow suprisingly slowly. It is probably safe to state that the average rate of growth of the gastrinoma is unknown, which makes a reliable clinical prognosis hazardous. This factor also makes the evaluation of various forms of treatment difficult.

The role of chemotherapy in the treatment of gastrinoma has not been well defined. In a series of 6 patients with evidence of metastases and high gastrin levels who were treated with streptozotocin, 5-fluorouracil (5-FU) and tubercidin in 1976[39], the clinical impression of results was favorable. However, 2 patients with advanced disease who had been predicted not to respond were dead within 1 and 4 years respectively. On the other hand, 4 patients with extensive metastases, including 1 who had metastasis removed from the left lobe of the liver, have survived for more than 5 years after the last treatment. While this is encouraging, other patients have survived longer than 5 years with multiple metastases to the liver and local lymph nodes without chemotherapy.

Moertel, Hanley and Johnson[21] reported results in 84 randomized patients with advanced islet cell carcinoma treated with streptozotocin alone or in combination with fluorouracil. They received 500 mg/m^2 body surface for 5 consecutive days. The dose was repeated every 6 weeks if the malignant disease improved or remained stable. White cell counts and platelet counts were assessed each week, and liver and renal function before each treament. Fluorouracil was reduced by 25% if leukopenia below 2000 cm^3 or thrombocytopenia below 50 000 cm^3 were present. The dose of streptozotocin was reduced by 50% if the patient had severe nausea and vomiting or presented evidence of renal toxicity, indicated by a creatinine of 1.5 mg/ml. If problems persisted, fluorouracil was given. A favorable response was reported in 3 of 8 patients in the group having a gastrinoma.

Streptozotocin may be given every 6 weeks in a bolus of 200 mg/m^2 body surface. The patients should be good risks and younger than 65 years of age. They should have significant symptoms, microscopic proof of a gastrinoma, and measurable serum gastrin elevations. The usual blood, renal, and liver function studies should precede each treatment.

Experience with patients with gastrinoma since 1954 gives support to the concept that perhaps chemotherapy should be considered routinely rather than sporadically, as in the past.

DISCUSSION

The pros and cons of the various policies of treatment of the gastrinoma cannot be fully evaluated until at least a 5-year follow-up of patients treated with cimetidine has been carefully documented. The 5-year survival of the pre-cimetidine era approximates 45% to 50% following total gastrectomy. Death has been related to extent of disease, complications, and other factors. Such a variety of surgical procedures, combined with varying degrees of aggressiveness in the attack on the tumor have been used that it is risky to quote statistics.

Our experience shows a 5-year survival of 50% for 14 patients having only total gastrectomy. When total gastrectomy was combined with hemipancreatectomy in 19 other patients who had identified tumor, the 5-year survival was increased to 68%. This suggests the value of aggressive tumor resection. However, 6 of 7 patients (87%) having less than a total gastrectomy are living after up to 12 years. Only 1 patient, who had removal of a large solitary pancreatic tumor, was symptom-free with a normal gastrin level 14 years afterwards, having had no gastric procedure performed. The remaining 6 patients had truncal vagotomy combined with gastroenterostomy, pyloroplasty, or antrectomy. One patient died of diffuse metastases 4½ years after truncal vagotomy, gastroenterostomy, and removal of a gastrinoma by hemipancreatectomy. A basophil adenoma of the pituitary was found at the time of autopsy. Another patient died 10 years after vagotomy and three gastric resections done elsewhere. He required cimetidine therapy for relief, and autopsy revealed extensive alcoholic cirrhosis of the liver and a tumor in the submucosa of the duodenal stump.

It should be emphasized that no gross tumor was discovered in 3 of the patients at the time of operation, but their gastrin levels have slowly increased each year. All have had elevated gastrin levels in response to the secretin perfusion test. Of the 6 patients, 5 have lived 7, 7½, 9½, 10 and 12 years, but have required cimetidine to relieve symptoms. One patient had recurrent ulceration with massive bleeding, but has been symptom-free for the past 3 years on regular cimetidine therapy.

It must be noted that 1 of the 2 patients in the original report is living 27 years after total gastrectomy and removal of two small lymph nodes containing metastatic islet cell tumor on the surface of the pancreas in November 1954. Ten years later, at the time of cholecystectomy, there was no evidence of tumor in the pancreas or of metastases. A blind left hemipancreatectomy revealed one small gastrinoma. Currently, after 27 years, liver and pancreatic scans remain negative, but the fasting serum gastrin levels show a steady rise (*Figure 10.4*). The secretin provocative test shows a modest increase in gastrin response each year, and the levels of the G-17 fraction have increased to 30% of total gastrin. As emphasized by Fabri *et al.*[11], the mounting of the G-17 fraction indicates increased tumor activity, and all but one of the patients who died had G-17 fraction levels of 20% or above. But this patient currently feels well, has maintained her weight, and has two daughters, both born after she underwent total gastrectomy in 1954.

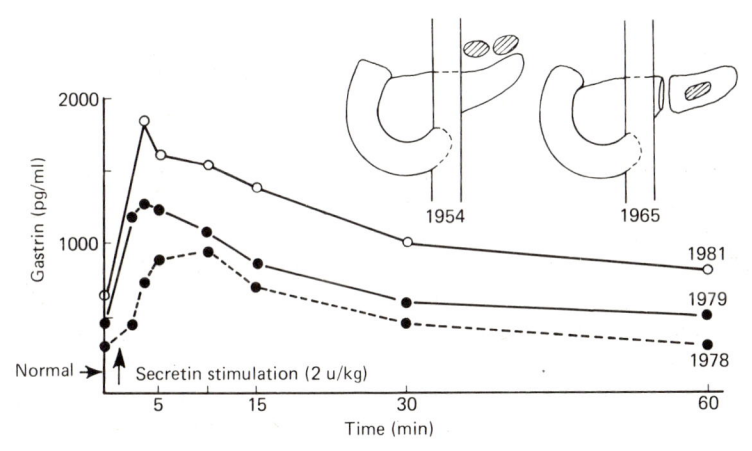

Figure 10.4 Gastrinoma follow-up. Continued growth 27 years after total gastrectomy and 16 years after hemipancreatectomy is evident from the elevated gastrin response to secretion stimulation. The patient is the survivor of the 2 patients described in the original report in 1955

Current concepts in the management of gastrinoma offer three modes of treatment. The first consists of initial management with cimetidine to relieve pain with safety while the diagnosis is confirmed, possible additional endocrine gland involvement is investigated, and the patient is evaluated as a surgical risk. Eventually, a decision must be made whether long-term medical treatment[20] will be continued indefinitely, or combined with conservative surgery or a radical approach consisting of radical tumor excision and total gastrectomy.

The medical-surgical viewpoint advises surgical intervention in all patients to confirm the diagnosis in the hope of finding and removing a solitary tumor and performing a conservative surgical procedure such as truncal vagotomy and pyloroplasty. Patients treated in this manner are likely to be committed to a lifetime of cimetidine therapy.

The radical surgical approach advises surgical exploration of every patient not only to establish the diagnosis, but to eradicate as much tumor as possible and perform total gastrectomy and possible left hemipancreatectomy. This procedure would be chosen when extensive tumor and metastases are found, when cimetidine therapy fails, or in the very young patients with a predictable long life span.

Chemotherapy should probably be more frequently considered for all patients with proved residual tumor or metastases to the liver and lymph nodes, especially those with mounting gastrin levels in response to secretin stimulation or those in whom the G-17 fraction surpasses 20% of the total gastrin.

Although future developments may well alter the methods of treatment, it seems logical to use both the H_2-receptor antagonists and surgery in the management of gastrinoma. There is no disagreement that surgery is indicated when cimetidine fails to control symptoms or the patient rejects the discipline of years of regular medication. There is also no disagreement when a catastrophic complication occurs, such as perforation or a persistent and recurrent massive hemorrhage. Surgeons have long accepted the challenge of solid intra-abdominal malignant tumors by exploring the patient in the hope of prolonging life by extirpating all or part of the tumor. Physicians, on the other hand, have been able to provide almost immediate relief to the patient with gastrinoma for the first time with the use of cimetidine, and the patient becomes asymptomatic even in the presence of a malignant lesion. It is becoming increasingly clear than an individualized approach, based on the history and laboratory and clinical evidence of each patient, is needed.

It is a departure from established tradition to treat a solid intra-abdominal malignant lesion by medical means rather than to attempt to eradicate it by surgery. The chance to cure the disease or prolong life in the presence of a resectable lesion grows less the longer the patient is treated medically without surgical exploration. The pros and cons of medical versus surgical treatment cannot be fully evaluated until a 5-year follow-up of patients treated with cimetidine or other H_2-receptor antagonists has been carefully documented.

References

1 BONFILS, S., MIGNON, M. and GRATTON, J. Cimetidine treatment of acute and chronic Zollinger-Ellison syndrome. *World Journal of Surgery*, **3**, 597–604 (1979)
2 BLOOM, S. R., POLAK, J. M. and WELBOURN, R. B. Pancreatic apudomas. *World Journal of Surgery*, **3**, 587 (1979)
3 CAMERON, D. and SPIRO, H. M. Zollinger-Ellison syndrome with multiple endocrine adenomatosis type II (letter). *New England Journal of Medicine*, **299**, 152–153 (1978)
4 CLARK, C. G. and BOULOS, P. B. Cimetidine and the gastric surgeon. *World Journal of Surgery*, **3**, 745–752 (1979)
5 DAMGAARD-PETERSON, K. and STAGE, J. G. CT scanning in patients with Zollinger-Ellison syndrome and carcinoid syndrome. *Scandinavian Journal of Gastroenterology*, Suppl. 53, 117–122 (1979)
6 DAVIS, C. E., Jr and VANSANT, J. H. Zollinger-Ellison syndrome: spontaneous regression of advanced intra-abdominal metastases with 20 year survival. *Annals of Surgery*, **189**, 620–626 (1979)
7 DESMOND, P. V., PATWARDHAN, R. V., SCHENKER, S. and SPEEG, K. V., Jr. Cimetidine impairs elimination of chlordiazepoxide ('Librium') in man. *Annals of Internal Medicine*, **93**, 266 (1980)

8 DOMSCHKE, W., LUX, G. and DOMSCHKE, S. Gastric inhibitory action of H_2-antagonists ranitidine and cimetidine. *Lancet*, **1**(8111), 320 (1979)

9 DUNN, E. and STEIN, S. Percutaneous transhepatic pancreatic vein catheterization in localization of insulinoma. *Archives of Surgery*, **116**, 232–233 (1981)

10 ELLISON, E. H. The ulcerogenic tumor of the pancreas. *Surgery*, **40**, 147 (1956)

11 FABRI, P. J., JOHNSON, J. A., McGUIGAN, J. E. and ZOLLINGER, R. M. Response of species of gastrin to calcium infusion in ZES. *Journal of Surgical Research*, **26**, 94–96 (1979)

12 FEELY, J., WILKINSON, G. R. and WOOD, A. J. J. Reduction of liver blood flow and propranolol metabolism by cimetidine. *New England Journal of Medicine*, **304**, 692–695 (1981)

13 FRIESEN, S. R. Zollinger-Ellison syndrome. *Current Problems in Surgery*. April (1972)

14 GOODMAN, L. S. and GILMAN, A. *The Pharmacological Basis of Therapeutics*, 6th Edn. New York, Macmillan (1980)

15 JACKSON, J. E. Reduction of liver blood flow by cimetidine (letter). *New England Journal of Medicine*, **305**, 99–100 (1981)

16 LEBREC, D., GOLDFARB, G. and BENHAMOU, J.-P. Reduction of liver blood flow by cimetidine (letter). *New England Journal of Medicine*, **305**, 100 (1981)

17 MA, K. W., BROWN, D. C., MASLER, D. S. and SILVIS, S. E. Effects of renal failure on blood levels of cimetidine. *Gastroenterology*, **74**(2, part 2), 473–477 (1978)

18 McCARTHY, D. M. Report on the United States experience with cimetidine in Zollinger-Ellison syndrome and other hypersecretory states. *Gastroenterology*, **74**, 453–458 (1978)

19 McGUIGAN, J. E. and WOLFE, M. M. Secretin injection test in the diagnosis of gastrinoma. *Gastroenterology*, **79**, 1324–1331 (1980)

20 MIGNON, M., VALLOT, T., GALMICHE, J. P., DUPAS, J. L. and BONFILS, S. Interest of a combined antisecretory treatment, cimetidine and pirenzepin, in the management of severe forms of Zollinger-Ellison syndrome. *Digestion*, **20**, 56–61 (1980)

21 MOERTEL, C. G., HANLEY, J. A. and JOHNSON, L. A. Streptozotocin alone compared with streptozotocin plus fluorouracil in the treatment of advanced islet-cell carcinoma. *New England Journal of Medicine*, **303**, 1189–1194 (1980)

22 PASSARO, E. Localization of pancreatic endocrine tumors by selective portal vein catheterization and radioimmunoassay. *Gastroenterology*, **77**, 806 (1979)

23 PEARSE, A. G. E. and WELBOURN, R. B. The apudomas. *British Journal of Hospital Medicine*, **10**, 617 (1973)

24 PEARSE, A. G. E. Common cytochemical and ultrastructural characteristics of cells producing polypeptide hormones (the APUD series) and their relevance to thyroid and ultimobranchial C cells and calcitonin. *Proceedings of the Royal Society of London, Biological Sciences*, **170**, 71 (1968)

25 PUURUNEN, J., ESOTANIEMI, J. and PELKONEN, O. Effect of cimetidine on microsomal drug metabolism in man. *European Journal of Clinical Pharmacology*, **18**, 185 (1980)

26 RICHARDSON, C. T., FELDMAN, M., McCLELLAND, R. N., DICKERMAN, R. M., KUMPURIS, D. and FORDTRAN, J. S. Effect of vagotomy in Zollinger-Ellison syndrome. *Gastroenterology*, **77**, 682–686 (1979)

27 RICHARDSON, C. T., FELDMAN, M., BRATER, C. and WELBORN, J. Tiotidine, a new long-acting H_2-receptor antagonist: comparison with cimetidine. *Gastroenterology*, **80**, 301–306 (1981)

28 ROBERTS, R. K., GRICE, J., WOOD, L., PETROFF, V. and McGUFFIE, C. Cimetidine impairs the elimination of theophylline and antipyrine. *Gastroenterology*, **81**, 19–21 (1981)

29 SIGEL, B., KRAFT, A. R., NYHUS, L. M., COELHO, J. C. U. and GAVIN, M. P. Identification of a parathyroid adenoma by operative ultrasonography. *Archives of Surgery*, **116**, 234 (1981)

30 SPENCE, R. W. and CELESTIN, L. R. Gynecomastia associated with cimetidine. *Gut*, **20**, 154 (1979)

31 STADIL, F. and STAGE, J. G. The Zollinger-Ellison syndrome. *Journal of Clinical Endocrinology and Metabolism*, **8**, 433–446 (1979)

32 STRAUS, E., GREENSTEIN, R. J. and YALOW, R. S. Plasma secretion in management of cimetidine therapy for Zollinger-Ellison syndrome. *Lancet*, **2**, 73–75 (1978)

33 VAN THIEL, D. H., GAVALER, J. S., SMITH, W. I. Jr and PAUL, G. Hypothalamic-pituitary-gonadal dysfunction in men using cimetidine. *New England Journal of Medicine*, **300**, 1012 (1979)

34 WELBOURN, R. B., PEARSE, A. G. E., POLAK, J. M. and JAFFE, S. N. The apud cells of the alimentary tract in health and disease. *Medical Clinics of North America*, **58**, 1359 (1974)

35 WELBOURN, R. B. Current status of the apudomas. *Annals of Surgery*, **185**, 1–12 (1977)

36 WILSON, S. D., SCHULTE, W. J. and MEADE, R. C. Longevity studies following total gastrectomy in children with Zollinger-Ellison syndrome. *Archives of Surgery*, **103**, 108–114 (1971)

37 WINTERS, S. J., BANKS, J. E. and LORSAIX, D. L. Cimetidine is an antiandrogen in the rat. *Gastroenterology*, **76**, 504 (1979)

38 ZOLLINGER, R. M. and ELLISON, E. H. Primary peptic ulceration of the jejunum associated with islet cell tumors of the pancreas. *Annals of Surgery*, **142**, 709 (1955)

39 ZOLLINGER, R. M., ELLISON, E. C., FABRI, P. J., JOHNSON, J., SPARKS, J. and CAREY, L. C. Primary peptide ulceration of the jejunum associated with islet cell tumors: twenty-five year appraisal. *Annals of Surgery*, **192**, 422–430 (1980)

Editors' commentary on Chapter 10

The introduction of effective histamine receptor antagonists into clinical practice has allowed the control of excess gastric acid secretion in patients with Zollinger-Ellison syndrome to become primarily pharmacological.

The approach in many centres is now to limit surgery to the complications of the disease or to patients in whom the syndrome cannot be controlled medically. Effective control of excess gastric acid secretion enables the patient's general condition to be improved and allows time for the accurate assessment and staging of the underlying tumour pathology, using modern techniques, including selective vein catheterization. Surgery, if required, can then proceed in fit patients with a greater degree of safety.

Brennan and his colleagues in New York have managed 26 patients with cimetidine primarily in a deliberate attempt to avoid surgery. Nine of these patients had metastatic disease and six had multiple endocrine neoplasia. Six patients (23%) required surgery during cimetidine treatment because of complications of their disease.

We have successfully maintained two patients with the syndrome with H_2-receptor antagonists for up to 6 years. Both patients have slowly progressive metastatic disease and have had numerous abdominal operations, including subtotal gastric resection. One patient with peptic ulcer disease relapses within weeks of stopping, or significantly reducing, his cimetidine treatment, but both have no digestive symptoms when on a full dose of cimetidine.

There are several problems, however, with long-term cimetidine. Some patients become resistant even to high doses while others develop complications or side effects. The incidence of gynaecomastia in patients on long-term high-dose cimetidine can be as high as 4% and impotence can also be a problem.

The second generation of H_2-receptor antagonists are now available. Ranitidine (Zantac) is as effective as cimetidine in controlling gastric acid secretion but appears to cause fewer side effects.

There are encouraging reports now of patients with the Zollinger-Ellison syndrome in whom treatment with ranitidine has led to an improvement in the cimetidine-induced gynaecomastia.

There is also evidence that ranitidine is effective in regaining control of the syndrome in patients who have become resistant to cimetidine.

The availability of a second powerful histamine receptor antagonist is another important advance in the control of the Zollinger-Ellison syndrome.

The chemotherapy for malignant gastrinoma has proved relatively ineffective, but direct infusion of drugs such as streptozotocin into the coeliac axis merits further investigation along with medical control of gastric hypersecretion.

11
Surgery of primary aldosteronism
Ivan D. A. Johnston

It was not long after the isolation of the hormone aldosterone that Conn[4] described a patient with hypertension, hypokalaemia, polyuria and intermittent episodes of paralysis who was found to have an adrenal adenoma and was cured by its removal.

Primary aldosteronism is responsible for less than 1% of all cases of hypertension. The uncontrolled secretion of aldosterone is the cause of the sodium retention, potassium depletion and hypertension found in patients with primary aldosteronism due to either adenoma or hyperplasia. In over 75% of patients a single benign, well encapsulated adenoma has been found. The remainder have bilateral hyperplasia. Excision of an aldosterone secreting adenoma almost invariably cures both the hypokalaemia and the hypertension. Excision of a multinodular or hyperplastic gland fails to cure, but aldosterone blocking drugs are effective in these patients. The number of patients with hyperplasia who are explored should be less than 5%. It is therefore very important to first identify patients with primary aldosteronism within a population of hypertensive patients, and then determine with considerable accuracy whether the aldosteronism is due to adenoma or hyperplasia.

A typical aldosterone secreting tumour is small, between 8 and 20 mm in diameter, and usually has a very distinct golden yellow colour. They may project from the surface of the gland, but they can be intraglandular and only found when the excised gland has been sectioned. The typical histological picture is of large lipid-laden or clear cells arranged in cords or lines and separated by fine fibrous tissue trabeculae.

Diffuse or nodular hyperplasia of the zona glomerulosa is usually a uniform feature of both glands when hyperplasia is the cause of the syndrome, but on occasion areas of focal hyperplasia may be visible on naked-eye examination as macronodules and it can be very difficult to distinguish these areas from small aldosterone secreting adenomas.

The symptoms of primary aldosteronism develop usually between the ages of 30 and 50, and many years may elapse before the diagnosis is confirmed[2]. Conn's syndrome is twice as common in women as in men and rarely occurs in childhood.

The most common symptoms are headache, dizziness, nocturia, polyuria, and muscle weakness which can be generalized or localized and intermittent. On occasion paralysis may supervene. Hypertension is usually found and may have been present for many years. The hypertension may be mild but can sometimes be severe and even be associated with complications before the diagnosis is made. Oedema rarely occurs; postural hypertension may occur when hypokalaemia is severe.

INVESTIGATIONS

A review of patients operated on at the National Institutes of Health identifies those patients who may be suspected of having Conn's syndrome and who merit more detailed investigation[2].

The preoperative blood pressure was high, 204/122 ± 49/22 (s.d.) mmHg. Serum potassium was decreased (2.7 ± 0.6 mmol/l) and CO_2 content was raised (31.6 ± 4.7 mmol/l). This triad of findings in patients who are not taking diuretics is sufficient to indicate the need for further investigation.

Aldosterone secretion should be determined initially during a standard sodium intake (110 mmol/day) and later during a high intake (250 mmol/day). Plasma renin activity should be measured after overnight bed rest and following 3 hours of standing or walking. Plasma renin levels will be less than 1 µg/dl in patients with adenoma[8]. These measurements are extremely accurate in confirming the diagnosis and in separating primary from secondary aldosteronism.

The secretion rate of aldosterone is between 30 and 15 µg per day when the sodium intake is around 120 mmol per day. The secretion rate is measured by an isotope dilution technique. Metabolites of aldosterone are isolated from the urine and the specific activity of one of these is calculated; from this information the aldosterone secretion rate can be measured.

A low plasma renin level is a reliable indicator of primary aldosteronism, and very low or unrecordable plasma renin activity which does not respond to diuresis or the assumption of the upright posture is important in the diagnosis[8].

The development of a reliable radioimmunoassay for plasma aldosterone was of great importance and allowed the diagnosis to be made with considerable accuracy. A disproportionate increase in plasma aldosterone activity over plasma renin activity is diagnostic of primary aldosteronism.

Plasma levels of aldosterone are not affected by the administration of deoxy-corticosterone in primary aldosteronism.

The biochemical diagnosis of primary aldosteronism can now be made with precision and it is possible to establish the probability of adenoma or hyperplasia on the basis of biochemical measurements alone. Patients with adenoma generally have more profound biochemical disturbances than those with hyperplasia.

The mean plasma concentrations of aldosterone, sodium and total carbon dioxide tend to be significantly higher, while mean concentrations of renin and potassium are much lower in the adenoma group compared to the hyperplasia patients[5]. Ganguly et al.[6] observed that plasma aldosterone concentrations fell in the majority of the adenoma cases after a few hours in the upright position whereas it remained unchanged or even increased in patients with hyperplasia. These observations have been confirmed by others. An analysis of these reports shows that no patient with proven hyperplasia showed a postural fall in plasma aldosterone whereas there was a significant fall in 77% of patients with adenoma. Considerable overlap in each of the variables can occur, and straightforward analysis may not produce a clear separation of the two groups[5]. However, a multidimensional computer assisted analysis enabled complete separation of tumour and non-tumour groups. These calculations and the subsequent use of localization methods allow an accurate diagnosis of the cause of the disease to be established in almost every patient. It can, however, be difficult to apply the quadric analysis in all centres, and more and more reliance is being placed on localization to confirm the presence of an adenoma.

LOCALIZATION

An aldosterone secreting adenoma is relatively avascular and appears as a well defined negative image on a selective adrenal arteriogram, but the accuracy is poor and this invasive technique should only be used if other methods have been unsuccessful[1].

Adrenal venography will also delineate quite small aldosterone secreting adenomas, but venous disruption can occur and the extravasation of dye and adrenocortical haemorrhage can damage the gland and cause adrenal dysfunction[1]. A number of centres have now abandoned this investigation. It must also be remembered that a tumour found at venography is not necessarily functioning.

Transfemoral catheterization of the inferior vena cava allows the right and left adrenal veins to be entered and the venous effluent sampled so that aldosterone levels can be measured simultaneously in the region of both adrenals[3]. A marked increase in aldosterone concentration localizes an adenoma on that side, while hyperplasia is present when high levels are recorded at the same time on both sides. The accuracy of this method of localization is approaching 100% in most series at this time, but its reliability depends on accurate positioning of the catheters in the adrenal veins.

The use of [^{131}I]19-iodocholesterol and an external photoscanner or γ-camera can provide confirmation of an adenoma in many patients[9]. The results can be improved by the simultaneous administration of dexamethasone. Photoscans taken several days after the injection of the radionuclide will show a hot spot at the site of an adenoma. Adenomas between 1 and 2 cm in diameter will be pinpointed by this non-invasive technique, but its accuracy for smaller tumours is poor, and at the moment radionuclide scanning and selective venous catheterization are complementary investigations and should be performed on all patients.

Recent advances in methods of localization have been so rapid and the incidence of primary aldosteronism is so low that it is difficult for one centre to evaluate different methods of localization. Measuring of adrenal vein aldosterone levels has been reported as more effective than iodocholesterol scanning or adrenal venography in most series.

Granberg and his colleagues at the Karolinska Institute in Stockholm have provided very important information by comparing six different methods of localizing adrenal lesions as reported in the literature[1]. Their survey includes the results of 495 patients from 39 reports (*Table 11.1*).

Table 11.1 Primary aldosteronism: results of localization studies in 495 patients from 39 reports

	Adenoma		Hyperplasia	
Venography	106/173	61%	7/16	43%
Successful selective vein catheterization	144/150	96%	17/25	68%
Scintigraphy	60/76	79%	1/7	14%
Scintigraphy and dexamethasone	35/56	63%	15/20	75%
Postural fall in plasma aldosterone	53/74	72%	23/24	99%

The differentiation between hyperplasia and adenoma was best predicted by measuring the diurnal rhythm of plasma aldosterone and its response to posture[6]. Aldosterone levels in adrenal veins during selective catheterization confirmed the diagnosis of hyperplasia in 70% of cases.

Correct localization of aldosterone secreting tumours was obtained in 91% of patients by selective vein catheterization and measurement of aldosterone levels in samples of plasma. It is, however, not always possible to catheterize the adrenal veins, and success rates as low as 50% are recorded. Renal vein samples on the left side are less accurate and of little value on the right when the adrenal veins cannot be entered. When only renal vein and vena cava samples can be obtained the ratio of aldosterone to cortisol in each sample can be helpful, as the production of cortisol from a tumour-bearing gland is unaffected. Venography and iodocholesterol scanning have a much lower diagnostic accuracy. Computerized tomography is ineffective because of the small size of most tumours, and even relatively large aldosterone secreting tumours have not been detected.

It is concluded that measurement of peripheral aldosterone levels, the response to posture, and aldosterone concentrations in the venous effluent of the adrenals should be sufficient and will in 98% of patients be the only investigations required to localize an adenoma or confirm hyperplasia.

HYPERTENSION

It is suggested that the hypertension in primary aldosteronism is usually mild. Experience in one English region showed that the mean diastolic pressure was 125 mmHg[3]. Eight patients presented with complications of hypertension while two were found at routine medical examination.

Primary aldosteronism should therefore be considered in hypertension of all grades of severity[10]. The search should perhaps be limited to those patients who have hypokalaemia (plasma potassium 3.5 mmol/l) at first examination or who develop hypokalaemia at subsequent follow-up, whether or not diuretic therapy has been used. It may be that such a policy will miss normokalaemic hyperaldosteronism but then this is probably a very rare condition. The claim of Conn that 20% of patients with normokalaemic essential hypertension are harbouring aldosterone secreting adenomas has not been substantiated.

CONTROL OF SYNDROME

The aldosterone blocking agent spironolactone will correct the hypokalaemia and lower the blood pressure effectively, and most patients can tolerate the treatment although a few male patients will develop gynaecomastia. A dose of 200–400 mg per day is usually effective in controlling hypokalaemia and lowering blood pressure. Some workers have found that a distal tubular diuretic is as effective as spironolactone and more acceptable to some patients.

It is suggested by some that, as the hypertension is mild and the medical treatment acceptable, prolonged medical management is the treatment of choice since the results of surgery are unpredictable.

Recent experience would refute this approach and indicate that once the diagnosis is made strenuous efforts at localization are required. The results of surgery for adenoma are excellent and many patients will require no maintenance therapy following surgery. The fact that the hypertension is often significant and increases the risk of complications suggests that surgery to remove the source of excess aldosterone secretion is the treatment of choice in preference to a lifetime of medical treatment with its problems of side effects, drug compliance, doctor dependence and complications for employment.

The finding that very mild hypertension persists in about 30% of patients after surgery is confirmed in a number of series, but only about 10% are likely to require any antihypertensive treatment after operation.

Patients with hyperplasia are treated with spironolactone (Aldactone) either alone or in combination with other antihypertensive drugs. Bilateral adrenalectomy is occasionally recommended in male patients in whom the hypertension does not respond well and when the side effects of spironolactone, such as gynaecomastia and impotence, are intolerable.

All patients should be treated initially with spironolactone 300 mg per day and oral potassium supplements 50 mmol per day[7]. This treatment reduces blood pressure and restores biochemical equilibrium within 2 weeks. The total body potassium content is thus restored prior to surgery although the blood pressure may not be controlled completely.

SURGERY

Single adenomas are best removed by unilateral adrenalectomy[7] using the posterior approach, but the lateral approach is used by some surgeons. The incision is vertical and the twelfth rib is excised and the pleura swept upwards before dividing the posterior part of the diaphragm. The small adenomas are surprisingly close to the surface with this approach, but great care is required in identifying and tying the adrenal vein on the right side as it joins the vena cava. Troublesome bleeding from this source is difficult to control through a posterior approach.

If preoperative localization studies are inconclusive then both adrenals should be exposed, and this is probably simpler through an anterior transabdominal approach by one operating team. If one gland is larger than the other then only one gland is removed. If both glands are enlarged and the biochemical diagnosis is not in doubt then bilateral adrenalectomy should be performed.

The option of subtotal adrenalectomy, leaving a fraction on one side, was used for a while before accurate localization became possible, but the results were not satisfactory. The aim, therefore, is to operate only for adenoma, but if forced into a situation where both glands are exposed and there is an element of doubt about any difference, even after mobilization of the glands, then bilateral adrenalectomy is likely to be the most effective way of dealing with the problem. Morbidity and mortality have been reduced to insignificant levels by careful patient selection, preoperative control with spironolactone and accurate localization.

There is sometimes a suppression of aldosterone activity from the remaining gland after an adenoma has been removed, and sodium conservation may be poor for a number of weeks. A good sodium intake is important under these circumstances. There is a complete and permanent remission in over 90% of patients after operation.

The important developments in the management of Conn's syndrome can be summarized as

(1) the recognition that primary aldosteronism due to bilateral hyperplasia responds poorly to surgery
(2) the ability to diagnose accurately the presence of an adenoma and localize it precisely
(3) the preparation for surgery with spironolactone to reduce hypertension, correct hypokalaemia and reactivate the renin–angiotensin system.

A number of fascinating problems remain unanswered: for example, what are the stimuli which cause hyperplasia of the zona glomerulosa when renin is suppressed? Do hyperplastic nodules ever become adenomas? Is there really a fundamental difference between a small adenoma and a large nodule in hyperplasia? Careful review and repeated studies in patients with hyperplasia may answer some of these questions.

References

1 ADAMSON, U., EPENDIC, S., GRANBERG, P. O., LINDVALL, N., INIS, P. E. and LOW, H. Preoperative localisation of aldosterone secreting tumours. *Acta Medica Scandinavica*, **208**, 101–109 (1980)
2 AUDA, S. P., BRENNAN, M. F. and GILL, J. R. Evolution of the surgical management of primary aldosteronism. *Annals of Surgery*, **191**, 1–7 (1980)
3 CLARKE, D., JOHNSTON, I. D. A., WILKINSON, R., HACKING, P. M. and HAGGITH, J. W. Severe hypertension in primary aldosteronism and good response to surgery. *Lancet*, **1**, 482–485 (1979)

4 CONN, J. W. and LOUIS, L. H. Primary aldosteronism – a new clinical entity. *Transactions of the Association of American Physicians*, **68**, 215–218 (1955)

5 FARRIS, J. B., BROWN, J. T., FRASER, R., NEVILLE, A. M., O'MUIRCHEARTAIGH, I. G., ROBERTSON, J. I. S., SYMOYTON, T. and LEVER, A. F. Hypertension with aldosterone access and low plasma renin preoperative distinction in patients with and without adrenocortical tumour. *Lancet*, **2**, 995–1000 (1970)

6 GANGULY, A., DOWDY, A. J., LUESCHER, J. A. and HELADA, G. A. Anomalous postural response of plasma aldosterone concentration in patients with aldosterone producing adrenal adenoma. *Journal of Clinical Endocrinology and Metabolism*, **36**, 401–404 (1973)

7 HUNT, J. K., SCHAMBELAN, M. and BIGHERI, E. G. Selection of patients and operative approach in primary aldosteronism. *Annals of Surgery*, **182**, 353–357 (1975)

8 KATZ, F. H. Primary aldosteronism with suppressed plasma renin activity due to bilateral nodular hyperplasia. *Annals of Internal Medicine*, **67**, 1035–1039 (1967)

9 SEABOLD, J. E., COHEN, E. I., BIERWALTES, W. H., HINERMAN, D. L., NISHYAMA, R. H., BOOHSTEIN, J. J., ICE, R. D. and BALANCHANDRAW, P. Adrenal imaging with ^{131}I 19-iodocholesterol in the diagnostic evaluation of patients with aldosteronism. *Journal of Clinical Endocrinology and Metabolism*, **42**, 41–45 (1976)

10 THOMPSON, N. W. Adrenal lesions causing hypertension – surgical treatment. *Urologic Radiology*, 1–4 (1982)

Editor's commentary on Chapter 11

In the quarter of a century since primary aldosteronism was first described by Conn, much has been learned about the disease. It is now apparent that the incidence of Conn's disease is much lower than originally predicted. New cases are less frequent than were found during the first decade after recognition of the syndrome.

As emphasized, differentiation of adenomas from hyperplasia is critical in the selection of patients who should be subjected to adrenalectomy. This can be done with a high degree of accuracy in most cases. Only those with macronodular hyperplasia continue to present a problem in specific diagnosis and it remains to be determined whether they are best treated by adrenalectomy or long-term spironolactone.

The noriodocholesterol (NP-59) scintiscan after dexamethasone suppression (1 mg every 6 hours for 7 days) has been very accurate in localizing aldosteronomas larger than 1.2 cm in diameter. Localization was positive in 28 of the last 30 patients proven at operation to have adenomas. Although the accuracy of selective adrenal vein sampling for aldosteronomas approaches 100% when simultaneous cortisol levels are obtained, the technique is limited to patients in whom the right adrenal vein can be successfully catheterized and this can be a difficult manoeuvre. Selective venous assay studies should really be carried out only in patients in whom NP-59 scintiscan localization is equivocal or negative.

12
Recent developments in the management of phaeochromocytoma

John R. Farndon, Lennart Fagraeus
and Samuel A. Wells, Jr

INTRODUCTION

In 1896 Scipone Riva-Rocci described an instrument which enabled 'the blood pressure' to be determined in the human subject. Harvey Cushing visited the clinic of Riva-Rocci and later wrote an amusing account of the incident, but urged that blood pressure should be recorded during surgical operations[12].

The term 'phaeochromocytoma' was first used by Pick[40] in 1912 and is derived from the histological characteristic of the tumour cell to take on a dusky colour on staining with chromium salts (from the Greek 'phaios' meaning dusky and 'chroma' meaning colour. 'Cytoma' designates the lesion, a tumour).

In 1946 Ulf Svante von Euler[16] discovered that noradrenaline was the neurotransmitter of the sympathetic nervous system. He went on to elucidate the biochemistry and pathophysiology of phaeochromocytomas[17]. For these contributions to the understanding of catecholamine metabolism he shared the Nobel Prize for Physiology in 1970.

L'Abbé, Tinel and Doumer[30], in 1922, were the first to observe a paroxysmal hypertensive crisis associated with a phaeochromocytoma. Four years later Roux[45] in Switzerland and Charles Mayo[33] at the Mayo Clinic successfully removed phaeochromocytomas and coincidentally cured episodes of paroxysmal hypertension that were occurring in their patients. Dr Mayo commented with prophetic accuracy that 'epinephrine acts quickly on arterial and capillary vessels, and the suprarenals probably have much to do with quick vascular changes in this region of the abdomen'. Pincoffs[41] was the first to make a preoperative diagnosis of a phaeochromocytoma (in 1929), and later that year Shipley[49] successfully removed this right-sided adrenal lesion.

Hypertension, phaeochromocytoma, catecholamines, and their interrelationships are therefore newly described in this century. As with most endocrine tumours, new advances continue to be made and long-term results are only currently becoming available.

THE DIAGNOSIS OF PHAEOCHROMOCYTOMA

Phaeochromocytoma is a rare tumour. Large consecutive autopsy studies (more than 15 000 cases) suggest an incidence of less than 0.1%[35,46], but in smaller series (around 3000 autopsies) Blacklock et al.[4] found no tumours, and Berkheiser and Rappaport[3] reported an incidence of 0.25%. Screening within hypertensive populations reveals an incidence of between 0.32% and 2.2%[23,24,26,29]. This variation can be accounted for by the use of different screening procedures and varying degrees of patient preselection. The cost-effectiveness of screening even a population at risk has recently been questioned[39]. The cost of measuring only a single urinary catecholamine metabolite on one occasion in an Australian clinic dealing solely with hypertensive patients was estimated at £21 000 (US$42 000) per phaeochromocytoma (allowing for inflation and conversion rates to present-day terms).

The true incidence and prevalence of phaeochromocytoma is therefore not known. It is clear, however, that a significant number of persons die each year from complications of the disease, without prior recognition of the tumour[44]. Manger and Gifford[32] have calculated that, in the United States, about 36 000 persons may be harbouring a phaeochromocytoma.

Diagnosis of this uncommon tumour therefore depends on a constant awareness of its existence and its ability to mimic many other conditions. Confirmation of the diagnosis is made by the measurement of free catecholamines, 3-methoxy-4-hydroxy mandelic acid (VMA) or metadrenalines in 24-hour collections of urine. Different medical centres and hospital laboratories place varying degrees of reliance on these various determinations. At the Mayo Clinic, for example, greater reliance is placed on urinary metadrenalines[43], whereas free catecholamines are measured at Vanderbilt[54]. It has been shown that measurement of noradrenaline excretion rates during sleep provides as effective a diagnosis as a full 24-hour collection[21]. The availability of an easier method of measuring plasma catecholamines (adrenaline, noradrenaline and dopamine)[52] should theoretically provide a more direct measure of adrenal medullary function and thus a more effective diagnostic tool in detecting overactivity due to a phaeochromocytoma. In practice, however, divergent results have been obtained. Bravo et al.[5] found measurement of plasma catecholamines more useful than 24-hour urinary VMA or metanephrines, or both, but the obverse was reported by Plouin et al.[42]. Brown et al.[7] have recently reported that the sensitivity and accuracy of phaeochromocytoma diagnosis can be increased by measuring plasma adrenaline levels during a pentolinium suppression test. Increased plasma adrenaline concentrations were not suppressed by intravenous injection of 2.5 mg pentolinium in 18 patients with a phaeochromocytoma, whereas in 8 non-tumour cases elevated levels were lowered to the normal range.

Clearly, further evaluation of the efficacy of direct measurement of plasma catecholamines in the diagnosis of phaeochromocytoma is required.

PERIOPERATIVE MANAGEMENT

We have recently shown that determination of the 24-hour urinary VMA both helps in the diagnosis of phaeochromocytoma and allows a prediction of expected tumour mass[18]. This relationship was seen in three independent groups of patients, and pooling of data allowed the establishment of a 95th percentile lower limit for tumour mass. Despite numerous localizing modalities, failure can still occur, and it is well documented that phaeochromocytomas can be single, bilateral, extra-adrenal and any combination of these in any of the paraganglionic tissues[15, 22, 28, 32, 34, 36]. Any discrepancy between the least preoperative predicted tumour size and that found at surgery should therefore alert the surgeon to a thorough search for bilateral or additional extra-adrenal tissue.

'Blind' exploration of both adrenals, the retroperitoneum and the pelvis would be associated with considerable morbidity and, perhaps, mortality. It is customary therefore to attempt to localize phaeochromocytomas preoperatively, and many techniques are available. Their use varies from centre to centre, depending on availability, but, as a rule, progresses from the least invasive techniques to the more difficult and invasive procedure until the site of the lesion is demonstrated. Palpation, grey scale ultrasound, negative adrenal imaging in iodocholesterol scintigraphy, plain abdominal radiographs, intravenous urography with or without tomography, aortography, venography with or without blood sampling for catecholamine estimations, and computerized axial tomographic scanning have all been used. Pneumatography is very rarely used these days.

The most significant recent contribution to the management of patients with phaeochromocytoma has been the development of a specific radionuclide for catecholamine precursors in the adrenal medulla. [^{131}I]metaiodobenzylguanidine (MIBG or 'hot Guano' as the compound is sometimes affectionately labelled) concentrates selectively in the chromaffin cells of the adrenal medulla of dogs and rhesus monkeys[55, 56]. Initial clinical studies have shown that the isotope is capable of localizing phaeochromocytomas, found within the adrenal gland and in ectopic locations, of benign and malignant nature, of greatly differing size, and with various hormonal secretory patterns[51]. Loading MIBG with larger doses of isotope could theoretically help ablate or reduce functional tumour burden in those patients with inoperable or metastatic phaeochromocytomas in whom sufficient uptake can be demonstrated within the tumour mass. Early efforts with this therapeutic modality have been encouraging (Beierwaltes, personal communication).

Kahn et al.[27] have recently described four cases of phaeochromocytoma of the bladder. Awareness of this site of chromaffin tumour formation must be maintained and any patient in whom symptoms are associated with micturition should undergo cystoscopy and intravenous urography. Other localization procedures should be directed specifically toward the pelvis, as well as the conventional tumour sites, e.g. sampling catecholamines in internal iliac veins.

A firm biochemical diagnosis of phaeochromocytoma is often established concurrently with localization procedures. The obvious demonstration, by less invasive techniques, of an adrenal mass sometimes lends credence to an otherwise unconvincing biochemical profile. It must be emphasized, however, that the exposure of a patient to arteriography, venography and cystoscopy might stimulate a phaeochromocytoma to release potentially fatal amounts of catecholamines. This awareness must extend to tumours not producing sustained hypertension. At the appropriate time of investigation or diagnosis, therefore, attention must be turned to the effective blockade of the effects of high circulating levels of catecholamines. It was this concept, introduced about 15 years ago, that significantly reduced the operative and perioperative mortality of this physiologically malignant tumour. The data of Crandell and Myers[11] are typical of patient management before the advent of preoperative blockade. Postoperative blood transfusion and treatment with vasopressor agents such as ephedrine, phenylephrine or noradrenaline (levarterenol) were required in 8 of 11 patients. Regimens of blockade vary from centre to centre, but that described by Freier, Eckhauser and Harrison[20] is representative. It is usual to initiate blockade with the long-acting, non-competitive α-adrenergic blocker phenoxybenzamine in an initial dose of 10 mg three times each day. The dose is gradually increased, while measuring supine and standing blood pressures, until mild orthostatic hypotension is noted. This allows expansion of the contracted blood volume and may unmask an anaemia which requires preoperative correction by packed cell transfusion. Any residual tachycardia after correction of the anaemia might be indicative of unopposed β-adrenergic effects. This is more likely if biochemical investigations have shown that the tumour secretes predominantly adrenaline. Most centres would advocate control of the tachycardia by the addition of a β-adrenergic blocking drug such as propranolol. It is said to be safer to institute α- before β-blockade to avoid the consequences of unopposed agonist, pressor α-effects. As well as restoring blood pressure to normal or near normal levels, blockade allows the patient to feel better, often restores euglycaemia, and reduces the incidence of ventricular extrasystoles. The efficacy of this preoperative preparation, carried out over a period of 1 to 3 weeks, has substantially reduced the operative mortality. We have shown that in a series of 17 patients undergoing 17 operations before the advent of blockade there were 3 deaths (18%), whereas in 41 patients undergoing 45 operations with blockade there was only 1 operative death (2%), and this was probably related to overzealous β-blockade[36].

Despite patient preparation with seemingly adequate α- and β-adrenergic blockade, surgery provides the most critical period in the management of patients with a phaeochromocytoma[6]. Most centres have a team of anaesthetists experienced in the preoperative management of cardiovascular crises. *Figure 12.1* demonstrates the phenomenal increases in circulating levels of all three amines measured during the removal of a large benign phaeochromocytoma and the concurrent perturbations in the systolic and diastolic blood pressures. Such findings are not uncommon in patients who are receiving apparently adequate preoperative blockade, and careful perioperative monitoring with arterial and central venous pressure lines is therefore mandatory. Peroperative control of hypertensive crises is advised and a variable infusion of sodium nitroprusside is recommended for this purpose. This drug, available since the turn of the century, has only recently found clinical acceptability and is ideal in the regulation of hypertension encountered during the removal of a phaeochromocytoma. It has several advantages[10, 31]:

(1) It causes direct and specific relaxation of arterial and venous smooth muscle, with subsequent vasodilatation and hypotension

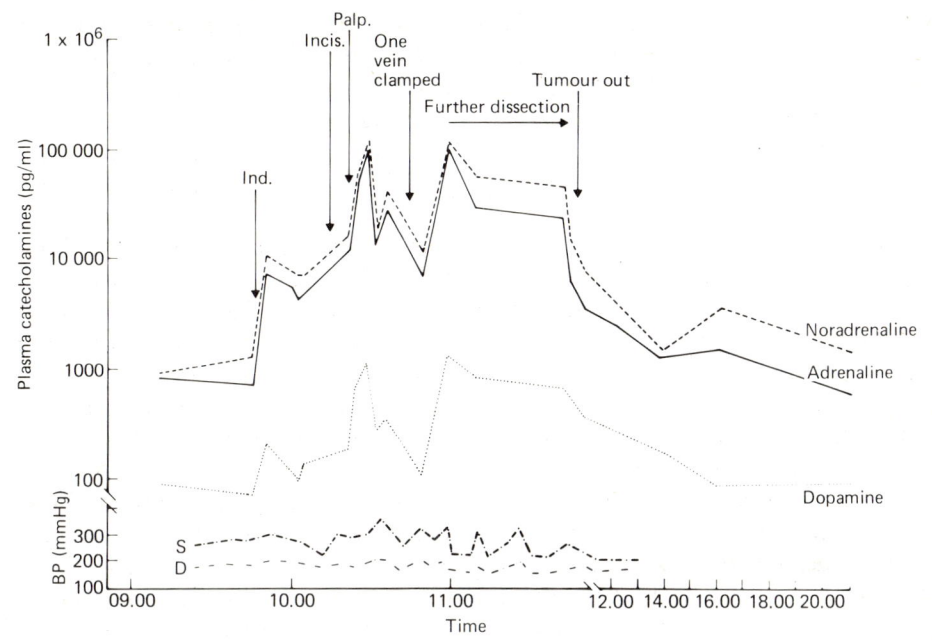

Figure 12.1 Perioperative changes in blood pressure and plasma catecholamine concentrations (noradrenaline, adrenaline and dopamine) during the removal of a benign phaeochromocytoma from a male aged 38 years. BP = blood pressure; S = systolic; D = diastolic; Ind. = induction; Incis. = incision; Palp. = palpation

(2) It exerts its effects independently of α- and β-adrenergic receptors
(3) It acts upon various vascular beds to a similar degree and therefore regional distribution blood flow is little affected
(4) Its effects are of rapid onset and short duration.

The technicalities of tumour removal are straightforward and well described elsewhere. Awareness of the possibility of malignancy in phaeochromocytomas must be emphasized. The malignant tumour is not always apparent during excision and even histological examination does not always clarify the situation. Nuclear atypicality, pleomorphism and mitotic figures exist in benign tumours, and capsular and vascular invasion and penetration have been documented in tumours subsequently proved to be benign[37]. Tumour invasion of adjacent tissues, with or without metastatic spread to sites normally devoid of chromaffin tissue, constitutes a criterion of malignancy, and others have suggested that metastases should retain functional capability[13]. A recent case report of a malignant phaeochromocytoma, including a review of the cases documented in the English literature, demonstrated that one third of these tumours arose in the urinary bladder[14]. Metastases occurred to the lymph nodes, lungs, liver, bones and brain, but in some instances prolonged survival was not precluded. Because of the uncertainty regarding the behaviour of these tumours, long-term follow-up is recommended and recurrence of symptoms or recrudescence of hypertension might herald metastases as the first signal of a malignant tumour.

IS HYPERTENSION A PROBLEM AFTER SURGICAL EXCISION OF A PHAEOCHROMOCYTOMA?

Because phaeochromocytomas are rare tumours which have only been recognized and removed by surgeons during the past 50 years there has been little opportunity to accumulate significant information about the efficacy of surgical treatment. It is appropriate that the Mayo Clinic (Dr Charles Mayo was the first to successfully remove a phaeochromocytoma) should be one of the first institutions to describe its experience[43]. In an unparalleled series of 138 patients the actuarial survival curve for 120 patients with benign tumours was not significantly different from that of the normal population, but no long-term follow-up was obtained. Blood pressure measurements, which were available for 103 patients 1 year after excision of a benign tumour, showed that 28 had residual hypertension (criteria not stated). Preoperatively 18 of these patients (64%) had sustained hypertension and 9 had paroxysmal disease.

Scott et al.[48] reviewed 25 patients from Vanderbilt with benign tumours from 1.5 to 20 years after surgery and found that 36% had residual hypertension, but criteria were again not given.

Long-term results have recently been reported in 58 patients followed from 1 to 20 years after operation in three United Kingdom centres[36]. Rigorous criteria were applied to the definition of hypertension: a patient was hypertensive if (a) the mean of several systolic or diastolic readings was greater than the mean for subjects of the same age and sex in the general population, or (b) hypertensive crises were observed and recorded. On these grounds only 1 patient was normal, 10 (17%) had sustained hypertension, 28 (48%) had paroxysms alone, and 19 (33%) had sustained hypertension with superadded paroxysms before surgery. The degree of hypertension was severe in the group as a whole, but most severe in females.

Paroxysms of hypertension were relieved in all cases – objective evidence to support the surmise of Öhman et al.[38]. At follow-up only 6 patients were normotensive without specific surgery and, at the other extreme, 13 patients required antihypertensive therapy. The results of the comparisons are given in Table 12.1.

Table 12.1 Long-term follow-up of blood pressure following surgery for phaeochromocytoma

	Measured pressure (mmHg)*	Actuarial pressure (mmHg)*	Probability value
Male systolic	156 ± 13	136 ± 3	0.1
Male diastolic	89 ± 6	83 ± 1	0.2
Female systolic	144 ± 7	132 ± 3	0.09
Female diastolic	89 ± 4	81 ± 1	0.07

*Mean of groups ± s.e. (mean) – paired analyses.

The well documented correlation between advancing age and increasing blood pressure was seen in actuarial systolic and diastolic pressures for the whole group (current age versus actuarial systolic pressure; $r = 0.94$, $P < 0.01$; and current age versus actuarial diastolic pressure; $r = 0.81$, $P < 0.01$). This relationship was less well demonstrated in the observed systolic pressures ($r = 0.55$, $P < 0.01$) and was not seen in the observed diastolic pressures.

Observed systolic pressures tended to be greater than corresponding actuarial figures at any particular age, but the difference in the gradients did not achieve significance except at the mean age of the group (50 years), where confidence limits were tightest (pressure difference 14.3 mmHg, $P < 0.01$).

The concept that residual or recurrent hypertension is related to prolonged exposure of the cardiovascular system to catecholamine excess is difficult to prove in a clinical study. Longitudinal studies of patients with *in situ* phaeochromocytomas are neither feasible or ethically justifiable. There is, however, no correlation between the length of history and the degree of systolic or diastolic hypertension. It cannot, of course, be assumed that the duration of symptoms correlates directly with the functional life of tumours or that all tumours secrete uniform and equal amounts of the various catecholamines throughout their existence. We have, however, demonstrated that catecholamines in the dog support renal vascular resistance during carotid sinus stimulation[1]. There is thus some laboratory evidence of a catecholamine-mediated response that could be implicated in the pathogenesis of residual or recurrent hypertension after surgery for phaeochromocytoma.

The responsible physician should therefore be prepared to enjoy the challenge of diagnosing, localizing and removing a phaeochromocytoma as safely and expeditiously as possible. He must also be prepared to follow his patients for many years, being aware that in a minority unexpected malignancy will declare itself and that in a majority he will have to evaluate and treat significant hypertensive disease.

ADRENAL MEDULLARY DISEASE IN MULTIPLE ENDOCRINE NEOPLASIA TYPE II

The clustering of phaeochromocytoma, thyroid tumours, and parathyroid adenomas or hyperplasia in a single patient is known as multiple endocrine neoplasia type II, or MEN II. It is sometimes eponymously called Sipple's syndrome[50]. The thyroid tumour is of the medullary type (MTC)[25]. MEN II can occur in a familial setting with an autosomal dominant pattern of inheritance[47], and it is in this situation that economically and clinically justifiable screening for phaeochromocytomas might be feasible.

Carney, Sizemore and Tyce[8] described the pathology of both adrenals removed from an asymptomatic girl aged 12 from an MEN II kindred whose urinary VMA excretion was suggestive of a phaeochromocytoma. Adrenal medullary hyperplasia was found, but no evidence of tumour formation. The hyperplasia was characterized by increased adrenal weight, decreased corticomedullary ratios, increased medullary mitotic activity and increased catecholamine content of the left adrenal. In a retrospective, largely histopathological study, Carney, Sizemore and Sheps[9] postulated that diffuse and nodular adrenal medullary hyperplasia was the precursor of phaeochromocytoma in the MEN II syndrome. They recommended that symptomatic or asymptomatic patients with biochemical evidence of adrenal medullary disease should have bilateral adrenalectomy because:

(1) synchronous bilateral involvement was likely
(2) there were risks of local recurrence if the entire glands were not removed
(3) this component of the syndrome was associated with a high mortality.

Valk et al.[53] have used metaiodobenzylguanidine (MIBG) imaging to confirm this evolving spectrum of adrenal medullary disease in MEN II patients, correlating degree of isotope uptake with degree of biochemical abnormality.

Freier et al.[19] reported 15 patients with the syndrome and found that none of the 3 deaths within this group could be attributed to a phaeochromocytoma. They felt that available data did not support the conclusions of Carney and his colleagues, but suggested that 'the biology of untreated adrenal medullary hyperplasia within the MEN II syndrome is unknown'. There would appear to be little or no justification to committing a patient to lifelong corticosteroid replacement therapy and its attendant risks if at least some years could be gained for a patient with a single 'normal' gland, without danger from significant adrenal medullary disease.

We have studied 30 patients from six kindreds who have undergone adrenal surgery for phaeochromocytoma in the MEN II syndrome. Medullary thyroid carcinoma (MTC) is diagnosed and treated earlier than adrenal medullary disease, but it is not clear whether this is due to evolutionary patterns within the syndrome or our ability to detect MTC before adrenal medullary disease. Sporadic, non-familial phaeochromocytomas are diagnosed within an even older population (*Figure 12.2*).

Once a biochemical diagnosis has been confirmed our operative strategy has been less aggressive than that of others, and if no palpable phaeochromocytoma (i.e. a nodule of more than 1 cm in diameter) is present within the contralateral gland, it is left *in situ*. Histopathology of the excised glands supports the theory of Carney, Sizemore and Sheps[9], i.e. bilateral disease was present in 21 patients (70%), and in 4 of these bilateral phaeochromocytomas occurred in a background of medullary hyperplasia. The incidence of multiple foci in the glands removed was 45.5%. A total of 9 patients have been followed annually for a minimum of 5 years and a maximum of 14 years (mean 8 years) after unilateral adrenalectomy. All 9 patients have undergone total thyroidectomy for MTC and all remain fit, well and asymptomatic. One male has mild sustained hypertension readily controlled with medications, but all 9 patients have normal 24-hour urinary excretions of VMA, catecholamines and metadrenalines. Annual computerized tomographic scanning of the remaining adrenal gland has shown one female who has 'a fullness' but no obvious tumour. We have not encountered a single malignant phaeochromocytoma within the MEN II syndrome. These clinical data therefore support a more conservative approach to adrenal surgery within the MEN II syndrome, but thorough and frequent patient review is mandatory.

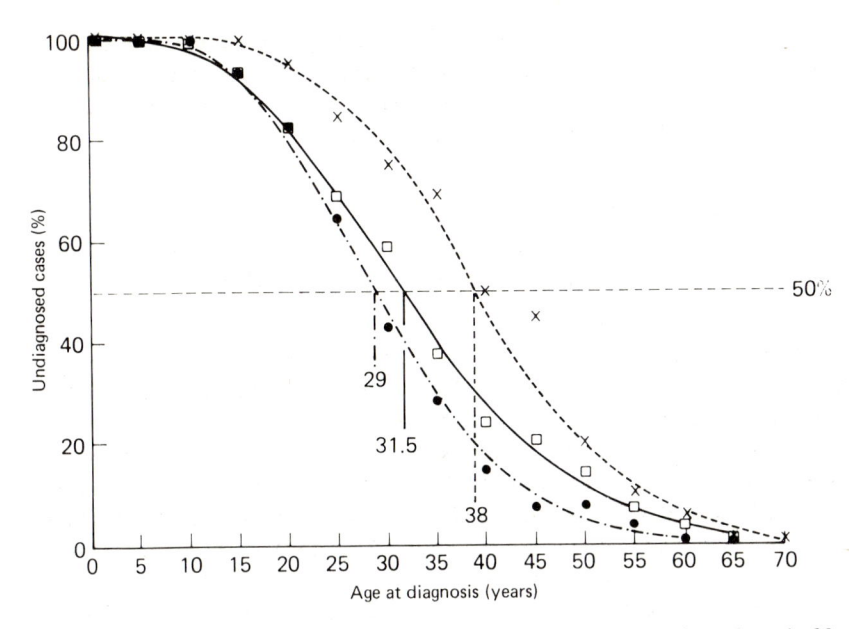

Figure 12.2 The percentage of cases not yet diagnosed as a function of age in 30 patients with MEN II syndrome and 20 patients with sporadic, non-familial phaeochromocytoma. (●) Medullary thyroid carcinoma in MEN II; (□) phaeochromocytoma in MEN II; (X) sporadic, non-familial phaeochromocytoma

It is possible that longitudinal clinical and physiological studies within kindreds affected by the MEN II syndrome will increase our understanding of the rare, elusive and potentially lethal phaeochromocytoma.

Acknowledgements

The authors thank John F. Seaton and Jakob D. Peuler, Department of Surgery, Milton S. Hershey Medical Center, Pennyslvania State University, for plasma catecholamine determination. They are grateful to Professor Timothy S. Harrison, Department of Surgery, Milton S. Hershey Medical Center, Pennsylvania State University, for his advice and review of the manuscript.

References

1 BADDER, E. M., SEATON, J. F. and HARRISON, T. S. Adrenal catecholamines support renal vascular resistance stimulated by the carotid sinus. *Journal of Clinical Surgery*, **1**, 87–92 (1982)

2 BEIERWALTES, W. H. (personal communication)

3 BERKHEISER, S. W. and RAPPAPORT, A. E. Unsuspected phaeochromocytoma of the adrenal: report of 5 cases. *American Journal of Clinical Pathology*, **21**, 657–665 (1951)

4 BLACKLOCK, J. W. S., FERGUSON, J. W., MACK, W. S., SHAFAR, J. and SYMINGTON, T. Phaeochromocytoma. *British Journal of Surgery*, **35**, 179–197 (1947)

5 BRAVO, E. L., TARAZI, R. C., GIFFORD, R. W. and STEWART, B. H. Circulating and urinary catecholamines in pheochromocytoma. Diagnostic and pathophysiologic implications. *New England Journal of Medicine*, **301**, 682–686 (1979)

6 BROWN, B. R. Anesthesia for pheochromocytoma. In *Anesthesia and the Patient with Endocrine Disease*, edited by B. R. Brown, pp. 185–196. Philadelphia, F. A. Davis (1980)

7 BROWN, M. J., JENNER, D. A., ALLISON, D. J., LEWIS, P. J. and DOLLERY, C. T. Increased sensitivity and accuracy of phaeochromocytoma diagnosis achieved by use of plasma-adrenaline estimations and a pentolinium suppression test. *Lancet*, **1**, 174–177 (1981)

8 CARNEY, J. A., SIZEMORE, G. W. and TYCE, G. M. Bilateral adrenal medullary hyperplasia in multiple endocrine neoplasia, type 2. The precursor of bilateral pheochromocytoma. *Mayo Clinic Proceedings*, **50**, 3–10 (1975)

9 CARNEY, J. A., SIZEMORE, G. W. and SHEPS, S. G. Adrenal medullary disease in multiple endocrine neoplasia type 2. *American Journal of Clinical Pathology*, **66**, 279–290 (1976)

10 COHN, J. N. and BURKE, L. P. Diagnosis and treatment. Drugs five years later. Nitroprusside. *Annals of Internal Medicine*, **91**, 752–757 (1979)

11 CRANDELL, D. L. and MYERS, R. T. Pheochromocytoma – anesthetic and surgical considerations. *Journal of the American Medical Association*, **187**, 112–116 (1964)

12 CUSHING, H. W. Fashions in surgery. *Surgery, Gynecology and Obstetrics*, **52**, 266–268 (1931)

13 DAVIS, P., PEART, W. S. and VAN'T HOFF, W. Malignant phaeochromocytoma with functioning metastases. *Lancet*, **2**, 274–275 (1955)

14 DOW, C. J., PALMER, M. K., O'SULLIVAN, J. P. and KIRKHAM, J. S. Malignant phaeochromocytoma: report of a case and a critical review. *British Journal of Surgery*, **69**, 338–340 (1982)

15 ENGLEMAN, K. and SJOERDSMA, A. A new test for pheochromocytoma: pressor responsiveness to tyramine. *Journal of the American Medical Association*, **189**, 81–86 (1964)

16 EULER, U. S. VON. Presence of a substance with sympathin E properties in spleen extracts. *Acta Physiologica Scandanavica*, **11**, 168–186 (1946)

17 EULER, U. S. VON and STRÖM, G. Present status of diagnosis and treatment of pheochromocytoma. *Circulation*, **15**, 5–13 (1957)

18 FARNDON, J. R., DAVIDSON, H. A., JOHNSTON, I. D. A. and WELLS, S. A. VMA excretion in patients with pheochromocytoma. *Annals of Surgery*, **191**, 259–263 (1980)

19 FREIER, D. T., THOMPSON, N. W., SISSON, J. C., NISHIYAMA, R. H. and FREITAS, J. E. Dilemmas in the early diagnosis and treatment of multiple endocrine adenomatosis, type II. *Surgery*, **82**, 407–413 (1977)

20 FREIER, D. T., ECKHAUSER, F. E. and HARRISON, T. S. Pheochromocytoma. A persistently problematic and still potentially lethal disease. *Archives of Surgery*, **115**, 388–391 (1980)

21 GANGULY, A., HENRY, D. P., YNNE, H. Y., PRATT, J. H., GRIM, C. E., DONOHUE, J. P. and WEINBERGER, M. H. Diagnosis and localisation of pheochromocytoma. *American Journal of Medicine*, **67**, 21–26 (1979)

22 GIFFORD, R. W., KVALE, W. F., MAHER, F. T., ROTH, G. M. and PRIESTLEY, J. T. Clinical features, diagnosis and treatment of pheochromocytoma: a review of 76 cases. *Mayo Clinic Proceedings*, **39**, 281–302 (1964)

23 GITLOW, S. E., MENDLOWITZ, M., KRUK, E. and KHASSIS, S. Diagnosis of pheochromocytoma by assay of catecholamine metabolites. *Circulation Research*, **9**, 746–754 (1961)

24 GOODALL, McC. and STONE, C. Adrenaline and noradrenaline producing tumours of the adrenal medulla and sympathetic nerves. *Annals of Surgery*, **151**, 391–398 (1960)

25 HAZARD, J. B., HAWK, W. A. and CRILE, G. Medullary (solid) carcinoma of the thyroid: a clinicopathological entity. *Journal of Clinical Endocrinology*, **19**, 152–161 (1959)

26 HUME, D. M. Pheochromocytoma in the adult and in the child. *American Journal of Surgery*, **99**, 458–496 (1960)

27 KAHN, O., WILLIAMS, C., CHISHOLM, G. D. and WELBOURN, R. B. Phaeochromocytomas of the bladder. *Journal of the Royal Society of Medicine*, **75**, 17–20 (1982)

28 KEHLET, H., BLICHERT-TOFT, M., HANCKE, S., FOG PEDERSEN, J., KVIST KRISTENSEN, J., EFSEN, F., DIGE-PETERSEN, H., FOGH, J., LOCKWOOD, K. and HASNER, E. Comparative study of ultrasound, ^{131}I-19-iodocholesterol scintigraphy, and aortography in localising adrenal lesions. *British Medical Journal*, **2**, 665–667 (1976)

29 KVALE, W. F., ROTH, G. M., MANGER, W. M. and PRIESTLEY, J. T. Pheochromocytoma. *Circulation*, **14**, 622–630 (1956)

30 L'ABBÉ, M., TINEL, J. and DOUMER, E. Crises solaires et hypertension paroxystique en rapport avec une tumeur surrénale. *Bulletin de la Société Médicine Hôpital*, **46**, 982–990 (1922)

31 LIPSON, A., HSU, T-H., SHERWIN, B. and GEELHOED, G. W. Nitroprusside therapy for a patient with a pheochromocytoma. *Journal of the American Medical Association*, **239**, 427–428 (1978)

32 MANGER, W. M. and GIFFORD, R. W. *Pheochromocytoma*. New York, Springer-Verlag (1977)

33 MAYO, C. H. Paroxysmal hypertension with tumor of retroperitoneal nerve. Report of a case. *Journal of the American Medical Association*, **89**, 1047–1050 (1927)

34 MELICOW, M. M. One hundred cases of pheochromocytoma (107 tumors) at the Colombia Presbyterian Medical Center, 1926–1976. A clinicopathological analysis. *Cancer*, **40**, 1987–2004 (1977)

35 MINNO, A. M., BENNETT, A. W. and KVALE, W. F. Pheochromocytoma. A study of 15 cases diagnosed at autopsy. *New England Journal of Medicine*, **251**, 959–965 (1954)

36 MODLIN, J. M., FARNDON, J. R., SHEPHERD, A., JOHNSTON, I. D. A., KENNEDY, T. L., MONTGOMERY, D. A. D. and WELBOURN, R. B. Phaeochromocytomas in 72 patients: clinical and diagnostic features, treatment and long-term results. *British Journal of Surgery*, **66**, 456–465 (1979)

37 NEVILLE, A. M. The adrenal medulla. In *Functional Pathology of the Human Adrenal Gland*, edited by T. Symington, pp. 217–324. Baltimore, Williams and Wilkins (1969)

38 ÖHMAN, U., GRANBERG, P-O., HJERN, B. and SJÖBERG, H. E. Pheochromocytoma. *Acta Chirurgica Scandanavica*, **140**, 660–666 (1974)

39 PHILLIPS, P. J., COLES, M. E. and WISE, P. H. Cost of diagnosis of phaeochromocytoma. *Medical Journal of Australia*, **2**, 406–407 (1975)

40 PICK, L. Das Ganglioma embryonale sympathicum (Sympathoma embryonale), eine typische bösartige Geschwulstform des sympathischen Nervensystems. *Berliner Klinische Wochenschrift*, **49**, 16–22 (1912)

41 PINCOFFS, M. C. A case of paroxysmal hypertension associated with suprarenal tumor. *Transactions of the Association of American Physicians*, **44**, 295–299 (1929)

42 PLOUIN, P. F., DUCLOS, J. M., MENARD, J., COMOY, E., BOHUON, C. and ALEXANDRE, J. M. Biochemical tests for diagnosis of phaeochromocytoma: urinary versus plasma determinations. *British Medical Journal*, **282**, 853–854 (1981)

43 REMINE, W. H., CHONG, G. C., VAN HEERDEN, J. A., SHEPS, S. G. and HARRISON, E. G. Current management of pheochromocytoma. *Annals of Surgery*, **179**, 740–748 (1974)

44 ROSS, E. J. The management of cases of phaeochromocytoma (Clinical Staff Conference, University College Hospital, London). *Proceedings of the Royal Society of Medicine*, **55**, 427–436 (1962)

45 ROUX, R. Thesis, Lausanne (1926). Cited by Barbeau, A., Marc-Aurèle, J., Brouillet, J., Vityé, B., Leboeuf, G., Cartier, P., Mignault, G. and Genest, J. Le phéochromocytome bilatéral: Presentation d'un cas et revue de la littérature. *Union Médicale du Canada*, **87**, 165–178 (1958)

46 SCHLEGEL, C. G. VON. Neurofibromatose Recklinghausen und Phäochromocytom. *Schweizerische Medizinische Wochenschrift*, **90**, 31–39 (1960)

47 SCHIMKE, R. N. and HARTMANN, W. H. Familial amyloid-producing medullary thyroid carcinoma and pheochromocytoma. A distinct genetic entity. *Annals of Internal Medicine*, **63**, 1027–1039 (1965)

48 SCOTT, H. W., OATES, J. A., NIES, A. S., BURKO, H., PAGE, D. L. and RHAMY, R. K. Pheochromocytoma: present diagnosis and management. *Annals of Surgery*, **183**, 587–593 (1976)

49 SHIPLEY, A. M. Paroxysmal hypertension associated with tumor of the suprarenal. *Annals of Surgery*, **90**, 742–749 (1929)

50 SIPPLE, J. H. The association of pheochromocytoma with carcinoma of the thyroid gland. *American Journal of Medicine*, **31**, 163–166 (1961)

51 SISSON, J. C., FRAGER, M. S., VALK, T. W., GROSS, M. D., SWANSON, D. P., WIELAND, D. M., TOBES, M. C., BEIERWALTES, W. H. and THOMPSON, N. W. Scintigraphic localization of pheochromocytoma. *New England Journal of Medicine*, **305**, 12–17 (1981)

52 TASSERON, S. J. A., FIOLET, J. W: T. and WILLEBRANDS, H. F. Evaluation of a radio-enzymatic kit for determination of plasma catecholamines. *Clinical Chemistry*, **26**, 120–122 (1980)

53 VALK, T. W., FRAZER, M. S., GROSS, M. D., SISSON, J. C., WIELAND, D. M., SWANSON, D. P., MANGNER, T. J. and BEIERWALTES, W. H. Spectrum of pheochromocytoma in multiple endocrine neoplasia. *Annals of Internal Medicine*, **94**, 762–767 (1981)

54 VAN WAY, C. W., SCOTT, H. W., PAGE, D. L. and RHAMY, R. K. Pheochromocytoma. In *Current Problems in Surgery,* edited by M. M. Ravitch, Chicago, Year Book Medical Publishers (1974)

55 WIELAND, D. M., BROWN, L. E., TOBES, M. C., ROGERS, W. L., MARSH, D. D., MANGNER, T. J., SWANSON, D. P. and BEIERWALTES, W. H. Imaging the primate adrenal medulla with [^{123}I] and [^{131}I] metaiodobenzylguanidine: concise communication. *Journal of Nuclear Medicine,* **22,** 358–364 (1981)

56 WIELAND, D. M., WU, J., BROWN, L. E., MANGNER, T. J., SWANSON, D. P. and BEIERWALTES, W. H. Radiolabelled adrenergic neuron-blocking agents: adrenomedullary imaging with [^{131}I] iodobenzylguanidine. *Journal of Nuclear Medicine,* **21,** 349–353 (1980)

Editors' commentary on Chapter 12

At present the biochemical diagnosis of pheochromocytoma can be made with certainty in virtually all patients. Traditionally 12- or 24-hour urinary catecholamine levels have been considered the most reliable measurement to establish the diagnosis. However, the availability of plasma catecholamines by immunoassay and high pressure liquid chromatography has made it questionable whether reliance on these studies alone is sufficient to confirm the diagnosis in most cases. The answer is not yet known. At present, elevated urinary catecholamines are still considered necessary for establishing a firm biochemical diagnosis.

Localization of most pheochromocytomas can be achieved by CT scan when the tumor is within the adrenal gland. The [^{131}I]MIBG scan is also proving very reliable and provides the additional information that the mass identified by CT scan is functional and in fact the suspected pheochromocytoma. It has the additional advantage of identifying unsuspected metastases or a second, perhaps benign, extra-adrenal tumor. Its greatest value has been in localizing primary extra-adrenal pheochromocytomas, metastases and medullary hyperplasia in the MEN II syndromes even before catecholamine levels are elevated. Since August 1980, when this agent was first introduced clinically, more than 40 patients with surgically proven pheochromocytomas have been evaluated with [^{131}I]MIBG. Only three tumors have failed to image by scintigraphy within 48 hours after administration of this agent. These three tumors were all extra-adrenal and in the right renal hilum. Seven other occult extra-adrenal tumors were readily demonstrated, however. Currently [^{131}I]MIBG is being evaluated for the treatment of metastatic pheochromocytoma and has been administered to 5 patients thus far. The preliminary results are encouraging in that several patients have had a noticeable decrease in the size of their tumors.

A controversial area is the surgical management of the adrenal glands in the MEN II syndromes. Their experience in following nine patients after unilateral adrenalectomy for 5 years or more is unique. The accumulating pathological and surgical evidence has demonstrated that the adrenal involvement is always bilateral although the extent of disease may be asymmetrical, with pheochromocytomas and hyperplasia in one gland and only medullary hyperplasia in the opposite. In our experience with 12 cases, bilateral adrenalectomy was done in each. Pheochromocytomas were present in both glands in all but one patient. This last patient had bilateral medullary hyperplasia. Perhaps, as the authors have shown, in some cases patients in whom careful follow-up is possible, total adrenalectomy can be avoided or at least delayed for a number of years.

Index

Adenocarcinoma, 92, 160
Adenoma, toxic thyroid, *see* Plummer's disease
Adrenalectomy,
  in adrenal medullary diseases, 196, 201
  in aldosteronism, 186–187
    bilateral, 186, 187
    unilateral, 186
  in Cushing's syndrome, 53–69
    autotransplantation, 64
    bilateral, 53, 66, 68
    complications, 54, 55, 63
    development of, 63–64
    indications for, 68
    operative approach, 63, 68–69
    results of, 54–56
    unilateral, 64
Adrenal hyperplasia,
  aldosteronism, 182, 188
  bilateral, in Cushing's syndrome, 54, 57, 63, 66, 68
  in MEN II, 195, 196, 201
Adrenaline, in phaeochromocytoma diagnosis, 190
Adrenal medullary disease, 195–197, 201
Adrenal venography, 184
α-Adrenergic drugs, 192
β-Adrenergic drugs, 5, 192
Adrenocortical tumours, 55, 57, 65, 68
  adenoma,
    aldosteronism, 182, 184–185, 188
    Cushing's syndrome, 54, 55, 57, 63
  carcinoma, 53, 54, 64, 65, 67
  diagnosis, 58

Adrenocorticotrophin (ACTH),
  in Cushing's syndrome, 53, 54, 57
  ectopic, syndrome, 57, 66, 67, 144
  secretion by insulinoma, 105
Alcohol, and hypoglycaemia, 112
Aldosterone,
  adrenal vein, 184, 185, 188
  in primary aldosteronism, 182, 183
Aldosteronism, primary, 182–187, 188
  adenoma, 182, 184–185, 188
  clinical features, 182, 183
  control of, 186
  hyperplasia, 182, 188
  hypertension in, 180, 185–186
  investigations, 183–184
  localization of adenoma, 184–185, 188
  surgery, 186–187
Aminoglutethimide, 60
Angiography, islet cell adenomas, 96–98, 113
Antibodies,
  antithyroid, 21
  thyroid stimulating (TsAb), 1, 2, 6, 9
Antilymphocyte serum (ALS), 132, 135
Antithyroid drugs, 2, 3, 4, 12, 13
Apud concept, 168
Arteriography,
  in hyperparathyroidism, 45, 46, 51
  in insulinoma localization, 96–98, 113
Azathioprine, 132, 135

Bendrofluazide, 119
Beta blocking drugs, 5, 192
Biopsy, needle, of thyroid, 19–20, 22, 23

Blood pressure,
    after phaeochromocytoma excision, 194
    age and, 195
Bone disease, 28, 44
Bromocriptine,
    in Cushing's syndrome, 60
    in MEN I syndrome, 160, 161
Bronchus, carcinoma of, 64

Calcitonin, in thyroid carcinoma diagnosis, 21
Calcium, (*see also* Hypercalcaemia; Hypocalcaemia)
    after parathyroid autotransplantation, 33
    balance, and parathyroid glands, 25
    therapy,
        in parathyroid autotransplantation, 26, 30, 33
        in parathyroid reoperation, 48
Calcium gluconate, 167, 169
Carbimazole, 4, 5
Carbohydrate control in diabetes, 125–126
    in pancreatic transplantation, 128, 132, 135
Carcinoid syndrome, 95
    insulinoma with, 105
    localization of tumour, 95–96
Catecholamines, in phaeochromocytoma, 189
    blockade, preoperative, 192
    free, in diagnosis of, 190, 201
    in residual, recurrent hypertension of, 195
    in surgical removal of, 192, 193
Children,
    adrenalectomy in, 69
    hyperthyroidism in, treatment, 3, 12, 13
Cimetidine, 164–181
    in gastrinomas, 164, 165–166, 170–180
        postoperative, 174
        preoperative, 170–171
        vs. surgical treatment, 170, 176–178, 180
    in MEN I syndrome, 153, 155, 157
    side-effects, 165, 181
Computed axial tomography,
    in hyperparathyroidism, 46
    in islet cell tumours, 98, 116
        gastrinomas, 168
Conn's syndrome, 183–187, 188
Corticosteroids, in pancreatic transplantation, 132, 135
Cortisol, in Cushing's syndrome, 53
Cortisone, 55, 69

C-peptide, 108–110
    after pancreatic transplantation, 135
    test, 110
Cushing's syndrome, 53–69
    adrenalectomy in, *see* Adrenalectomy
    adrenal exploration, indications, 66–68
    causative lesions, 57
    diagnosis, 57
    drug therapy, 58, 59–60, 65
    in MEN I syndrome, 161
    pituitary adenoma, removal, 62–63
    radiotherapy, 60–61, 67
    treatment selection, 64–68
Cyclosporin A, 128, 132, 135
Cyproheptadine, 60

Diabetes mellitus, 125–126
    juvenile, 125, 126
    pancreatic transplantation in, 126–136
        (*see also* Pancreas, transplantation)
    renal failure in, 125, 133, 136, 142–143
Dialysis, continuous ambulatory peritoneal, 143
Diazoxide, in insulinomas, 116, 117, 118, 119
DiGeorge syndrome, 31
Dihydrotachysterol, 33
Disseminated intravascular coagulopathy, 129, 130
Doege-Potter syndrome, 112
Drug therapy, (*see also specific drugs*)
    of Cushing's syndrome, 58, 59–60, 65

Echography, of thyroid gland, 18
Embolism, pulmonary, 54, 63
Exophthalmos, 4

5-Fluorouracil (5-Fu), 175

Gastrectomy,
    indications for, 170, 177
    in MEN I syndrome, 157
    postoperative care, 174
    preoperative preparation, 170–171
    technique, 171, 172–174
    in Zollinger-Ellison syndrome, 155, 157, 169–177
    vs. medical treatment, 170, 176–178
Gastrin, 83 (*see also* Hypergastrinaemia)
    distribution, portal venous system, 83
    in hypersecretion syndromes, 91–95, 175

Index

Gastrinoma, (see also Zollinger-Ellison syndrome)
  chemotherapy, 175–176, 178, 181
  cimetidine in, 164–166, 170, 176, 178, 180
  hormone distribution in, 83, 85
  malignant potential, 155, 157, 166
    treatment, 170, 172, 175, 178
  in MEN I syndrome, 82, 92, 93, 99, 152–158, 168
    management, 155, 157, 158
  site localization, 91–95, 167
  surgery of, current views, 164–178
    indications, 168–171, 177
    operative techniques, 171–174
    postoperative care, 174–175
    preoperative preparation, 170
    results, evaluation, 176–178
  surgery vs. medical therapy, 170, 176–178, 180
Gastrocolic trunk, 77, 83, 88
Gastroentero-pancreatic (GEP) tumours, 76 (see also specific tumours)
  hormones, distribution, normal, 79–85, 115
  localization by THVS, 85–98 (see also Venous sampling)
    gastrinoma, 91–95, 167
    insulinoma, see Insulinoma
    mixed insulin/GEP hormone, 91
  in MEN I syndrome, see Multiple endocrine neoplasia venous anatomy in, 77–78
G cell hyperplasia, 78, 83, 91, 167
  gastrin concentration pattern, 93, 95
Glucagon, 83
  distribution, portal venous system, 83, 84
  -like immunoreactivity (GLI), 84
  in mixed insulin/GEP hormone tumour, 91
  test, 108
Glucose,
  after insulinoma surgery, 117
  after pancreatic transplantation, 135
  in insulin release, 109
  tolerance test (GTT), 107, 123
Glucose: insulin ratios, 108–110, 123
Goitre, 1
  diffuse toxic, see Graves' disease
  toxic multinodular, treatment, 1, 2–3, 4, 6, 8, 12, 15
Graves' disease, 1, 2, 12
  diagnosis, 1
  exophthalmos in, 4
  postoperative care, complications, 7–8, 10
  preoperative preparation, 4–6

Grave's disease (cont.)
  results of surgery, 8–9
  surgery, 6

Hashimoto's disease, 21
H$_2$-receptor antagonists, 164, 165, 170, 180–181 (see also Cimetidine)
Hurthle cell neoplasm, 20
Hyperaldosteronism, primary, 182–187 (see also Aldosteronism)
Hypercalcaemia, (see also Hyperparathyroidism)
  familial hypocalciuric, 26, 30, 36, 43, 148
  in graft-dependent hyperparathyroidism, 33–35
  in MEN I syndrome, 147–150, 152
  postoperative, in hyperparathyroidism, 26, 27, 35, 41, 47, 150
  assessment, diagnosis in, 42–44
Hypergastrinaemia, 82, 91–95 (see also Gastrinoma)
  diffuse, 92, 157, 158
  localization by THVS, 91–95
  in MEN I syndrome, 82, 92, 93, 99, 152–158
  parathyroidectomy and, 152, 153
Hyperinsulinism, organic, 81, 90–91, 96, 98, 104–119
  glucose: insulin ratio, 109
Hyperparathyroidism, (see also Parathyroid gland)
  diagnostic tests, 43, 149
  familial hypocalciuric hypercalcaemic (FHHH), 26, 30, 43, 148
  gastrinoma with, 153, 168
  graft-dependent, 28, 30, 33–34, 36
  in MEN I syndrome, 147–150
  Zollinger-Ellison syndrome of, 153
  persistent, recurrent, 28, 35, 41–49, 149–150
    after autotransplantation, 33
    assessment, diagnosis of, 29, 42–44, 51
    autotransplantation for, 25, 28, 36, 48, 51, 149–150
    complications of reoperation, 49
    localization studies in, 29–30, 44–47, 51
    in MEN I syndrome, 149, 150
    operative aspects, 29–30, 35, 41, 47
    reoperation, results, 30, 47–48
  primary, 26, 29, 35
    surgery, autotransplantation, 26–28
  secondary, 25, 27, 28, 36
  tertiary, 28 (see also Hyperparathyroidism, persistent)

Hypertension,
  aldosteronism and, 182, 185–186
  paroxysmal, phaeochromocytoma and, 189
    after phaeochromocytoma excision, 194–195
    preoperative control of, 192
Hyperthyroidism, 1–2 (*see also* Thyrotoxicosis)
  bone turnover, resorption in, 7
  in children, 3
  in elderly, 4
  recurrent, after surgery, 4, 8
  solitary thyroid nodules, 18
Hypocalcaemia, after,
  parathyroid autotransplantation, 26, 28, 32, 34, 35
  parathyroid reoperation, 47–48
  thyroid surgery, 7, 29
Hypocalciuria, with hyperparathyroidism, 148
Hypoglycaemia, 91
  alcohol and, 112
  alimentary, 111–112
  causes of, 107
  essential reactive, 107, 112
  factitious, 111
  insulin levels in, 109
  in insulinoma, 91, 104, 106, 117
    malignant, 118, 119
    postoperative, 119
    prevention, 117
  in suppression tests, 110
  tumour, 112
Hypokalaemia, in aldosteronism, 182, 183, 186
Hypoparathyroidism,
  after parathyroid autotransplantation,
    latent, 34
    persistent, 34
  after reoperation for hyperparathyroidism, 29
  iatrogenic, allotransplantation in, 31
Hypophysectomy, 56, 66, 67
Hypothyroidism,
  after surgery for Graves' disease, 9
  transient, postoperative, 10

Immunosuppressive agents, 128, 131, 132
Insulin,
  concentrations in insulinomas, 85, 98
  in diabetes mellitus, 125
    after pancreatic transplantation, 136

Insulin (*cont.*)
  in diabetes mellitus (*cont.*)
    extraction, by liver, 114–115
    in factitious hypoglycameia, 111
    in gastrinomas, 84
    glucose ratio, 108–110, 123
    hypersecretion, diffuse, 90–91
    mixed GEP tumours with, 91
    peaks, normal pancreatic, 115
    release,
      inhibition by diazoxide, 117
      stimuli, 109
    suppression tests, 110, 124
    synthesis, half-life, 108
Insulinoma, 76, 104–119
  diagnosis, 106–112, 123–124, 159
    current methods, 108–111
    differential diagnosis, 111–1123
  hormone distribution in, 83, 85, 89
  incidence, 104
  localization, 98, 112–116 (*see also* Venous sampling)
    by imaging methods, 96–98, 116
    indications, role of, 116
    intraoperative venous sampling, 115
    in MEN syndrome, 159
    by THVS, 85–87, 98, 113–115, 159
  malignant, 104–105, 118–119, 159
  in MEN I syndrome, 106, 119, 124, 152, 158–160
  pathology, 104–104
  postoperative assessment, 119
  pre-, postoperative care, 117
  size, 76, 96, 105
  surgical removal,
    after negative laparotomy, 76, 98, 117–118
    complications, 76, 117
    in MEN I syndrome, 159
Iodine, radioactive
  in thyroid nodule diagnosis, 17
  in thyrotoxicosis treatment, 1, 2, 3, 12
Iodocholesterol, 184, 188
Islets of Langerhans,
  hyperplasia, 158
  isolated, preparation, 126–127, 129
  transplantation, *see under* Pancreas
  tumours, localization, 78–99, 113–116 (*see also specific tumours*; Venous sampling)
Isotopic imaging, 45, 116
Isthmusectomy, thyroid nodule, 22

Kocher manoeuvre, 171

Laryngeal nerve, recurrent (RLN)
  paralysis of, 16, 19, 22
Laryngoscopy, in thyroid surgery, 5, 7
Liver,
  disease and cimetidine, 165
  GEP hormones, extraction, 83, 84, 114–115
  malignant insulinoma metastases, 104, 118
  metastatic disease, in MEN I syndrome, 152
  in metastatic disease diagnosis, 84
Lobectomy, thyroid, 6, 7, 22

Metadrenalines, 190
[^{131}I]Metaiodobenzylguanidine (MIBG), 191, 196, 201
3-Methoxy-4-hydroxy mandelic acid (VMA), 190
Methylene blue, in hyperparathyroidism, 46
Metiamide, 164
Metyrapone, 59–60, 65
Microadenomatosis, 104, 105, 124, 157, 159
Microangiopathic lesions in diabetes, 125–126
Mitotane (o'p-DDD), 60
Motilin, 83
  distribution, portal venous system, 83, 84
Multiple endocrine adenomatosis (MEA), see Multiple endocrine neoplasia
Multiple endocrine neoplasia (MEN), 78, 91
  type 1, 26, 104, 144–161, 168
    angiography in, 98
    case histories, 144–145, 153, 154
    clinical features, 144–147
    hypergastrinaemia in, 82, 92, 93, 99, 152–158, 168
    insulinoma in, 106, 119, 124, 152, 158–160
    malignant gastrinoma, 157, 158
    pancreatic islet cell disease, 151–160
    parathyroid involvement, 147–150, 168
    pituitary involvement in, 160–161
    PPoma in, 151–152, 159–160
    Zollinger-Ellison syndrome in, 144, 148, 151–158
  type 11, 168, 195–197, 201
    surgical management, 196
  type IIa, 26
  type II B, 43
Muscle weakness, in hyperparathyroidism, 44

Neck massage, 45
Nelson's syndrome, 55, 62, 64, 69

Neoprene, 132
Nephrolithiasis, in hyperparathyroidism, 44
Nesidioblastosis hyperplasia, 78, 91, 104, 124, 159
Nodular hyperplasia, 57, 68
Noradrenaline, excretion rate, 190
Nuclear magnetic resonance (NMR), 116

Occluding agents, pancreatic grafts, 132
Oedema, laryngeal, 7
Osteodystrophy, renal, 28, 31, 34, 35

Pancreas,
  blind resection, insulinoma, 117–118
  islet cell tumours localization, 76–99, 113–116 (see also specific tumours)
  in MEN 1 syndrome, 151–160
  normal hormone distribution, 83–85, 114
  venous anatomy, 77–78, 114, 131
  weight, blood flow, 115
Pancreas, transplantation of, 125–136
  delayed graft, 133
  experimental, tissue, 126–128
    results, 127–128
  fetal, extraction technique, 127, 130
  future prospects, 136
  human islet, 128–130, 136, 143
    allograft, unpurified, 130
    autograft, 129
    fetal allograft, 130
  neonatal tissue, 127
  organ transplantation, 130–132, 143
    ductal drainage, 131–132, 134
    duct occlusion, 132
    experimental vascular technique, 131, 143
    rejection, 132
  segmental grafting, current methods, 132–136
    kidney transplantation, 133–134
    metabolic effects, 132, 135, 136
  tissue implantation, 126–128
  tissue preparation, 126–127, 129
Pancreatectomy,
  in gastrinomas, 171–172, 176
  in insulinomas, 118, 159
  in MEN 1 syndrome, 157, 158, 159, 160
Pancreatic hormones, 77
Pancreatic polypeptide (PP), 83
  distribution, portal venous system, 83
  in gastrinoma, 89, 91
  in insulinoma, 105
Pancreatitis, chronic, 129

Index

Paraendocrine tumours in Cushing's syndrome, 57, 64, 68, 69
Parathyroidectomy, 4
  hypergastrinaemia and, 153, 168
  in MEN 1 syndrome, 149–150, 152, 153
  prior to gastrinoma surgery, 153, 168–169
  reoperation for hyperparathyroidism, 41, 47, 51
  3½-gland, 26, 28, 35
  total, autotransplantation, 28, 30, 31, 33, 36
Parathyroid glands, (see also Hyperparathyroidism)
  allotransplantation, 31
  autotransplantation, 8, 25–36, 149
    clinical indications, 25, 26–29, 48
    deferred, 30, 48–49, 52
    deferred, technique, 32
    graft sites, 29, 32
    postoperative management, 32–34
    at reoperation, 29–30, 48, 52
    technique, 31–32
  cryopreservation of, 30, 32, 36, 48, 52
  hyperplasia, primary, 26–28, 35
    asymmetrical, 150
    in MEN 1 syndrome, 147–150
  hyperplasia vs. adenoma, 148, 149
  in MEN 1 syndrome, 147–150, 168
  parenchymal fat test, 149
  reoperation, see under Hyperparathyroidism
  supernumeray, in MEN 1 syndrome, 150
Parathyroid hormone (PTH),
  in parathyroid transplantation, 25
  venous sampling, 46, 51
Pentolinium, 190
Peptic ulcer,
  cimetidine in, 164, 165
  in MEN 1 syndrome, 145, 151, 153
Phaeochromocytoma, 189–197, 201
  diagnosis, 190, 201
  malignancy in, 193, 201
  in MEN II, 195, 196, 197, 201
  MIBG therapy, 191
  perioperative management, 190–193
    α-, β-adrenergic blockade, 192
    catecholamine concentrations, 192, 193
    localization, 191, 201
  removal, hypertension after, 194–195
Phenoxybenzamine, 192
Photon irradiation, 61
Pigmentation, Addisonian, 55
Pituitary tumours, 53
  after adrenalectomy, 55
  in Cushing's syndrome, 53, 54, 56, 57

Pituitary tumours (cont.)
  diagnosis, 53, 57, 160
  hypophysectomy, 56, 66, 67
  in MEN 1 syndrome, 151, 161–162
  microadenoma, size, 160
  radiotherapy, 60–61, 65, 69
  surgical removal, 62, 68
    microsurgery, 62, 65
    yttrium-90 implantation, 63, 65, 67
Plummer's disease, 1, 2, 6, 8
Portal venous system, 77–78
PPoma, 151–152, 159–160
Pregnancy, hyperthyroidism in, 3–4, 13
Pro-insulin, 108, 123
Prolactin cell adenoma, 160
Propranolol, 5, 7
Proton irradiation, 61
Pyloroplasty, 172

de Quervain's disease, 1

Radiosurgery, closed stereotactic, 61
Radiotherapy, of pituitary, 60–61
  external irradiation, 61
  interstitial irradiation, 61, 67
Ranitidine, 181
Renal failure, in diabetes, 125, 131, 136, 142–143
Renal osteodystrophy, 28, 31, 34, 35
Renal stones,
  in gastrinomas, 169, 175
  in MEN 1 syndrome, 145, 148
Renal transplantation, 28, 31, 126, 142–143
  pancreatic grafts and, 133–134
Roux-en-Y anastomosis, 170, 173

Sarcomata, retroperitoneal, 112
Scintiscans,
  iodocholesterol, 184, 188
  selenomethionine, 45–46, 116
  thyroid, 16–18
Secretin stimulation ('push') test, 166–167, 175
Selenomethionine scan, 45–46, 116
Serotonin, in carcinoid syndrome, 95, 96
Sipple syndrome, 168, 195–197
Sodium nitroprusside, 192
Somatostatin, 83
  distribution, portal venous system, 83, 84
  in mixed insulin/GEP hormone tumours, 91

Spironolactone, 186, 187
Sternocleidomastoid muscle, 29, 32
Streptozotocin, 118, 175–176
Substance P, 96
Sulphonylurea, 111

Technetium-99 pertechnetate ($^{99}Tc^m$), 17
Thionamide drugs, 4
THVS, see Venous sampling, percutaneous transhepatic
thyroglobulin assays, 21
Thyroidectomy, (see also Thyrotoxicosis)
  parathyroid autotransplantation after, 29
  subtotal lobectomy, 6
  thyroid carcinoma, 22
  total lobectomy, 22
Thyroid gland,
  adenoma, 1, 2, 6, 8
  carcinoma, 14
    diagnosis, 15–16, 20, 21
    implants with needle biopsy, 19
    incidence, 15, 23
    medullary, 15, 20, 21
    in MEN 11 syndrome, 196
    operative treatment, 22
    parathyroid autotransplantation after, 29
    radiation exposure and, 15
    thyroid suppression, 21
  cysts, 18
  stimulating antibodies (TsAb), 1, 2, 6, 9
  surgery, 6–10, 14–23
Thyroiditis, viral subacute, 1
Thyroid nodule, solitary, 14–23
  diagnostic studies, 15–21
    needle biopsy, 19–20, 22–23
    scintiscans, 16–18
    TSH suppression, 20–21
    ultrasonography, 18
  incidence, 14–15, 23
  operative treatment, 22
Thyroid stimulating hormone (TSH),
  suppression test, 16, 20, 21
  thyroid nodule with, 16
Thyrotoxicosis, role of surgery in, 1–10, 12–13
  contraindications, syndromes, 1, 4
  follow-up, 9–10
  heart disease with, 4
  indications, syndromes, 1, 2, 12
    special cases, 3–4, 12, 13
  operation, 6–7
  postoperative care, complications, 7–8
  preoperative investigations, 5–6

Thyrotoxicosis, role of surgery in (cont.)
  preoperative preparation, 4–5
  results of, 8–9
Tolbutamide test, intravenous, 108
Toluidine blue, 115
Total lymphoid irradiation, 132
Transhepatic portal venous sampling, see Venous sampling
Transplantation, see specific organs
Trilostane, 60

Ultrasonography,
  in islet cell tumours, 98, 116, 168
  of parathyroid glands, 45, 51
  of thyroid gland, 18, 51

Vagotomy, 157, 170, 172, 176
Vasoactive intestinal polypeptide (VIP), 83
  distribution, portal venous system, 83, 84
  tumours, 84
Venous anatomy, gastroentero-pancreatic axis, 77–78, 114
Venous sampling,
  aldosterone secreting tumours, 185
  intraoperative, 115
  parathyroid hormone, 46, 51
  percutaneous transhepatic portal (THVS), 76, 77–99, 113–115, 124
    advantages, 98–99
    catheterization procedure, 78–79, 84, 114, 167
    diagnostic criteria, conditions, 115
    in GEP hormone tumours, 85–98, 114–115, 167
    hormone distribution, normal, 79–85, 115

Water clear cell hyperplasia (WCCH), 26
Wermer's syndrome, see Multiple endocrine neoplasia type 1

Yttrium-90 implantation, 63, 65, 67

Zollinger-Ellsion syndrome, in MEN 1 syndrome, 144, 148, 151, 152–158 (see also Gastrinoma)
  diagnosis, 153
  gastrectomy, 155, 157
  malignancy in, 153, 155
  parathyroidectomy, 152, 153–154